PLANET
MEDICINE

Modalities

RICHARD GROSSINGER

North Atlantic Books
Berkeley, California

Published by
North Atlantic Books
P.O. Box 12327
Berkeley, California 94712

Cover art by Sergei Ponomarov
Cover and book design by Paula Morrison
Typeset by Catherine E. Campaigne

Printed in the United States of America

Planet Medicine is sponsored by the Society for the Study of Native Arts and Sciences, a nonprofit educational corporation whose goals are to develop an educational and crosscultural perspective linking various scientific, social, and artistic fields; to nurture a holistic view of arts, sciences, humanities, and healing; and to publish and distribute literature on the relationship of mind, body, and nature.

Library of Congress Cataloging-in-Publication Data
Grossinger, Richard. 1944–
        Planet medicine / Richard Grossinger.—7th ed.
            p. cm.
        Includes bibliographical references and index.
        Contents: — v. 2. Modalities
        ISBN 1-55643-391-3 (paper).
        1. Holistic medicine.   2. Alternative medicine.   I. Title.
R733.G76   2002
615.5—dc21   2002022196

7   8   9   10   11   12   13   MALLOY   08   07   06   05   04   03

I dedicate this book to those whose vision, compassion, and acts of healing made it possible:

Paul Pitchford

Randy Cherner

Amini Peller

Elizabeth Beringer

Richard Strozzi Heckler

Ron Sieh

Cybèle Tomlinson

John Upledger

Frank Lowen

Michael Wagner

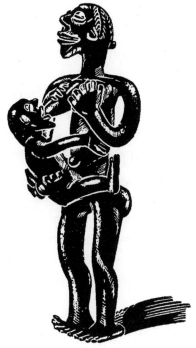

ACKNOWLEDGMENTS

THE PEOPLE WHO helped me the most with the material in this book are noted in the dedication and throughout the book. Here I would like to acknowledge those colleagues who contributed directly to the preparation of the text.

I acknowledge and thank Amy Champ for her research on the "Practical Ethnomedicine" chapter of *Origins;* Don Hanlon Johnson for his thorough reading and comments on the entire manuscript; Michael Salveson, Elizabeth Beringer, John Upledger, Bonnie Bainbridge Cohen, Judyth Weaver, Fritz Smith, and Dana Ullman for their reading and comments on particular sections of the text; Kathy Glass for her thoughtful and patient editing; Victoria Baker for her exceptional index; Paula Morrison for her elegant and spirited design; Catherine Campaigne for her technical work in the preparation of the finished book; Janna Israel for her updating of the bibliography; Jay Kinney and Richard Smoley of *Gnosis* for their assistance in finding artwork; and Sergei Ponomarov, Spain, Kathy Park, Alex Grey, and Kathy Maguire for drawing images specifically to fit in the text.

We come from an unknown place and go to an unknown place. These do not concern me. But the trajectory of my life, which I share with this body, does.

I want us all to participate in reconstructing the temple, to heal the planet, which is a masterpiece in danger.

—Jean Louis Barrault (the mime in *Les Enfants de Paradis*)

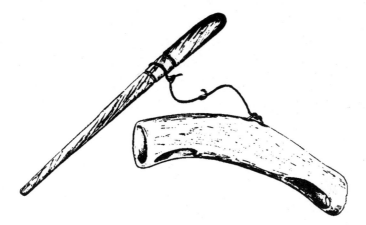

TABLE OF CONTENTS

*Table of
Contents*

MODALITIES

TABLE OF ILLUSTRATIONS

Many of the illustrations in this book are used in clip-art style from a wide variety of sources. They include rock art, cave paintings, indigenous graffiti, religious woodcuts, amulet insignias, pottery motifs, codex glyphs, illustrations from herbals and old medical books, and traditional totemic designs from the different regions of the Earth. Because some of this material was collected from secondary and tertiary sources, complete citations are not always possible. The artwork in the Introduction is made up of animal motifs used in African decorations (plus an assortment of Australian kangaroo glyphs).

*Table of
Illustrations*

Table of Illustrations

*Table of
Illustrations*

FOREWORD

IN THIS NEW REVISED EDITION OF *Planet Medicine: Modalities* Richard Grossinger tackles the difficult task of providing an accessible charting of the myriad of "alternative" health-care approaches and systems, many of them superficially similar but functionally quite different, and others seemingly different while sharing principles and sources. In taking on this monumental challenge Grossinger is encyclopedic, thorough, and scholarly. While this book will be invaluable for those seeking health and wholeness for themselves, the text is much more than that. Particularly, it is a critical recording of an evolutionary development in health care itself and should, as well, be valuable to physicians from a wide range of professional background and interests, including doctors who want to understand what alternative methods are and how they work. It should also be useful to patients attempting to understand the history and rationale of methods of diagnosis and treatment being applied to them.

The modern evolution of health care is most likely in its beginnings and, as it matures and tests itself against changing disease and trauma over coming years and decades, a completely new model of medicine will arise in the West. Since healing addresses fundamental mind-body issues, its transformation will likely contribute to a new human philosophy and new cultural institutions not only for dealing with illnesses but for generating values, ethics, and meanings.

Perhaps the core of this research is Richard's ability to capture the essential components of diverse systems, to relate them to one another and to overall conceptual vectors, and to put them in the context of values and meanings. No one could possibly be exhaustive in this important task. However, it would be difficult to imagine anyone being more lucid and effective than Grossinger is, as he leads the reader through systems as diverse as Reiki, Taoist breathing, cranial osteopathy, visceral manipulation, psychotherapy, body electronics, and color therapy. In particular Richard does a splendid job in tracking the development and offshoots of the Osteopathic model and its somatoemotional approach to healing, an undertaking that would challenge any historian of this field. To a somewhat lesser degree, he applies this level of discrimination and tracking to a number of other therapeutic categories such as Acupuncture/Oriental medicine and Bodywork/Somatics itself.

For those seeking direction in their individual health needs, I would suggest an overall skimming of the book, however daunting. Doing this, I believe, will give the reader a compass and coordinates for further in-depth reading. In addition, Grossinger provides an appendix to help people locate professional and dietary resources they are seeking. It is quite thorough, if not in listing every major or obscure resource, then in providing an overall strategy for locating tools and practitioners from any starting point.

Sometimes, while reading, I wondered what the target audience is for this book. It is certainly, first of all, meant for the health-care consumer (now well over fifty percent of the American public seeking alternative health practitioners), offering them a unique guide for making informed and intelligent choices. Then it is a trusted companion for alternative practitioners, a reference to their own broad network of fields. And finally it is a guide for "mainstream" medical and health-care workers to begin to access the potential benefits and applications of particular complementary treatments.

"Modalities," although complex in its vocabulary and structure, is clearly written. It invites disciplined reading, offering a rich exploration into a field that is rapidly changing the landscape of medical care worldwide. It may even be seen as contributing to a narrowing of the bridge

between mainstream medicine, which has its own well-documented history, traditions, and empirical components, and those alternative treatments that arise from a variety of different histories, cultures, and applications of human skills and intuitions. Since we are all human beings in bodies with consciousness, one day there may be a true "planet medicine" rather than a reigning and sanctioned paradigm shadowed by a sortless variety of alternatives.

Peter A. Levine, Ph.D.
Author of *Waking the Tiger: Healing Trauma*

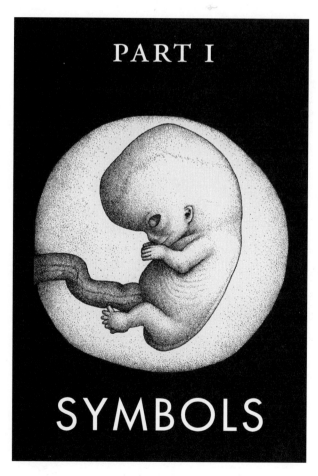

PART I

SYMBOLS

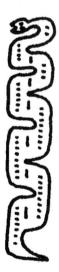

The Multicultural Basis of Medicine

The Fallacies of Indigenous Medicine

IN THE PRECEDING VOLUME of this book I explored the origins of systems of diagnosis and healing. Drawing from ethnographic accounts, historical documents, and the extant versions of ancient therapies, I constructed a possible evolution of medicine as both a social institution and a philosophical category. The former has given rise to guilds of doctors and healers, while the latter has spawned epistemologies of disease and cure. Medicine has always been both a therapeutic profession and an alembic of preconscious symbols.

I showed that the myths arising from our partial recovery of indigenous non-Western medicines inspire two quite contrary fallacies—one, that modern medical science represents an improvement over aboriginal medicine of almost incalculable proportions; and, two, that a majority of indigenous medicines continue to be practiced (or have been revived) in their original forms.

The first fallacy is a common misunderstanding of the sycophants of technological progress. It overlooks the distinction between medicine as a branch of natural science and the art of healing (which does not require doctors and was practiced aboriginally). It also overlooks the fact that scientific medicine is merely the contemporary status of prehistoric lineages of herbalists and manipulators; its core methodology was established by the time of the Greeks.

The second fallacy overlooks the fact that many of the ancient and indigenous medicines to which we have access have been reinvented according to contemporary notions of holism, shamanism, and archetypal psychology and no longer exist in their traditional forms. Many New Agers believe that they can appropriate the gist of any culture simply by borrowing its artifacts and declaring their allegiance to cosmic harmony.

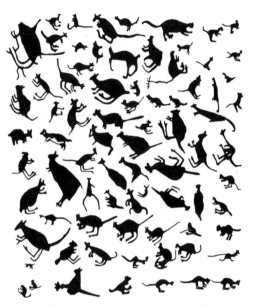

Indigenous systems of healing are closer than we think, for they are woven into the fabric of modern society at both conscious and preconscious levels, and they contribute historically to a variety of medical and nonmedical institutions. On the other hand, they are further than we think, for, even as we study and reenact their remnants, their original mechanics and phenomenology have been lost, likely forever.

Categories of Healing

IN THE THE first volume I divided medical practice into the following broad systems:

- simple mechanical, surgical, and herbal techniques and etiologies of disease based on natural and supernatural progressions; these formed the basis of tribal ethnomedicine and led (notably in the Middle East and Asia) to the technological medicines of Neolithic civilization, flowing ultimately into the Hippocratic-Galenic synthesis;

- diverse branches of shamanism, embracing psychic healing, symbolic and ritual transfiguration, visualization, voodoo, divination, sympathetic magic, and primitive psychoanalysis, all based on mythodrama, transference, abreaction, and sleight-of-hand

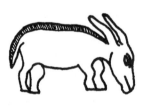

reifications and detraumatizations of abstract diseases through objects (e.g., a bolus, lightning in a sand painting, a bloody down);

- modes of massage and manipulation, originating in folk traditions of bone-setting, physical adjustment, and palpation and giving rise to the nineteenth-century American outlaw sciences of chiropractic and osteopathy;

- elemental cosmology combined with internal and external alchemical medicines, specifically the scientific theories that incubated therapeutic pantheons in India, Tibet, and China (including Ayurvedic medicine, the Taoist healing treatises assigned to the Yellow Emperor, and the coction—fever and fermentation—principles of early Greek medicine);

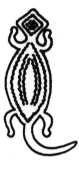

- language-oriented and symbolic medicine, based on psychosomatically derived self-knowledge and flowering in the system of psychoanalysis propounded by Sigmund Freud and transformed by Carl Jung and Wilhelm Reich, and providing a cognitive basis for treating mind and body as an integrated whole; and

- reincarnational medicine, proposing a karmic origin for disease and practiced through heterogeneous systems tapping disembodied spirits, transpersonal channels, and cosmic energies as super-curative agents.

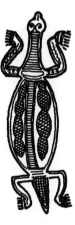

These categories exist only as my device for defining ancient, non-Western, and holistic medical systems (and their interrelationships) in contemporary terms. They help distinguish major differing principles of healing. Yet in almost every culture their expressions overlap and generate one another. It may be said that in any active medical system some of these categories are dormant while others are active. In orthodox scientific medicine most of them are suppressed, but that hardly obliterates their influences, which are sustained unconsciously.

"Disease" is a purely subjective event (especially when applied as a concept to something less concrete than chicken pox or malaria). Each medical system struggles with contradictory and paradoxical elements to produce a makeshift doctrine that satisfies its clients and institutions. The development of both modern scientific medicine and its holistic alternatives has depended on antitheses of levels of concretization and latent structures and beliefs.

I WILL BEGIN with a discussion of the most inexplicable of all medical systems—those that treat patients without an anatomical model, without drugs, and often without a palpable space-time connection between the physician and the patient. Faith healing illuminates the frontier of mind over matter. I have no idea what faith healing actually is—what paraphysics it represents. I believe it is either a portal into another dimensionality or an emergent property of mind, body, and symbol. I hope that elsewhere in the universe it has become a fully developed esoteric science. Mind medicine gives us a baseline. If healing can be transmitted without any direct contact or pills, manual and herbal modalities can certainly transmit cures.

Treatments in all systems may be little more than methods of conducting pure healing energy through the labyrinths of a densely materialized world (though not so dense and opaque as to be made of anything but atoms, thought, and space). Each discrete medical nuance may be not so much a departure from healing by "faith" as an avenue for engaging a knot of psychosomatic resistance.

When an act of faith is inadequate to stop a malignancy or plague, we encounter the nitty-gritty of infection, predation, and worldstuff. Our substantial embodiment requires real material transformation. Faith healing may prove that mountains can be sometimes moved in

6

the blink of an eyelid, but it does not change the fact that armies trample through vineyards daily, machine-gunning the inhabitants and burning their homes.

I WILL MOVE FROM psychic healing to palpation and examine the wide range of somatic modalities that have developed under rubrics of physical therapy, bodywork, osteopathy, manipulation, manual medicine, and adjustment. I will also explore a broad spectrum of other healing modalities* including martial arts, sexual therapies, meditational practices, prayer, esoteric medicines, color and sound medicines, and dietary and herbal medicines as well as aspects of healing that lie beyond category and are indistinguishable from art, sports, war, politics, economics, and crime.

I AM ADDRESSING DIRECTLY our global perception of a malaise, a sickness transcending any conventional notion of disease, that has come to include environmental despoliation, genocide, poverty, institutionalized greed, slavery, child armies, forced prostitution, pornography, and other social pathologies. Certainly the nuclear and chemical arsenals and toxic industries of nations, the sheer number of land mines from wars, are as much diseases as smallpox, schizophrenia, and AIDS. Any paradigm the Earth invents must find a way of addressing them.

If we are to heal ourselves and this world, there can be no exceptions. We must heal guns, money, factories, armies, governments, laws, prisons, schools, and medical institutions. Insofar as these are the projections and externalizations of unresolved pathologies in us, they too must be treated by a "planet medicine."

---

*Many modalities are described primarily or substantially in the first volume *(Origins),* among them: shamanism, Traditional Chinese Medicine, Ayurvedic medicine, herbalism, and shamanic psychoanalysis. Homeopathy is treated thoroughly in *Homeopathy: The Great Riddle,* a third volume (or subvolume) in this series.

Empiricism, Rationalism, Vitalism, and Science

EMPIRICAL HEALING SYSTEMS treat patients by intuitive trial-and-error guesswork, preserving methods that succeed, regardless of their rationale or plausibility. Most herbal medicines (those using animal and mineral compounds too) arose empirically. Without microscopes where else could Stone Age peoples have learned pharmacy except in trance visions from ancestors, goddesses, and gods?

Divination, symbolic medicines, and healing ceremonies were likely the outcome of disease conversion by jackpot—guessing what aspects of a sacred ritual were also curative. These differ from herbal medicines in that they treat sick people by totems and "thought objects" rather than by natural substances.

All prehistoric medicines had substantial empirical aspects, for that was how treatments originated. The Hippocratic Corpus systematized some of their popular surviving elements. These premises were later formalized by the ancient Roman doctor Galen and gradually expanded into a formal profession during the Middle Ages and Renaissance. Medicine became an organized body of theories, rules, and applications.

Empirical doctors do not seek scientific or theological confirmations in order to prescribe a remedy. They require only hunches confirmed by successes. They are less concerned with the theoretical or esoteric nature of disease and more with the art of healing. Thus, many contemporary "medical" systems (acupuncture, much of Ayurveda, chiropractic, homeopathy, prayer, and Navaho sand-painting among them) continue to be practiced not because there is proof that they work but because (for whatever reasons) patients improve after their enactments. In fact, in most of the above cases, there is scientific "proof" that they *could not work.*

RATIONALIST SYSTEMS, CONVERSELY, extrapolate from prior theory and experiment to treatment. Models of the body and its functions are used to develop suitable methods of attacking disease processes

MODALITIES

8

(which are also modeled mechanically). All modalities are now developed according to biochemical and thermodynamic logic and implemented often regardless of side-effects or deleterious consequences. Resting on centuries of laboratory experiments, modern scientific medicine is the pinnacle of Rationalism. It is sustained by theories of natural law and the cumulative work of physicists, chemists, and biologists. It denounces as quackery all cures that cannot be explained by its materialistic sequences of cause and effect.

V ITALISM COMPRISES A variety of practices, all of them based on an intrinsic life force or transpersonal energy field that provides a catalyst for healing. Taoist and Ayurvedic modalities locate the source of energy in the body's *chakra* system, auras, *chi* and *prana,* and meridians; other canons (orgone therapy, astrological medicine, and to some degree Polarity) claim an extrabodily ether or resonance. Alchemical and homeopathic medicines place the vital force in potentized substances.

Darwinian science refutes the existence of any intrinsic synergistic or vital energies and bases its treatments solely on the recognized thermochemistry of living systems.

Energy Medicine

T HE ADHERENTS OF most holistic systems have at one time or another defined their own field as either energetic or as something more concrete (mechanical, skeletal, verbal, integrative, cognitive, or neuromuscular). Craniosacral and Polarity therapists, *Chi Gung* and Reiki practitioners, and homeopaths usually (but not always) refer to their methods as energy based. Although they do not deny corporal components, they usually interpret those as secondary to the movement of energy—and energy can be defined in a range of ways, from the passage of feeling, to *chi*-flow, to the intercession of paraphysical fields. Likewise, Rolfers, herbalists, chiropractors, instructors of the Alexander Technique, dieticians, Body-Electronics practitioners, and a diverse range of other healers view their work as thermodynamic and structural to one degree or another (even when they purport to move something they call "energy"). An individual structural practitioner might even emphasize the energetic component of his or her work, but the system rests on its anatomical logic.

Despite any rhetoric to the contrary, all systems are energy based and all systems are topokinetic (anatomical). We are in bodies, and bodies are organized by something ineffable. The reason Rolfing or trace minerals get results is that energy is moved and continues to build on itself after the treatment is concluded.

At the same time, all systems have a material logic even if the practitioner of them is not aware of that logic—sometimes the hands are more intelligent than the brain. I would argue that except in instances of channeled and other mind, sound, or color healing, practitioners are better off with a knowledge of anatomy, even if their system does not make direct use of such a map. Anatomy provides a path to energy. It also offers an equation of relative degrees of fluidity and congestion at any given moment. It allows the practitioner to work in terms of material structures and molecular events even while honoring their vital and metabolic flow.

The physical anatomy of the body is an energetic outcome and expression; the energy of life travels in a network of fractal tissue mazes, suspensory visceral structures, projections of forces through hollower and denser spaces, and cellular adhesion and gliding—organ by organ. Energy must pass through these layers and lattices while being therapeutically absorbed.

Moshe Feldenkrais routinely deconstructed "energy" when people used it in the context of his work. Citing his own background in physics, he would remind them that there is a quite precise thermodynamic definition of energy.

Certainly no one can pin down exactly what "energy" means in a therapeutic context; hence, "energy medicine" can become a jargon by

which some systems may claim superiority over others (which are "merely mechanical"). In that sense, "energy" is a subtext for the claim to "psychospiritual" or <u>quantum medicine</u> and is used to place dibs on a kind of futuristic super-modality.

Yet, there is no way I can describe the healing systems in this book without using the discriminations of energy and structure they adduce in defining themselves. Despite my repetition of certain terminology (resonance, transduction, transfiguration) to describe mysterious types of processes, their "energies" are in many cases invisible and undetermined, and the terminology is merely a device by which to instruct trainees or provide a way of discourse. At core, we may be talking about some manner of healer transference, molecular organization, or cell-DNA signaling and embryogenic triggering—the stuff and forces that hold atoms, cells, life forms, and lives together; we may be talking about unknown paraphysical energies; or we may be talking about a combination of these.

One time while he was lecturing in San Francisco, I met John Upledger, a pioneer of healing touch, for dinner at a Thai restaurant. In the course of our discussion before the food arrived, I told him that I first realized I "got" the rhythm of cerebrospinal fluid when, while sitting in a class, I began unconsciously probing the carpet with my left hand, trying to find its pulse. "It didn't have any. Suddenly I understood what craniosacral therapy was."

"If you had felt more sensitively," he said, "you would have discovered that it *did* have a pulse—not a cerebrospinal rhythm, of course, but a vibration. Everything has a vibration. Feel the table. Like this [capping his fingers over the table cloth]. Can you pick up that vibration? In inanimate objects it's very slow. If it didn't have a pulse, it would fall apart."

And there it was, just as he described it, oscillating under my own cupped fingers at a rate so deliberate with vibrations so fine it could have been absolutely impalpable and still—but then, as John observed, without a pulse it would have collapsed.

Modalities

ENERGY AND MATTER may be universal, but treatments occur within cultures, languages, and healing tropes.

In the first volume I proposed six underlying core holistic principles: Reiki (energy), osteopathy (palpation), herbology (catalysis), iridology (hologram), shamanic psychoanalysis (transubstantiation), and homeopathy (potentization). Their rival is allopathy (linear thermodynamics and genetic algorithm).

Allopathic medicines cure diseases by application of sophisticatedly forged tools. They are in ascendancy now. Other medicines "succeed" by little more than the informed touch of a healer's hand or directed thought. Some such medicines operate by language and dialogue, some by lessons and exercises, some by chanting, some by silent internalization. There are medicines that use symbolic matrices, medicines that generate symbols, and medicines that annihilate symbols. All of these are viable. Their individual successes depend on a range of subtle factors linking healer, patient, disease, and environment. Discerning the outlines of such factors "through a glass darkly" is a major goal of this book. My hope is to discover the premises that underlie each of these variations and to propose ways of explaining and accommodating their divergences.

I am dealing more with cultural categories of disease and social meanings than with anatomical loci or the raw stuff of pathology. That is why my text rarely addresses actual disease processes or allopathic reversals of tissue damage. Such is already the fare of enough medical texts.

The objection will arise at some point that none of these alternative systems are really medicines; "real" medicine treats diseases scientifically, whereas these various other modalities are only self-improvement techniques, placebos, or pseudo-psychotherapies.

Whatever one chooses to believe, it is important to keep in mind that holistic treatments are directed toward individuals and imagined synergies of their fields, not toward diseases or anatomies as such.

Of course, alternative medicines are *all of the above:* self-improvement, auto-suggestion, hocus-pocus, psychoanalytic transference, "wine into blood," etc. But that does not stop them from being medicines. Treatment along holistic parameters may influence the *entire* organism (the life field), and the transmission of a "meaning" will be assimilated at many physical and psychological levels, including those where infections, viruses, tumors, and the like are located. Thus, holistic disciplines *are* real, though for rationales of an entirely different order from those of scientific medicine.

Allopathy treats diseases and cures at the level of infection, malignancy, and biochemistry. All other "pathological" conditions entail metastases of esoteric events in raw tissue: symbolic representations, mind-body grids, vibrations and resonances transcending concrete organ masses, presymptomatic and miasmatic stages of sickness, and karmic and archetypal disease states. Holistic systems engage the manifestation of disease at a level of mind-body synergy, potentized symbol, and the intrinsic intelligence of life. This is a critical distinction without which the book you are reading makes little sense.

Molecules and Symbols

IDEOLOGICAL CONFLICTS AMONG medical methods represent conflicts within and among ourselves. I believe that we suffer ambiguities of healing because we have lost a sense of who we are. We experience constantly shifting identities and boundaries of bodies, minds, desires, and destinies. As long as we do not not know ourselves, it is difficult to treat our diseases in any substantial or authentically consistent way. In fact, we are condemned to treating mostly metaphors, however palpable and concrete such metaphors may seem in Magnetic Resonance Images and lab reports.

In the medical environment of early twentieth-first-century Western civilization, one type of modality obviously predominates. As essen-

the diagnosis
lightman.

13

tially inert and nonsentient motes, neither molecules nor the cells they comprise which conduct their metabolism can be altered other than by concrete interference in their patterns. These patterns are considered entropic and inevitable unless deterred and allopathically reprogrammed. A patient expects a doctor to externalize the random material genealogy of his or her malaise and to apply a rational cure based on scientific premises. The sick person thinks of his disease as a natural event, arising circumstantially, and treatable most efficaciously by an objectification of his body in the operant paradigm. Invariably he is unaware of the cultural prejudices he brings to the doctor's office or the role that those prejudices play in his either improving or failing to improve from the remedy given. The dance of symbols about and through him truly eludes him.

Mainstream medical science emphasizes programs of diagnosis and treatment that conceptually dismember the human organism (and life itself) into smaller and smaller machinelike bits. A clinician or researcher is presumed to be most modern and closest to first causes when he or she is operating on a cellular or molecular level. Diseases are often considered untreatable or incurable for reasons of genetic determinism or metabolic fatalism. Treatment has little to do with internal biofeedback or experience. It is the slave of objectification, limited to direct attacks upon sites of pathology. Human beings become repositories of chance, dissociative, exogenous ailments—reversible mechanically. There is no link between our sentience and our metabolic functioning.

From computer analyses of bodily fluids and radiation images, doctors purport to know everything about a person—her past, her future, her propensity to disease. Since everyone is contaminated in one way or another, there is always a bad omen somewhere.

In many instances, it is difficult to know what to treat, when to interfere therapeutically, and when treatment of overly concretized disease images is more dangerous and unhealthy than the threat disclosed by these images. Should every malignancy be attacked with the most

powerful drugs or surgeries despite the consequence to the organism

14

as a whole? When does a system that made itself reorganize naturally and heal itself? When is allopathic medical intrusion too gross for the signaling parameters of endemic psychosomatic networks? When does machine analysis miss the active living factors?

Now, with DNA analysis and chromosome mapping, not only are people's present bodies turned into medical images but their entire destinies have become algorithmic quantifications, the implacable outcomes of myriad inevitable preordinations. All diseases are, at root, DNA mistakes. Even desire (sexual orientation) has been assigned to a genetic locus, along with bird calls, spider webs, and reptile egg-laying routes.

Such medicine is meant for life forms that totally lack mind and spirit, and lack homeostatic energy processes and synergistic reintegration as well. In an era in which advanced technology alone is considered progress, an integral and componential bodily infrastructure rules the medical profession, and any treatment that is holistic is considered suspect and soft because it does not get down to a microscopic and subcellular level, does not reduce the organism to its source atomistic parts. When cures do arise from alternative treatments (whether herbs, palpations, emotional gestalts, or vital energy), they are ascribed to misinterpretation or placebo effect. This entails (as well, by the way) a total misunderstanding of "placebo" and its crucial role in *all* cures.

Though it was never the intent of the benign Hippocratic guilds to take over lives, their unequal alliance with technology has yielded the whole of human existence as the spoils. The truth is that both capitalist and communist world-views of the twentieth century sought ruthlessly to turn everything into products—animal, vegetable, mineral alike—products to be exploited, consumed, and taxed, all in the name of greater collective welfare and prosperity, always in the guise of progress, equity, and justice. As the more obvious products became depleted, newer and more abstract ones were invented. This is now the unstated agenda of cyberspace and the genome.

The subtext of medicine has been to turn us into consumers (literally customers) of our own body/minds. We get to buy ourselves piece by piece—fertility, birth, immunity, beauty, and life insurance. The license to hold organs and body-parts is renewed annually. As the subliminal messages of Big Brother have it, we license our health, our sexuality, our right to live from one maintenance organization or another. We are not conceded these things by birth.

Cosmetic accoutrements, alcohol, and street drugs are insidious enough in their erosion of self into product. But the big pay-off is industrial medicine which, by a seeming trick of mirrors, has convinced a majority of the populace that they must petition it for an okay body. We don't get to live automatically and go into our own depths from there. Instead we are repeatedly called from our ground to confront our existence as mere burlap and bricks. Life is no longer a fusion of nature and spirit or an alchemy through which we arrive on this plane to ride the karma of our spirit. It is hospital garbage.

Existence has become the most marketable commodity of all, for without a life, a consumer can make little use of the other luxuries for sale. This is what medicine now offers first and foremost—not health but ransom to buy a life.

I make no argument with the validity and usefulness of a great majority of medical procedures; they find and remediate pathologies and speed recovery from injuries. But the overall way in which they have been institutionalized leads people to presume on an implicit level that their bodies are not their own.

How can people whose bodies are not their own heal them through their minds? How can people whose bodies are not their own take responsibility for the hungers and crimes of those bodies?

As long as the medical establishment claims not only the omnipotence of its procedures but the exclusive key to the provinces of healing and sanity, people will not even begin to seek intrinsic sources of healing or explore what they can train themselves to do. They will constantly look outside themselves, for maintenance as for amusement. They will excuse misdeeds as chemical imbalances and genetic flaws.

Orthodox medicine may well bequeath its technology and millennial scientific quest to a sustainable future society—these are great works—but it must give back the essential right of people to their own bodies and the responsibility of their own lives.

IT IS PARTICULARLY DIFFICULT for people to conceive alternatives once they are sick. They tend to externalize their oppressive disease event and hunt for a sanctioned modality to make them demonstrably and symptomatically better. Even when they patronize the alternative medical kingdom, they select natural cures that are the seeming equivalents of pharmaceutical and surgical ones—a bottle of herbal pills rather than a bottle of antibiotics, an adjustment rather than a scalpel. Perhaps they decide to improve their overall health by a regimen of exercise or a more conscious diet. What is harder for them is to address the persona of the disease in themselves and to turn toward it for a cure. If they were capable of this, any medicine they chose would be more effective. In fact, at this level the most widely divergent treatments are not all that different from one another.

The goal of medicine should be to creatively disorganize an overly rigid or false organismic structure/belief such that the body, mind, and spirit of the life form can reorganize themselves in a healthier, more synergistic fashion. The block to healing lies in an immobilized, often inscrutable bond between psychosomatic resistance and metabolism, an impasse that requires fresh energy and transduction.

The language of cells communicating with one another is intrinsic to the healthy functioning of tissues and organisms; yet that communication system is nonlinear and not necessarily penetrable by pharmaceutical intervention or acts of bioengineering (such as implanting stem cells in diseased tissue to grow replacement parts). Since all cells originated in multipotentiated, holographically projected forerunners, all cells are potentially stem anyway; all cells can respond therapeutically to the invocations of an inner physician; all cells can be reintegrated in the complex signaling networks of the body-mind. A creative dialogue, especially one using touch or "energy" rather than words (or in conjunction with words), might rearrange the biological codes binding organ systems and life force together and thus catalyze a healing agency.

Everything counts—the intention behind the scalpel as well as the scalpel, the thoughts and hidden agendas of a physician, words spoken in the presence of languageless newborns or patients under supposedly full anesthesia, and the mythologies and belief systems lodged in the patient's not only conscious but unconscious mind. These are not superfluities and superstitions; a medicine proposed in terms of fluid disease totems approaches the arcane, subatomic bond between mind and body, matter and energy, form and meaning. In that sense, a modernized shamanism might be millennia ahead of both physical medicine and biotechnology in understanding that symbolized entities rule every level of organism and consciousness, every level of cell communication; otherwise, sentient, autonomous agents made of cells and organelles could not arise in a biosphere.

M UCH OF OUR ILLNESS arises from global pathology at such an archetypal and psychospiritual level that we must employ new models of healing to begin to restore our human balance and the environment of this planet—though it will take many generations of self-discovery and accretion to accomplish this. My "planet medicine" proposes a revision of therapeutic philosophy and institutions so that a more inclusive paradigm of healing can guide our species through the intricacies of its present crisis.

Various alternative healing systems, by providing energetic and behavioral definitions of health, confront the problem of our global "health" more effectively than morally absolutist domains of allopathic medicine. In this farflung stalemate of values and resources, a new phenomenology would be far more useful than a new ideology.

A disease of commoditization is ruled by false symbols and quite
deadly pathologies that attach to those symbols. The desecrations

assigned to AIDS, cancer, Alzheimer's, and other catastrophic ailments are quite real indeed, but they are also driven into human anatomy by ghosts that attack the deep systems of meaning that keep cells in harmony and creatures healthy and alive. We can probably also break into those systems by intuitive and mysterious means.

It would be astonishing to most people to consider that they could be healed effectively by a Bear shaman or Zen priest. Some might acknowledge this as a poetic fancy or an unattainable ideal, but few are able to take it seriously and act on it.

It would be even more astonishing to learn that on a symbolic (and morphogenetic) level their body/minds already impose the cellular equivalents of Bear shamans and Zen priests in an attempt to self-heal and sometimes to mediate and effectuate sterile cures of science. In a realm of molecules and ciphers, latent alchemists and philosophers trade robes and empower each other inside us. The true cure is at once magically more available and fundamentally more elusive than the average person imagines. It is certainly of a different order from the cure our society presently valorizes.

T HE PRIMARY FUNCTIONAL DISTINCTION is not between orthodox scientific medicine and the array of holistic therapies and modalities of faith healing. It is between understanding disease as a process in oneself and regarding disease as an outsider. As long as diseases are reified as exogenous entities, they can never be totally cured. Their most painful and explicit symptoms may be alleviated in the name of cure, but their core will give rise to new manifestations. Most of the systems I describe in this book seek to find and touch the actual roots of disease and to stimulate a systemic cure. Some of them may represent brilliant conjectures that will be part of the science of the future. Others are probably a good part placebo and metaphor.

By presenting so many discrete modalities in such detail, I mean to demonstrate the wide range of alternatives available, both of practical therapies and meanings. By going into depth in each modality and comparing them at their most essential levels, I hope to provide readers with a key to the different aspects of themselves represented by each of these medicines. Thus, together we will begin to regain our human capacity to travel among meanings and redefine ourselves in terms of unlimited possibilities.

There are no right or wrong medicines *per se;* there is only a dichotomy between rigidity of thought and freedom of action, between biological restriction and resiliency. Limitation inevitably means fear of disease and reduction of one's body/mind to a commodity in the medical marketplace. Freedom may still incur anguish and doubt, but a body/mind is one's own, deeded from what gods there be, and one can go on whatever healing journey enhances depth of experience and personal growth. Healing may represent anything from a quick fix to a diagnosis of incurability to a miraculous remission. We are on the great road of life and death, and the path not the endgame is the true aspiration of medicine. Everyone gets to die.

"If I want a life that lasts a thousand years," Korean Zen Master Seung Sahn told his students, "it's not possible. Before one thousand years, already you are dead. So, if you understand what human beings are—what this world is really like—then you understand that you cannot decide anything. You have only this moment. If this moment is clear, then your whole life is clear."[1]

Each act toward cure is a moment becoming clear—no more, but no less.

Beyond Medicine

BETWEEN THE FOURTH and fifth editions of this book (in January 1990) I participated in a Native American ceremony conducted by a Western woman who had trained with a Cheyenne medicine man. Well into the rite she took up a small hoop-shaped drum I hadn't noticed and began beating it in rhythmic sequences punctuated by distinct pauses. We had already burned cedar and chanted. She had shaken a rattle and held a hawk feather over me.

The drum could not be evaded. The seriality of its beat and texture of its thumps resonated at different levels of my being.

"I could see your mind being chased by my drum," the medicine lady told me later. "So slippery it is, so tricky; you have so many ways and places to hide, so many ways to pretend to my drum you are there when you are not."

"Right," I thought. "All through *Planet Medicine* as well, I run."

"Your mind does you no good at this point. You must turn, embrace the drum's sound, and carry it to your heart."[2]

She was right.

What distinguishes *Planet Medicine* is not so much that its subject is medicine as that its context is our planet-wide search for a new healing imperative. The subject of the book is "medicine" insofar as disease itself is a text written on the body of man- and womankind. But disease, like medicine, when approached through mind, is both a polity in search of laws and a gap (or gash) in search of meaning. Disease doesn't think text; it just is, brilliant and profound. It defines worlds and cultures by the absoluteness of its presence, its capacity to interrupt life and impose itself on the basis of existence. Any medicine that attempts to neutralize it must become textual (or nontextual) at the same depth with the same degree of subtlety.

W HEN SCIENTISTS LOOK across the vastness of the physical universe, they see mindlessness, arbitrariness, and the utter insignificance of human beings. Against fields of starry matter we are surely zero. Jupiter alone is 1,316 times the volume of the Earth. Any single star, perhaps trailing many Jupiters, is millions to billions of times the size of the Earth. The galaxies of the heavens contain untold numbers of such stars, stretching to eternity. The universe is not only beyond comprehension; any means of comprehending it is beyond comprehension.

How science calculates this state of affairs is to declare the human condition trivial in advance. We are temporary holograms of accidental

molecular accretion in a partial vacuum filled with immense fires that
go on forever.

This gargantuan universe has no extrinsic meaning or intelligence.
Its size is raw.

I understand the vastness and brilliance of the cosmos in precisely
the opposite context to traditional science. I see a giant wheel fashioned of pure murk, a baby yawning, a god in the process of being
born. Everywhere the wheel sets its cutting edge down amid Orions
and Cassiopeias, mind trembles through dust and mud.

Where we are, the universe has never been. It is exploring the possibility of its own nature through us. It is using our experience to make
itself alive. Thus, its profundity and scope are *our* profundity and scope.
We are its rough margin struggling at the frontier of dreams, and what
is becoming conscious as we are becoming conscious (we and all sentient beings everywhere) is the creation itself.

The fires and luminous clouds of the night mark how vast and
poignant we can become if we follow our destiny. They are raw intelligence. We are focused, incarnated intelligence. As long as we stare into
our diminishment, that long will we suffer not only an incredible sense
of hopelessness and loss but the diseases and depravities of denial and
suppressed spirituality.

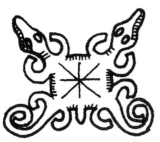

WHEN THE RIGHT hand of *t'ai chi* forming a needle
has been placed and taken from sea-bottom, then
one's arms are shot out like a fan from the roots, and one
is briefly an herb: intrinsic energy patterns change. But it
is difficult to keep this in mind, in heart—or to remember, as the old musical avowed (though not necessarily about
needles at sea-bottom), "The moon belongs ... to everyone."[3]

Notes

1. Zen Master Seung Sahn, in a talk at the Cambridge, Massachusetts, Zen Center, May 7, 1993.

2. Michelle Haviar, personal communication, Garberville, California, 1990.

3. "The Best Things in Life Are Free," words by B.G. De Sylva and Lew Brown; music by Ray Henderson, from the musical *Good News,* by Mary Lawlor and John Price Jones, 1927.

Introduction:
The
Multicultural
Basis of
Medicine

CHAPTER ONE

Spirit Healing

Disease will never be cured or eradicated by present materialistic methods for the simple reason that disease in its origin is not material. What we know as disease is . . . the end product of deep and long-acting forces.[1]
—Edward Bach

Healing in Absentia

SHAMANIC AND FAITH healing have a dynamic all their own. They defy any science which turns out doctors by a standard procedure from its medical schools, for they propose to accomplish the very same cures (or better and deeper ones) without any of the training or tools. That is, they intend the transmission (or channeling) of cures on the basis of mind alone or from a reservoir of elixir naturally abundant throughout the universe in pure energetic forms.

Successful healers have cured people long-distance merely by laying hands on letters written by them or by projecting positive mentations in their direction: Edgar Cayce's treatments by mail are legendary. He is rumored to have dispatched cures from the United States to "patients" on the other side of the world with only one known error (when he mistakenly "got" the twin of the person in France for whom he intended his remedy). ". . . [D]istance is not important, for there is no time or space in spiritual reality."[2]

The pony-tailed New Mexico healer taking the name Drunvalo Melchizedek is unequivocal about the accuracy of teleported energy:

> It doesn't matter *at all* if [the] person is physically in front of you or if they are on the Moon. They could be anywhere at all. Physical location means nothing for transfer of *prana* and thoughts. If they are physically there, then they're physically there, but if they're not there, then what I do is: I either visualize or bring in their essence (if I don't know exactly what they look like).[3]

Disciples of the Japanese art Reiki practice a rigorous protocol of long-distance healing, with both parties scheduling an appointment at which neither is *physically* present. According to one Reiki healer, "The results of absentee treatment are in no way inferior to those attained by the direct method, although patients will usually feel the effects of the latter more distinctly. In both cases, the energy will be the same. Many practitioners can feel the flow of Reiki energy in the various parts of the patient's body when they are treating with the absentee method...."[4]

A training manual instructs:

> ... [M]iniaturize the client, while holding him between your hands. You encapsulate the individual in *Christed Golden White Light*. The *Christed Golden White Light* looks like a glorious illuminated halo of vibrant crystalline shimmers of liquid white "mother of pearl" with sparks of gold floating through the depths and on the surface of the light.... When contact is established a fullness between the hands is felt. You are holding a ball of energy, a part of the etheric fabric of the healee's spiritual essence. You will physically sense the inability to close your hands, palm to palm, as long as energy is being received by the healee.... Keep in mind that subtle energies registering *from the Etheric Bodies* may not be known or obvious to the client.[5] (italics are the author's)

Is the image a holographic replica of the client, like a beneficent voodoo doll, or is it a symbolic device through which the healer shoots his initialled intention into the open paraphysical airways? In the latter

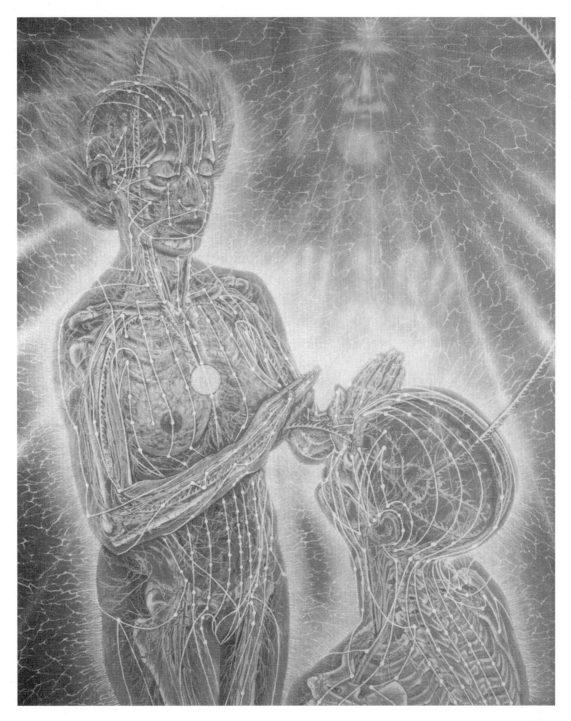

case, do his "effects" bounce off etheric "mirrors" like a pinball before connecting with some projected target? Or does a combination of synchronicity, signature, and sympathetic magic take them right to the intended recipient?

As in acts of sorcery, belief and even willing participation of the target do not appear to be prerequisites. Many faith healers recall "successfully" praying over "atheists" with life-threatening diseases at the request of worried family members.[6] Certainly projectors of black magic and malicious curses do not seek their subjects' consent.

In some instances, homeopaths have reported achieving the expected effects of a remedy just by intending to prescribe it, without ever actually dispensing a pill (which would have lacked material substance anyway!).[7]

This is not dabbling in Ouija boards. It is not idle fancying. It is meant to be practical long-distance medicine. The treatment is literally miniaturized and transported with no regard for limitations imposed by the laws of thermodynamics or the recognized topology of time and space. The sick person is supposed to receive the direct influence of the "session," even if he or she is unaware that it occurred, and be cured or altered in some concrete way.

Placebo Response and Other Mysteries

Much of what happens in the universe is spontaneous, self-organized, and autonomous. Life itself has no simple or purely physical explanation. If a patient is improved by an event, need its rationale matter? In absolute medicine, there can be no promises and no outlaws. If a psychosurgeon or Reiki master succeeds where a trained physician fails, this does not cheapen the cure. The cure, in fact, cannot be cheapened. The explanation, even the need for an explanation, is a residual issue for our intellect to resolve. People seek healers for cures, not

philosophical theory.

Spiritual healing is impenetrable to judgment or evaluation. How
can one know if an invisible or nonphysical energy lands accurately or
has a real existence at all? How can we distinguish its purported effects
from those of other spontaneous or random changes? What traits, if
any, distinguish the psychic imprint of one healer or sorcerer from
another?

If a patient is unimproved by a treatment, the healer can always
claim transcendental interference. On the other hand, if a cynical patient
derogates a particular technique being applied to him, he can attribute
any subsequent improvement to natural causes, notably the fact that
most illnesses are self-limiting and eventually improve. No matter how
many previous M.D.s might have tried unsuccessfully, no matter how
instantaneously and completely a miracle cure remedies the same condition, the skeptic always finds a way to presume that nothing happened. "No way," a rejected doctor might pout upon hearing his patient
had improved after laying on of hands; "it was prob-
ably only psychological in the first place." It probably was, but at an entirely different level than he
realizes.

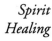

One homeopath told me about his sister who,
suffering from acute stomach pains for ten years,
had visited a number of specialists without any
cause being found. A disbeliever in homeopathy,
she saw no harm in honoring her brother's sugar
pills. When he didn't hear from her for several
months, he assumed that his medicine had flubbed.
Eventually he got a chance to ask her.

"Oh," she said. "The pains just went away."

"Was it when you took my medicine?"

She thought about it, then agreed it was right after slipping pellets
under her tongue. She hastened to add that it was a coincidence.

Recounting this sequence of events, the homeopath mused, "That's
the way it always is. The cure is so profound that the disease just slips

away. The person forgets that he was ever sick. The body knows something has happened to it; it changes. But the person doesn't make the connection in his mind."[8]

All medicine that works inexplicable cures runs into the same dilemma: there is no way of establishing a relationship between the treatment and the cure. No way now and no way in the foreseeable future.

How can needles inserted in an arm heal a stomach ulcer? How can pills with no substance in them have an effect on diarrhea? How can an adjustment of the spine improve a kidney function?

Many of the practitioners of medicines proposing such cures develop theoretical rationales based on energy transfer, scalar waves, electromagnetic fields, morphic resonance, and the memory of water. This is their post-scientific bias, even as the shaman's certainty of spirits and supernatural forces represents a pre-scientific bias. But any cure could equally well be explained by the curative benefit of plain old attention, the telepathic intercession of the doctor's unconscious, or a poltergeist.

In *The Alchemy of Healing*, Edward Whitmont recounts a case from the 1950s in which a placebo seemingly functioned as a long-sought cure for cancer. The story concerns a Mr. Wright who had developed a far-advanced lymphosarcoma. When a supposed miracle drug ("Kre-

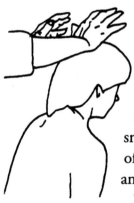

biozen") was dispensed at his hospital during a clinical trial, Mr. Wright was not even selected to receive it because of the critical state of his illness. However, the enthusiasm of the patient and his persistent begging finally persuaded the doctor to slip him this medicine against the rules. Not only did Mr. Wright rebound from the verge of death, but his "tumor masses had melted like snowballs on a hot stove, and in only [a] few days they were half of their original size."[9] Ten days after being a terminal patient with an oxygen mask, he flew home.

Two months later the results of Krebiozen trials from many different clinics were released, and it was found to be not only ineffective but inert. Upon hearing this, Mr. Wright had an immediate and complete relapse. He soon returned to life support.

With his patient's death all but certain again, the doctor decided to play a trick. He told Mr. Wright that the reason for his relapse was the rapid deterioration of Krebiozen over time. He offered him "a new super-refined, double-strength product"[10] which was actually just fresh water. Not only did the patient improve again, but this time the results were even more dramatic. Mr. Wright became quite healthy as he continued to receive water injections. Two months later, though, he read in the newspaper that the AMA had concluded that Krebiozen was useless in the treatment of cancer. In a few days he returned to the hospital in a terminal state and died less than forty-eight hours later.

Whatever else we might conclude about this unsettling course of events, it is clear that the dominant research protocol of our time, while searching relentlessly for one kind of explicit medicine (and spending billions of dollars annually in the process), is ignoring a whole other therapeutic modality that might have exponentially more value than any line of costly wonder drugs. The success of "nothing" is neither a fluke nor an outrage. It is the key to a science of transmutation and likely an aspect of the mystery behind cell-based life.

Medical educator Dana Ullman has observed that, "Homeopathy is either the most sophisticated way of stimulating placebo response, or it is a highly refined though mysterious way of stimulating powerful healing responses."[11]

If a placebo response is consistently this effective, why deprecate it? A whole new ontology of disease and health may be needed to explain the mechanism; far from indicating naiveté or fraud, "cure" by suggestion is an opening into an unexplored, unknown realm of meta-mechanical possibilities.[12]

Energy Fields

SOME SPIRITUAL HEALERS propose to be able to read life patternings around the body—that is, to "see" wavelengths invisible to the average human eye. These fields are associated with the historical aura, the electrical and magnetic pulses of the vital force, the astral body, the Hindu *chakra* system, the Egyptian *ka* "double," and the Pali Eckankar. Those who diagnose or cure by energy can "read" a disturbance in the field, usually as a separated pattern or color—bright chartreuse or yellow, a blob, sparkle, or loop of light. They warrant their method as "conducting pure energy" or "restoring the natural wavelength." The healer's life force penetrates the sheaths of the patient's various "bodies" to a depth at which it is received and distributed like breath. The change then becomes instantly visible in the energy field of the patient, though effects in tissue may not show up for some time.

Demonstrations of such events have not been left to mere assertions of believers. Kirlian photography, developed by Simeon and Valentina Kirlian just after World War II in the Soviet Union, is the most renowned among nemerous electrical enery-field recording methods on the fringes of science. When a proximate high-frequency spark generator (putting out 75,000 to 200,000 electrical pulses per second) is activated in the vicinity of a life-form—for instance, a finger or flower—in contact with a photographic plate, the processed image reveals a radiant field or corona. If a leaf is cut in half, the field of the whole will still show in a Kirlian image of the half, fading only gradually over time. Every life form possesses this invisible bioplasmic aspect.

Kirlian-derived cinema seems to reveal that a healer in the act of healing generates "radiation." Before the act, her field is bounded. At the moment of projection, plasma emits from her fingertips not unlike amoeboid surges of light from a bulb. Parapsychologist Thelma Moss calls this "a form of energy which emanates from people and interacts with other people or with objects. Of course," she continues, "if you put your hands on somebody, it's not supposed to do a bloody thing to them.... But we've done controlled experiments and obtained sometimes dramatic changes both in the person doing the healing and the one being healed—even if the healer's hands are held at a distance. It's not contact which produces the effect. It's an interaction of fields."[13]

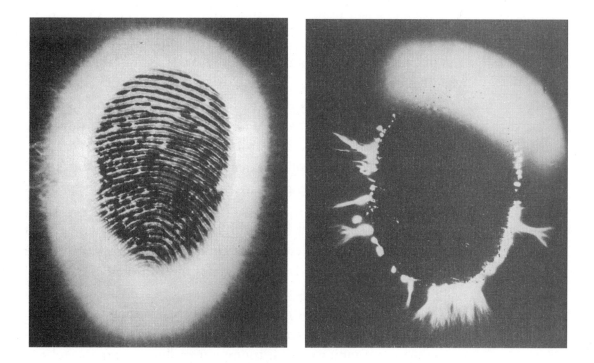

Harnessing of processes glimpsed in the Kirlian universe could give rise to a whole new paradigm of medicine. If "medicine" can be projected from auras or activated directly through a healer's hands, then other therapeutic modalities are artifice—elaborate mechanisms to accomplish what directed attention does alone.

Faith Healing

FAITH HEALING, the religious wing of spiritual medicine, is practiced in markedly divergent ways. It operates within the boundaries of traditional and evangelical Protestantism, e.g., Phineas Quimby, Mary Baker Eddy, Oral Roberts, and various Appalachian Fundamentalists, some of whom use radio shows to reach their patients, and others of whom dance with snakes draped around their bodies (according to their interpretation of Biblical injunction) to develop healing power.

Spirit Healing

Religious medicine has arisen independently inside Hinduism, Buddhism, Sufism, Shintoism, Christianity, and Judaism. It has famously been practiced by yogi Paramahansa Yogananda, Sufi musician Hazrat Inayat Khan, Reiki founder Mikao Usui, assorted Tibetan lamas, Persian Sufis, and countless others. It has also been "channeled" from "ancestors," or disincarnate beings—a newly popular revival in the United States during the latter part of the twentieth century.

The premise of faith healing is that all disease is spiritual at its roots. The healer is merely a messenger between cosmic energy and the patient's body/mind.

The context of channeled authority is cultural. Christian patients shake at the invocation of Jesus just as Haida patients resonate with the entry of the "killer whale." Biologically, it is the same vibration.

WHEN THE TRAINING of a healer or an actual healing is channeled, the "doctor"—remember—is "on the other side." Reincarnation is the most stunning possible triumph over illness—a transcendence of its direst effects through metamorphosis into an entirely new body. Hence, those who are already dead (and still petitionable) might well be the most powerful teachers and purveyors of healing. Theirs is power not over disease *per se* but over the intact passage between dimensions.

Of course, multidimensional beings, if they exist, have a more universal science than we do and can "touch" physical bodies in ways we cannot.

The signature of Jesus of Nazareth was his ability to cure major illness. He restored sight to the blind by the touch of a hand and summoned Lazarus back from death. Jesus' method was basic: he said you were healed, and you *were* healed. The particular disease or its origin hardly mattered. As the Son of God and the Holy Ghost, Jesus has power so great that not only do time and distance melt before him two thousand years later, but hack preachers in his name become spiritual "doctors" of the first magnitude. This is not a unique messiahism. Spon-

taneous timeless healing in other cultures also derives from ancestors,

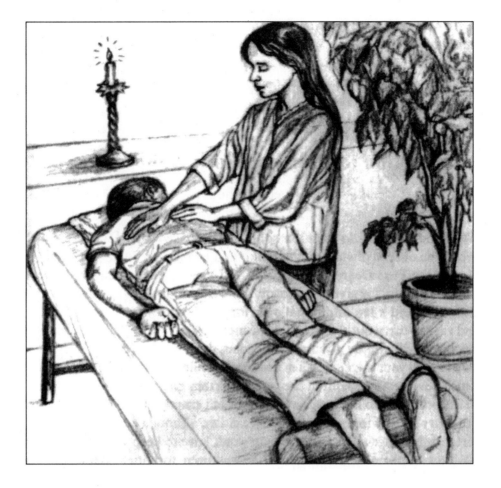

spirits, and legendary beings.

To a large degree, the *New Testament* is the singular inspiration and injunction for faith healing in the West. Practitioners need only claim lineage from Jesus (or faith in him) to be able to banish disease from cells under his aegis. Chapters and numbers of verses from the Bible are draped from walls at sporting events or held aloft on signs, reminders of sponatenous channeled effect; these numerological totems are direct invocations of power.

The Training of a Spiritual Healer

ORTHODOX MEDICINE TRAINS pharmacists and doctors, not healers. Healers gain their power and skill from *not* going to medical school: either they are "born" with it (however one explains that), or they develop it through personal discipline, prayer, vision quest, and/or initiation. The ability usually transcends any individual system. A healer is able to use the particular coda in which he or she is trained, or, in some cases, can work the universe without portfolio. Quesalid, a Kwakiutl shaman, became proficient in the very system he was poised to expose as a fraud! His investigative "apprenticeship" led to such miraculous cures that he became a renowned healer before he got a chance to spill the beans—that the disease object he extracted from sick people was just a bloodied clot of feathers. He was finally forced to bow before a magic greater than his reason and accept the bidding of spirits and totem beings (see Volume One, pp. 170–176).

A notable percentage of successful healers were average individuals who likewise discovered their talent spontaneously. Herbert Barker, the early twentieth-century British bone-setter, was prevailed upon to treat the dislocated elbow of a fellow passenger on a sea voyage to Canada. He was astonished by his own success. He had had no training at all at the time, but a cousin later taught him rudimentary medical methods. He then proceeded to realign bones, joints, and ligaments on the spot with such success that the British War Office employed him *sub rosa* during World War I.

Barker could not defend himself against an onslaught of medical criticism, and he was unable to explain his own method. He said he was not even sure how he did it. Unable to train successors, he left no system behind.[14]

Oral Roberts, the American TV evangelist, though widely suspected of fraud, convinced enough people of his gift that he built an empire upon it and even ended up underwriting branches of the medical establishment and national sports teams! He describes hearing an inner voice when he was young that told him simply to "be like Jesus." Several months earlier he had been healed by a preacher laying hands on him (he had tuberculosis). His own first success occurred during a public test he set for himself before twelve hundred people. During his sermon, an old woman's withered hand seemed to come alive. With that sign, he began treating others in the room.[15]

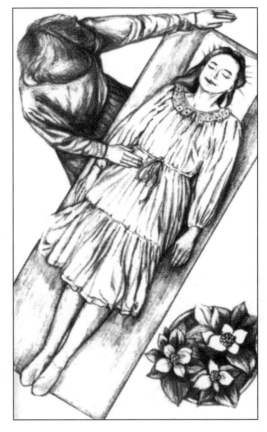

Thomas Johanson, a contemporary British healer, was "chosen" by a Roman Catholic monk in a trance as a man with healing ability. He was placed, against his own protests, in a Catholic clinic where he figured, since he was there, he might as well put his hands on patients and pray. Although he felt nothing, people reported a heat emanating from his touch. A decade later he was treating between eight hundred and a thousand people a year. By 1974 he was the head of the Spiritualist Association of Great Britain (SAGB), which had overseen the addition of spiritual-healing sections to more than 2,000 medical clinics.[16]

Harry Edwards, another contemporary British spiritualist, began his career as a confirmed skeptic. He had been told by several mediums, independently of one another, that he had a gift of healing. Curious, he began to try out his reputed magic on people who were seriously ill. The first time he touched a sick person, he felt a strong charge passing along his fingers, as though the cure were percolating through him. Years later, in an interview, Edwards summarized his conversion:

> Spiritual healing is a *science.*... It indicates that an intelligence superior to man's is operating. Therefore, it also implies that the spirit intelligence who carries out the healing has a knowledge far superior

Spirit Healing

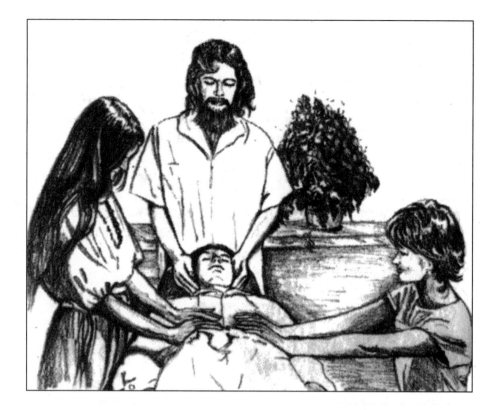

to human science. It also means that it has a much more extensive knowledge of the laws that govern physical science, energies, and things like that.[17]

This would cover the intercessions of paraphysical entities like Seth, Ramtha, Thoth, Babaji, and others by whom successful healers have claimed to be guided in their practices.

John Lee Baughman, a contemporary American healer, graphically describes four spiritualists and a doctor praying together to rid the doctor's wife of cancer:

> We saw these cells under the influence of God, and the action stemming from the subconscious to the cells, wherever they were, and they were being fed their proper direction again, and their form, and their movement.[18]

When healers suggest that they communicate directly with the etheric and astral levels and that these messages are then enacted on a physical plane through the genesis of new cells in the patient, we understand only that this is something like what *must* happen—likewise, when a patient actualizes his own spontaneous cure. That is, whether it happens or not, it is a cover story for an appearance.

We might like to believe, with the optimistic homeopath, that matter can be spiritualized and then communicated to the Intelligence of DNA. But that is mainly still our apologia. We can entertain whatever models of powers or channels we want, but our general world remains in quarantine from them. Such models are projections of our own isolation relative to such a condition. Unfortunately, the idea (and hope) of translating mind or matter into spirit is not the same as the concrete fact of it.

The fact walks the streets with the anonymous masses. The world goes on oblivious, preferring to trade its futures in abstractions of otherwise material substances like pork bellies and gold. In that sense, channeled medicines prove everything and nothing. Each act of cure is discrete and, as advertised, without reference to time and space.

Psychic Surgery

F EW HEALING METHODS are as idiosyncratic and inexplicable as the psychic surgery of Tony Agpaoa of the Philippines and José Arigo and Thomaz Morais Coutinho of Brazil. Their treatments are sleight-of-hand, placebo, telekinesis, or some combination of these. In any case it is unclear what they actually do and whether what observers see and what has been recorded on film is the real event or a mirage. These doctors "cut open" flesh with a small penknife or a motion of their hands, quickly alter the tissue, and then close the wound without a scar. At least this is what is reported by thousands of visitors. Psychic surgeons have been accused of fraud and stage magic, and quackbusters have routinely dismissed both the concept and routine as ridiculous to the point of not even meriting rebuttal. However, other onlookers have found no evidence of trickery and expressed wonderment at what they observed. John G. Fuller's description of Arigo includes an account of the first time Andrija Puharich, an American physician, and his friend Henry Belk witnessed the Brazilian's surgery:

> Puharich and Belk watched incredulously as the people moved up in line to the table, rich and poor, of all ages. Arigo would barely glance at them. For most, his hand began almost automatically scribbling a prescription at incredible speed, as if his pen were slipping across a sheet of ice. Occasionally he would rise, place a patient against the wall, wipe the paring knife on his shirt again, drive it brutally into a tumor or cyst or another eye or ear, and remove whatever the offending tissue was, in a matter of seconds.
>
> There was no anesthesia, no hypnotic suggestion, no antisepsis—and practically no bleeding beyond a trickle.[19]

Bloody down, chicken entrails, or real disease object? Symbolic transfiguration or mind over matter, or both?

At one point Arigo asked Puharich to perform the operation himself on a patient's eye. Puharich was terrified even to wield the knife, certain he would slash the eyeball. He hesitated but Arigo said, "Do it like a man!" He plunged the blade against the eye.[20] Expecting the worst, instead he experienced a repelling force coming back from the tissue. He never actually penetrated the physical eye.

Mechanically, physiologically, it makes no sense. It is not credible physics; it doesn't belong in this universe, certainly not on this planet, where a biosphere (at its own speed) makes life, cell by cell, tissue by tissue. But what about the Navaho patient who walks from the labyrinth of a sand painting cured? What about the lame who throw down their crutches and stride from the revival meeting?

The only thing that stands *for* these events is that they *happen.* Then their protocol vanishes like spring snowflakes. They cannot be replicated and no science can be fashioned from them. The idea itself of a faith healer is too hypothetical, too subjective, and too eccentric for any establishment to approach, let alone systematize. It is an uncomfortable prospect even in many holistic-health circles, where the general belief is that specific unorthodox techniques (like the palpation of tissue or the potency of herbs) are themselves the proximate causes of cures. Yet faith healing not only persists worldwide in a scientific era, in its manifold forms it may be the most popular medicine on the planet. Is it all wishful thinking, delusion?

The man restored by magicians or voodoo-masters takes his health home with him. His associates and family perhaps explain the cure by his faith or good luck (whatever *these* might be). The local doctor may of course question whether he was sick in the first place, or whether more comprehensive tests will reveal the disease still present.

Psychic surgeons have handed over gallstones extracted from patients who clearly had gallstones before their surgery and did not afterwards. The healers did not appear secretly to carry in gallstones that could then be substituted by the hand quicker than the eye; they presented their extractions immediately, and the stones were later chemically analyzed.[21] Of course any qualified stage magician will attest to an exhaustive range of tricks that can dupe intelligent and well-meaning but naive observers.

X-rays and diagnostic exams of people later treated by psychic surgeons have also shown tumors, cataracts, tuberculosis, etc., before the operation, then no evidence of these conditions afterwards. In one case (witnessed by a Brazilian neurosurgeon whose patient was the subject), a healer was eating dinner one mile away at the ostensible moment of carrying out his surgery![22] But what occurred? Teleportation of cure? Spontaneous healing? A shamanic form of Reiki?

Duplicity or sincerity?

*Spirit
Healing*

"You are doing what you are charged with, are you not?"[23] an exasperated judge asked Arigo at a trial in Congonhas, Brazil.

He answers with familiar words.

"I must say I don't even know myself whether I practice illegal medicine or not," replied the healer. "I am not the one who is doing this. I am just an intermediary between a spirit and the people.... All I know is that whenever anybody comes to me for material or spiritual help, I must try to help them. I will not turn them away."[24]

Reiki

REIKI IS A medicine which proposes to channel cosmic energy, the Source of creation in its immaculate, limitless state—prior to life forms, prior even to stars and planets. It is the finest and most absolute medicine available or imaginable. Since this energy is abundant, omnipresent, and undiminishable, one might ask why a system is needed to obtain it or, even more basically, why anyone gets sick in the first place.

These are esoteric questions whose answers lie at the heart of human existence. The fact is that the world of incarnate beings is a complex place with many pathways and interstices, some open, some convoluted, some impeded. Pure energy is deflected; obstacles develop; creatures become lost and misguided; they sabotage and suppress their natural cosmic bounty. Creatures are also mortal and in transition toward death at greater or lesser speed.

On this world, tapping bounteous energy requires learning how to regain one's original, untainted nature and working through the karmic labyrinths that separate each creature from the cosmic Source. Very few people can artlessly perceive the current of universal energy and draw on it. Most have to be trained (or retrained) and must develop a ritual mode of access—a set of visualizations or other protocols.

The healing modality of Reiki represents one possible training in cosmic energy. It is the outcome of a Japanese theologian's pilgrimage in the mid-nineteenth century for the grail of pure medicine in nature—

a quest paralleling Wilhelm Reich's orgone odyssey (described in Volume One), though differing from it in virtually every significant detail. Reich was assaying a precellular, physical life energy by scientific experiments using organic materials; Mikao Usui sought a divine transphysical, nonmolecular current by way of prayer and meditation. His countryman, Morihei Ueshiba, a century later would tap a different conduit of limitless cosmic force—converting the energetic feints and blows of fighters into maneuvers of self-protection and deflecting an opponent's aggressions into natural spirals that repelled and even spiritually transformed him. This became the martial art aikido.

A biblical scholar, minister, and principal of a Christian boys' seminary in Kyoto, Usui initially sought the lost healing modality of Christ. Unable to cultivate the power of miracle healing in himself, he committed himself to learning how Jesus healed. This research could not be carried out in Japan, so he left his homeland to attend a Christian university in Chicago. Studying scripture intensively for seven years, he earned a doctorate in theology, yet without finding the secret of Christ's healing.

At this point it becomes unclear how much of Dr. Usui's tale I am drawing on is legend.[25] An alternate version of his biography promulgated by Reiki researchers in the late twentieth century denies any Christian influence and refutes the entire biblical interlude as apocryphal history with the goal of making Reiki attractive to Westerners and recruiting practitioners from among those who would spurn a pure Japanese art.[26]

In the standard version Usui became convinced, only after studying it for years, that the Judaeo-Christian bible was not the best source for the original spiritual medicine; he realized, on the other hand, that Buddha and his disciples *had* employed a similar modality, so he switched to studying Buddhist sutras with equal perspicacity. He then traveled through Northern India and Japan, interviewing and training with monks, yogis, and other masters. Though he was met with a unanimous conviction that a Buddhist healing modality once existed, he found no one who knew how to practice it. Soon thereafter, he joined a monastery in Japan and, becoming a Zen monk, he absorbed himself in the subtle details of sutras, first in Japanese, then in Chinese and Sanskrit, to see if he could penetrate their multiple language barriers and get to the primordial symbols that activated cosmic energy.

By now both the legendary and actual Usui had saturated himself with holy scripture of at least two traditions and in six languages (including Hebrew and Greek). He had passed through all surface attributes and signs of text in a search for hidden core meaning and the key to an ancient healing system. His devotion and study had transported him outside of language and beyond conventional meaning. He was ready. Then something remarkable happened.

With the intention of discovering the secret or perishing in the attempt, Usui journeyed a few miles outside of Kyoto to a mountain site deemed especially holy and took up residency in a cave. Setting twenty-one stones outside it, he went deep into meditation and prayer, removing one stone each day to record his vigil. He had told the abbot that when the markers were gone, if he had not returned, they could come later and get his bones.

He fasted, meditated again on sutras, and chanted himself into various altered states of consciousness, but nothing earth-shattering happened. In the twilight before his twenty-first dawn he removed the last stone. As he stood and turned resignedly in the cave, he saw a tremendous projectile of light racing straight at him. Suppressing an impulse to flee, he faced it motionless, determined to receive its essence, even if it should obliterate him.

"It became bigger and bigger and finally hit him in the middle of the forehead. Dr. Usui thought he was going to die when he suddenly saw millions of little bubbles in blue, lilac, pink, and all the colors of the rainbow. A great white light appeared, and he saw the well-known Sanskrit symbols in front of him glowing in the shining gold and he said, 'Yes, I remember.'"[27]

At the moment of the bubbles he understood their meaning and, with it, the key to the universe's native healing modality. This lightning-bolt event is considered the first Reiki attunement of the modern epoch, a rediscovery of the miracle healing method of Christ and Buddha. Usui subsequently named it by a combination of the Japanese "rei" (universal) and "ki" (life energy or vital force).

On the path down the mountain we continue to skirt the realm of allegory. Stubbing his toe, Usui reached and clasped it, visualized the symbols he had just seen, and channeled a ray of energy through them. The pain vanished. Further along, he visited a roadside food stand. The face of his waitress, the owner's granddaughter, was swollen from an infected tooth. She allowed Usui to touch her cheek. He channeled the same energy through the same symbol with the same immediate result—a dissipation of pain, reduced swelling. Back at the monastery, he bathed, put on fresh robes, and then cured the abbot's longstanding arthritis.

Through the remainder of his life, Usui fostered Reiki and established its lineage. Since none of his lore was committed to writing, it is unclear how much of present-day Reiki derives from the initial lessons formulated by the founder and how much was contributed by later masters. It is likely that, as the years passed, Dr. Usui refined and complexified his original course of study, adding levels, degrees of proficiency, and new symbols—for instance, from self-healing (grade one) to healing others (grade two) to healing at a distance (grade three), and (finally) training other masters (grade four). The formal modern Reiki levels are organized somewhat differently. While level one is primarily self-healing, a practitioner can also use its symbols to treat those not physically present. Level two adds new runes and seals the path of energy from the head to the heart through the hands. The practitioner can treat others, both present and in absentia, and he or she is also permitted to charge money. Level three (the master level) provides additional symbols, a deeper connection to the source, and the responsibility to train neophytes to become practitioners.

At first Usui lived in Rei Jyutsu Ka, a spiritual community he founded, taking the example of Christ and his apostles. The members practiced Reiki daily. Later Usui decided to spread his discipline. For passing Reiki outside his spiritual group, he developed a process for directly transmitting his own attunement—a method of training, licensing, and empowerment that is still used today and that links every new Reiki practitioner back to the beam of light that initiated Dr. Usui on Mount Kyoto.

General belief is that Usui attuned seventeen Reiki masters outside his community; one of them, Chujiro Hayashi, a naval officer, succeeded him as grand master. Hayashi founded and managed many Reiki centers for both training and healing. His last disciple, in the early 1930s, was also the first woman attuned: Hawaka Takata. A Japanese immigrant to Hawaii and a recent widow, Mrs. Takata had developed a severe medical condition which proved (later) to comprise not only a stomach tumor but gallstones, appendicitis, and attendant respiratory and nervous problems. The death of her sister led her to return to Japan to bury the body in the ancestral cemetery. It was in a Japanese clinic that her serious conditions were first diagnosed. As she was prepared for surgery, a mysterious voice led her away from the table ("The operation is not necessary . . . the operation is not necessary. . . ."[28]).

She ended up at Chujiro Hayashi's clinic where she was ultimately bathed with Reiki energy by two men simultaneously. The degree of heat she felt coming from their hands caused her to search the room for electrical devices and wires from the ceiling to their pockets. There were none.

It took many months to cure Mrs. Takata by Reiki. She was so impressed by the results that she wished to become a practitioner herself. However, neither women nor foreigners were allowed to train. This obstacle was overcome by Hayashi himself who, foreseeing a major war, decided to use this new enthusiast to plant Reiki outside Japan where it could better survive. Mrs. Takata was attuned, and she returned to Hawaii to set up a practice in 1937. By her death in 1980 she had

attuned twenty-two masters. She also established the formalities and gradations of present-day Reiki and spread the system of healing to the world at large.

IN ITS MOST GENERIC FORM, Reiki is a system of nondiagnostic touch—the gentle laying of hands with fingers together on various parts of the patient's body. This version is akin to light bodywork. The potential healer first cleanses herself—physically of toxins and spiritually of doubts and anger, then cultivates compassion for all living things. While symbols are visualized and invoked, each position is held from three to

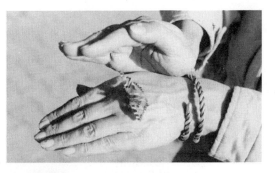

five minutes but sometimes (in problem areas) for as long as half an hour. Treatments are given four times a day for four days, although the regimen may vary. Reiki practitioners also treat animals, plants, stones, and bodies of water. One European healer regularly transmits to butterflies.

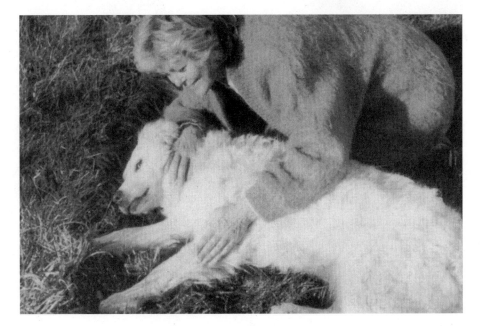

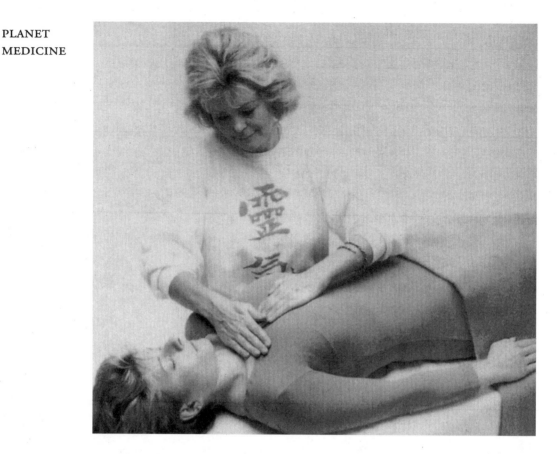

Reiki annoints an individual as a conduit for cosmic healing energy. This constitutes the reservoir of his own body/mind as well as energy from the divine and universal realms activating it. In Reiki a limitless force automatically streams from the ends of creation, outside of space-time, by an undiscovered Constant of Simultaneity, through the healer, to penetrate the area of the sick person's body most in need of remediation.

The physical hands do not conduct the flow, for Reiki is meant to be dispatched instantaneously and to other dimensions simply by intention. Before Mrs. Takata developed them as aids, there were no hand positions. In that sense Reiki is a ritualized form of faith healing or telekinetic cure.

Reiki transmission is not confined to life forms. Human-made machines draw on the same cosmic energy in the stepped-down form of electricity. One Reiki master describes using her art to recharge a flashlight whose batteries had burned out. As soon as she stopped channeling current (when the flashlight was no longer needed), it went off again.[29]

Reiki can also be integrated with dietary and psychological counseling, Chinese herbs or homeopathic medicines, and psychospiritual dialogue with the goal of learning the esoteric cause behind a disease condition (e.g., whether it is emotional suppression, withdrawal, separation of spirit and body, etc.).

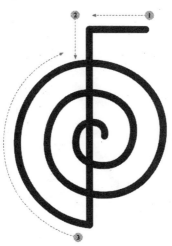

REIKI ENERGY IS specified and activated by a series of symbols that a practitioner memorizes through first drawing them in calligraphic fashion, then naming each one aloud and visualizing it; while treating clients, she revisualizes them repeatedly. The symbols may also be drawn in air discreetly with the nose or eyes when the hands are operating as contacts during a session.

The key runes include: Cho-Ku-Rei (a spiral penetrated by an upside-down L-shaped rod), Sei-He-Kei (a highly stylized dragon formed by two separate curved vertical glyphs), Hon-Sha-Ze-Sho-Nen (literally "no past, no present, no future,"[30] three or four separate characters in a vertical column involving a series of crossing lines, angles, and meeting curves), Dai-Ko-Myo (four separate glyphs with multiple triangles stacked in triangular fashion around curved marks), and Raku (a descending zigzag or lightning bolt). Cho-Ku-Rei is the initiator of resonance, a light switch; Sei-He-Kei the corridor into emotional and subconscious realms; Hon-Sha-Ze-Sho-Nen the transmitter of energy across time and space that enables channeling to overcome distance and separation; Dai-Ko-Myo (used in all healings and attributed specifically to Mrs. Takata) the spiritual first cause and attuning symbol; and Raku the grounder and stabilizer, required for attunements.

The symbols suggest the hieroglyphic circuitry of psychotronics, though they are fluid, immaterial runes rather than circuit boards (see Volume One, pp. 496–497).

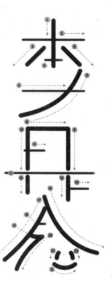

THE TRAINING PROVIDES precise positions in which to place the hands and methods of visualization for transmission:

> From your hand chakras and your 3rd eye you send a beam of Second Degree energy. The location is normally a specific part of the healee's anatomy. You activate the laser beam by visualizing the *Empowerment Symbol* directed from each hand and 3rd eye into the anatomical part and complete the *intoning* of the *sacred words*. . . . If you are knowledgeable in gross anatomy, have specific diagnostic information about a client's health challenges, and are capable of detailed visualization, you can work within the physical structure of an organ, gland, vascular or lymphatic duct, muscle, ligament or bone. . . .[31]

Reiki invokes anatomy as a way to tune and address the transfer to specific tissues. Physiology also provides a way to "name" and affirm results. A Reiki manual portrays the dialogue between healer and organs in vintage New Age skiffle:

> . . .[A]ll of a sudden you hear the *Adrenals* holler out, "I am really depleted, please laser in on me and recharge my batteries." When they are balanced, the *Liver* might speak up and say, "The body has overloaded me with toxins, how about a little additional Reiki to clear me out?" Then, when the *Liver* is happy, the *Spleen* might light up and say, "This stress has tired me down and the immune system needs strengthening before the body loses its ability to resist the emotional onslaught of a viral thought floating through its tired consciousness."[32] [italics are the author's]

In the person receiving energy, Reiki feels as soft and light as barely disturbed air, yet at the same time like dense, sticky waves and eddies. Energy seems to enter and swirl inside the body. There are occasional rivulets, trickles, and static shocks in the medium. The general sensation is a singular substanceless viscidity in the realm around and through the body. It is refreshing, inspiring, and generally delightful.

IN THE HIGHER degrees the Reiki healer attunes herself to deep-seated fear responses, psycho-emotional imbalances, and what is referred to as "the collective unconscious soul memory for this incarnation."[33] In this context healing in absentia is not merely an ability to project energy over a significant distance; it is access to the more ethereal levels of creation and karma—a fusion of religion and medicine in the greater Indo-European lineage of Christ and Babaji: transsubtantiation and yoga:

"*Absentia* is a direct contact through the mystical powers of the *Sacred Words* and *Symbols* from the healer to the Christ consciousness of the healee. We are making contact with the 5th Etheric Body, the Body of the 7th Chakra. . . . If the energy does not flow from your hands when you attune to the energy of *Absentia*, the healee's Christ Self is speaking to you saying, 'The lower desire consciousness will not utilize the energy for his highest good and is not ready to change his present consciousness, perception and vibrational energy level. . . .' It is his free will choice to continue as he is now. If you become emotionally involved or angered at his resistance, simply bless both you and him and surround each of you with unconditional love, forgiveness and light. When the time is right (Divine time), his free will shall desire to reunite with his 'I Am Christ Consciousness,' and no longer have the desire to be lonely and separate from God's promise to humankind: to be One with the Father."[34]

The goal here is quite a bit more ambitious than healing diseases and injuries; it is nothing less than opening the person to the Source of creation, the truth of his or her existence, and the harmony of all things. Ideally the recipient is then inspired to join the Reiki lineage.

Reiki attunement is technically an intellectual transmission of symbols, chants, hand positions, and sequences, and it is esoterically a permission to use cosmic energy to heal. The master opens the crown chakra of the student symbolically and, while entitling him or her as a Reiki practioner, provides a direct line back through Dr. Usui to the transdimensional beam of light. Whether such sanction is necessary to acquire Reiki power or merely a way of honoring tradition is a matter of dispute today. Certainly one can learn the extant Reiki symbols and sequences and cultivate them without a formal attunement. One can even invent one's own symbols and psychic circuitry; many practitioners do. (*"The stars belong to everyone;/they shine there for you and me. . . ."*[35]) The universe provides an infinite resource of runes and channels. If the Reiki force is as cosmic and nonsectarian as proposed, then permission could be obtained directly from any number of hyperdimensional guardian spirits or other transpersonal intelligences. If, on the other hand, Reiki was granted solely by divine beings to Dr. Usui and his enfranchised followers, then attunement through his lineage is crucial and may be something like getting an encryption removed from a piece of "software" so that the cosmic energy can flow through the initiate.

Attunement has also been described as a shortcut—an electric line back to the Source; the ritual itself is merely the circuit activator. Life forms are already "wired" or energy would not pass through them.

Licensing and money have been long-term dilemmas in Reiki. Dr. Usui claimed that when he gave Reiki away for free, people didn't respect and thus squandered it. There is nothing wrong with charging for medical training, but Usui's explanation sounds like self-justification.

When I discovered Reiki in the early 1980s, the first forms I encountered were quite ritualized, with large sums (up to $10,000 per level for three levels) being charged for attunements. Most of the practitioners I met behaved like New Age royalty, as though they held a monopoly on the disbursement of cosmic energy. For this reason I did not take Reiki seriously; I considered it almost a parody of New Age capitalism. Although I have gained new respect for it since then, my original attitude shows in my description in the previous edition of this volume. I wrote:

At its best, [Reiki] is psychic mediumship and anatomical astrology. At its worst, it is manipulative New Age psychobabble.

In theory, anyone can touch another person and attempt to transmit a healing force. Reiki formalizes and institutionalizes that process. Combining Christian mystical authority, the Hindu *prana* system, the theosophy of the etheric field, and the heightened awareness of Zen (with New Age marketing techniques), present-day Reiki projects an ambition to become global spiritual medicine. While offering a catchall disincarnate energy source for practitioners of all persuasions, it sets a standard for corporate faith healing.

After all, Reiki is also a church that charges substantial fees for initiating new practitioners while regarding a monetary arrangement as part of the symbolic union of healer and healee (Reiki tradition firmly states that there can be no healing without some prior exchange between the two parties). It justifies the expense in terms of an occult doctrine which regards money as a symbol requiring constant mutation and interchange. Money is simply another form of energy, a powerful catalyst in and of itself.

AFTER THAT EDITION was published in 1995, I met several masters who had little connection with the formal Reiki lineage and, though legitimately attuned, had paid and were charging quite reasonable sums. They also practiced a far more creative and improvisational version of Reiki, inventing their own techniques and symbols.

Suddenly the practice called Reiki intimated what universal cosmic healing should be—a community of practitioners of glyphs and rituals for drawing raw *prana* or *chi* out of nature.

In 2000, at my instigation as acquiring editor, North Atlantic Books served as the publisher for a self-healing Reiki book by Barbara Emerson, a master who sought not only to liberate "symbols, attunements, and techniques"[36] for everyone who wanted them but offered to attune all readers of her book by video. This would allow them to practice on others without direct physical conferring of power and license. It is her belief that no one owns Reiki, hence attunement can be by VCR or other electronic means: "It is not my position to limit Source by saying that something is impossible when dealing with the most powerful energy in the universe. If Reiki is for everyone, then there must be a way to attune everyone, even those not physically close to a Reiki master."[37]

You can't say that the Reiki church didn't ask for this. It furnished the rationale for its own obsolescence on a silver platter.

At this point, Reiki is not so much the Usui-Takata lineage as a millennial tradition of the transmission of cosmic healing reformulated anew in the protocols of Japanese Reiki and using its name. By now, at the dawn of the twenty-first century after Christ, Reiki has broken loose from the framework of Dr. Usui's orthodoxy, if in fact it was ever really confined to that, and its vernacularized name is fast becoming a euphemism for all universal channeled medicine.

By the time that practitioners let me know that they thought my description of Reiki in the previous edition was snide and disrespectful, I had come to my own fresh conclusion (see the companion Sixth Edition of Volume One, pp. 529–530); I honored Reiki as the epitome of harnessing timeless, delocalized, and unnamed energies by the signature of our human grace. Reiki is the sole medicine of a more perfect, nonsectarian world.

People all over the planet, in ever increasing numbers (and perhaps on other worlds as well), are visualizing versions of Reiki runes and glyphs as if they were wireless psychic-energy devices, individualizing and refining them, and conducting healing force from a variety of attunements, insights and visions, and an openness to the great mysterious and unknown beyond—the cosmic ocean.

There could be no Reiki without Dr. Usui and his long and arduous quest, but the form he discovered and named "Reiki" is likely attainable through myriad grails, journeys, and trainings. It would appear that more and more Reiki practitioners are going back to the equivalent of the beam of light and rainbow globules in the cave and, while

acknowledging and making use of symbols and positions that have proved effective, are also refurbishing Reiki as a general gateway to the vast healing forces of the universe.

Rebirthing

As taught by Leonard Orr and his disciples, rebirthing and its off-shoots—vivation, holotropic breathing, and transformational breathing—are self-generated spiritual and therapeutic cycles in which active breath becomes energy.* The legend of rebirthing places its origins in an accidental experiment. Feeling strong anxiety upon remaining too long in a bathtub, Orr decided to override his urgency to blast out and, by rapidly over-breathing, experienced tetany (paralysis) and a revisitation of the events of his life back to birth. As the rhythm of his breathing changed and its level deepened, he began to undergo emotional and somatic releases and what seemed to be actual birth and past-life memories.

Despite its name, rebirthing therapy is not limited to reliving birth. The breath cycle is meant to elicit a return of all moments not fully integrated at the time they were first experienced. The presumption is that the lack of integration was either amplified or locked into a repetitive pattern by a concomitant inhibition of breath. A fuller breath in the present allows the reexperience of the trauma in a relaxed, even joyous form; thus the blocks and illness patterns associated with it are released. Accumulated negative energy is processed, felt, and discharged. "Breathing is the basic healer," Orr acclaims. "We can clean ourselves inside and out with spiritual breathing. Our natural divine Breath of

---

*These should not be confused with any of a variety of other practices, many of them sloppy, dangerous, or both, that go by the name rebirthing. Some practitioners naively reenacting birth and its traumas have injured and even killed patients. In 2001 two such bogus "rebirthers" were sentenced to prison in Colorado for suffocating a ten-year-old girl in a blanket meant to represent the uterine canal.

Life can become inhibited at birth and throughout the School of Hard Knocks. Conscious breathing is a delight. It is more satisfying than fine food."[38]

As a technique, rebirthing teaches a strong, rhythmic breathing cycle guided by a positive imagery that may seem ingenuously affirmative to those outside the context of the therapy. As the patient breathes in and out, she gradually propagates a connected, resonant flow of breaths (the bathtub has become unnecessary, and dry rebirthing is now much more common).

Initially one's forced breathing is erratic and painful; it is difficult to establish any rhythm. One may feel as though he or she is drowning in oxygen. When a smooth cycle is finally established, one floats— the body through the passage of breaths, the mind through a panorama of images. In optimum circumstances, the journey takes on the ecstatic quality Orr described. The breaths come as waves. The oxygen becomes *prana,* pure life energy. The passage of time imparts a tinge of eternity. Stuck places and uncomfortable memories are experienced as bumps, or choppy surf, some of them barely more than blips. Occasionally there are breakers, which can be quite frightening. If a smooth breathing cycle is maintained, one passes through all this static not only unharmed but in some sense unburdened of the source traumas that are energizing it. Rebirther Bob Frissell explains:

> ... [T]his is not a regressive process to take you back to birth, early childhood and so on, even though memories of these experiences may come up for you in a session. What alone matters about these incompletions from the past is what you are currently carrying with you in a way that continues to manifest in present time.... What you are carrying with you in the form of stuck energy definitely feels like something, and you can access it in that way.... The process then is about breathing, relaxing, and tuning into feelings and shifting the way in which you have been habitually holding them in avoidance, resistance, and making wrong.[39]

One might add that in this regard feelings serve as markers for diseases. Obstructions and unresolved personal and emotional crises are germinations of colds, flus, allergies, asthma, and seeds of potential tumors. The flood of breath literally melts these knots in their earliest stage as thoughts or barely materialized intentions. If they are already materialized, it begins softening and dissipating their tissue. A person rides her knots as mere energy. Rebirthing is a process of cultivating one's own natural healing breath.

The exhale is forcibly shortened and swept up immediately in a new inhale (a priming of *prana* circulation sometimes trivialized as hyperventilation). In a simultaneous act of affirmation, one transforms this breath into an energetic seed. At the deepest possible level we acknowledge our basic situation and embody it fully and open-heartedly. Because our lesser mind is preoccupied with its egoistic concerns and tissue blocks, it is up to the Higher Self to "remember" who we are. We affirm that our experiences and sensations (however terrifying or painful) are positive, that the sublime forces of the universe are trying to heal us at every level (visceral, emotional, karmic), that we are meant to be healthy, that even pain or despair is exactly what we chose for ourselves right now.

As Higher Self, we invented this universe and willed it into being. Now that it is happening, we can't pretend to be its innocent victim.

With rebirthing, we are reclaiming the *pranic* base of ourselves, running our stagnant and impeded energy through a cosmic cleansing. If we do not constantly remind ourselves that this life is not only perfect but precisely perfect, the process triggers fear and withdrawal. Depth is initially intolerable. When it arouses terrors, by our immediately embracing them the sensations behind those terrors become joyful, as they link us to a larger cosmos.

We not only tell ourselves this in a series of resolutions or as a parable. We open all the pores and energy gates of our bodies to its rightness. More than simply to allow or believe it we *become* it. We try to feel as we would if we were this confident of our own birthright and the universe's good intentions. Then every event in the world and every experience inside ourselves becomes curative. (As an experiment, the reader might try a simplified version of this practice the next time he or she feels a recurrent stress pattern or anxiety, or awakes in the middle of the night and is unable to fall back asleep. Simply breathe and affirm every feeling, including discomfort, and, if that doesn't change things, breathe more consciously with a shorter exhale and make the affirmations more real and less merely "going along with the game." Believe them *literally.* Thank the universe for allowing you to come all the way here and feel it so deeply and poignantly.) Affirmation turns breath into *prana.*

The rebirther's cadence is not the jogger's engine of inhale/exhale; it is an overall kinesthetic, mind/body integration of sensations and feelings as they arise. Affirming is not just a matter of making adversity okay, as in the familiar Western process of toughing things out, finishing the marathon with gritted teeth. That won't accomplish anything in rebirthing. It is more a matter of: "This experience is perfect. If it does not feel perfect, I will make it so simply by declaring it. My word is unnecessary because the universe is saying the same thing. But my word is enough." Frissell adds:

> Fundamental to expanding your ability to relax into and feel the bodily sensations is the context in which you are holding your experiences. At the very least you need to be willing for sensations to be the way they are, even if you don't like them. This *will* work. Even more useful, however, is the willingness to hold everything you are feeling as a healing in process. By relaxing into and allowing your feelings on the deepest level you will create your own healing.[40]

One is never deemed deficient for having been sick or blocked in the first place. Guided by our Higher Self, each of us is simply involved in a protracted learning process which at this very moment has come to its fruition. That is why we are consciously breathing. Dynamite

affirmations in rebirthing are:

Pretend that you personally ordered whatever you are making wrong to be exactly the way it is.... See that whatever you are making wrong is part of being alive right now, and it is exactly the way it is. It is a miracle that whatever you are making wrong even exists and that it happened at exactly the right time for you, didn't it?[41]

While these can sound like the most sentimental and myopic New Age tripe, they can also be taken seriously precisely as stated. We can focus our attention on the all-too-stubborn facts of misery and disease and dismiss *prana* affirmation as wishful thinking, but then our problems become self-fulfilling prophecies. Cynicism, after all, affects the person who holds it (and has internalized it) more deeply than any person or event toward which it is directed. On the other hand, we can uncritically accept the sensations of connected breaths and breathe ourselves into another place, another body.

The subtlest forms of healing are often the ones with the fewest accoutrements and the simplest rituals. In the tradition of Jesus, say, "I am healed," and you are healed. Mean it. Make your word, your intention real.

A S BREATHING EXPANDS during rebirthing, one automatically returns to old unintegrated experiences and begins to reprocess them in a healthy fashion. This includes physical diseases, chronic conditions, and other acute maladies. Although one must be a skilled rebirther to heal viscera, in principle it is possible. Frissell describes it as house cleaning. "Who would want to live in a house that hasn't been cleaned for forty years?" he asks. "But," he says, "many of us live in exactly such dwellings." The rebirthing breath rips through the cellular-emotional house with the searing luminosity of *prana,* dislodging malignancies, traumas, nausea, indigestion, etc., in a single lucidifying breeze. All of these are swept away as cobwebs of shallow breathing.

The longer the breathing goes on, the more traumas and debilities are reclaimed—usually (according to traditional laws of cure) the deeper and older ones last. For those who hold a past-life belief system, the breathing cycle not only "rebirths" the most recent painful birth (and everything thereafter) but unfinished moments (including births and deaths) from other lifetimes.

The role of the rebirthing practitioner is that of guide and protector. She may occasionally give instructions to alert the breather to stay conscious of his breath cycle and to continue to allow experiences to arise and then to affirm them. Just by breathing fully in concert with her client, she reminds him of the journey they are on together. It is as though the pair were traveling through parallel internal landscapes, pulling each other along like mountain climbers on invisible ropes of energy. Skilled rebirthers learn to share (perhaps telepathically) the actual crises of their clients on the precise breaths during which they are undergoing them and thus to transmit their own breathing as part of the healing and repatterning cycle. They realign themselves and the stuck person in the same universal stream of energy.

Yet rebirthing is not bodywork. The rebirther does not use massage or even light touch. Orr's guidelines emphasize that since any person has the ability to rebirth naturally and will do so best if physically unaided, were a rebirther to assist the process (and here the birth metaphor prevails), she would be reinvoking the intrusive obstetrician who (in most instances) made birth a traumatic experience the first time.

ORR GRADUALLY CAME to view his guided breathing as much more than just a process of aerobicizing and healing with meditation and positive thinking. He suspected he was on the verge of a breakthrough in metabiology, a science of immortality, and he began training the deep breath as an agency of total bodily transmutation. If creatures naturally cycle *prana* as well as air, they should be capable of feats of cellular mutation. They should be able in fact to renew their basic anabolic energy. The opposite is also true: unless they expand to permit

prana flow into their systems, its nourishment is dissipated and lost—

or worse—transformed into an adversary which turns against them as fear, rigidity, and, ultimately, disease. Cut off from their natural healing energy and mistaking it as an enemy, they become sicker and their life-span is shortened.

By extension of this logic, traumas and pathologies do not just come to awareness randomly during rebirthing cycles. They return literally because *prana* is so powerful and pure that anything which is less pure is drawn immediately to the surface to be addressed by it. This is why the process of affirmation must be continuous and conscious and the accompanying breathing ever more precisely delegated. Unless the momentum of the breath is facilitated by the widest possible systemic assimilation and faith in one's own work, it begins to shrivel back into lower breathing. There is no middle ground: one is either expanding or contracting. If we are expanding, then every disease—mental, physical, spiritual—will eventually arise in its time and dissipate.

Orr ultimately came to promote his system as a rediscovery of a lost Vedic science:

> Rebirthing is an American form of prana yoga that is closest to Kriya Yoga. It may be called scientific breathing rhythm or spiritual breathing. Simply described, it is a relaxed, intuitive, connected breathing rhythm, in which the inhale is connected to the exhale, and the inner breath is merged with the outer breath. This merging of pure life energy with air sends vibrations through the nervous system and circulatory system, cleaning the body, the human aura, and nourishing and balancing the human mind and body.[42]

As his persistence in the bathtub proved, Orr was not one to take halfway measures. During a trip to India he purportedly met the immortal saint Babaji in an embodied form and received his permission to transmit the esoteric yoga of healing and immortality to the West. As Kriya Yoga, rebirthing takes the practitioner through the body to the limits of incarnation itself. Orr describes Babaji's talents:

For Jesus to go through physical death or for us to do it is a big deal, but Babaji is the total master of life and death. For Him physical death is a plaything which He uses to raise the consciousness of his Devotees.

He appears to me [now] almost daily as a bird, bug or as a human. At a certain point in your relationship [to him] you can tell the difference and, at another point, there is no difference. Babaji is all over. He is a particular historical person and also omnipresent.... He is mortal and immortal at the same time.[43]

Whereas rebirthing may have begun as a lay therapy for transforming a painful delivery from the womb (and is accepted as such under national healthcare systems as a medicine in many European countries), it has also grown into both an occult science and a theosophical religion. At an exoteric level it still functions as a breath journey for assimilating and transforming negative emotions and disease patterns; at an esoteric level it is a system fusing breath and mind to alter cell activity and assemble a new conscious body. From this standpoint, every human being is potentially Babaji, can master the physical realm, and thus can continuously heal, refresh, and rebuild his or her body at the organic base. Orr's destiny became a doctrine of immortality for the masses:

The belief that death is inevitable will kill you if nothing else does. But the truth is that your spirit is already eternal, you only have to move your mind and body into harmony with your eternal spirit.... Unless your parents are already immortal, you have probably inherited a death wish.... You kill it by unraveling your negative thoughts and feelings about death one at a time [like the waves experienced in rebirthing]. Death has no power except what you give to it in your own mind. Nobody can kill you but you. No one can kill you without your consent. Life is stronger than death.[44]

As religious metaphor this is neither unique nor new. But Orr didn't mean it as metaphor. He proposed immortality as an accessible technique on the level of learning to drive a car. Living forever is a natural

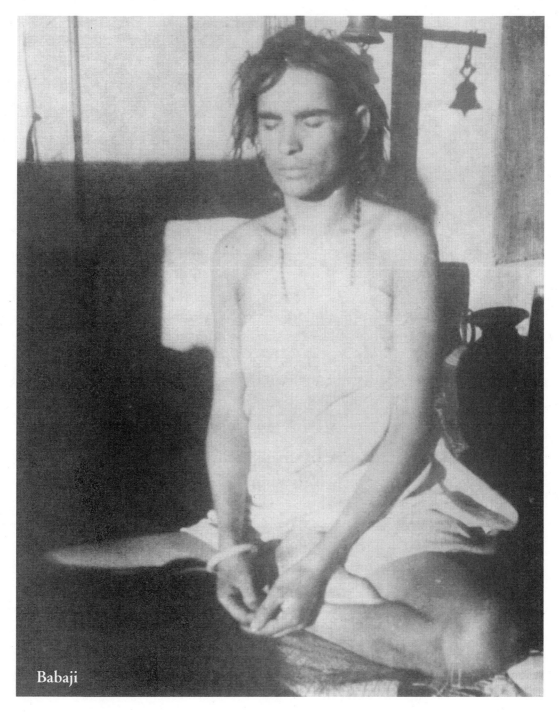

Babaji

skill to be cultivated. He argued that the only reason this hasn't achieved universal recognition yet is a profound species-wide death wish—that is, death is the most deep-seated and stubborn habit of the human race. People die because they assume they will die and are taught this from the beginning of life and because they refuse to change their minds and assimilate the energy that is available.

> The physiology of Physical Immortality is based on personal inner awareness of our energy body. It is learning how to clean and balance our energy body on a daily basis with earth, air, water and fire.[45]

Whatever judgment one may have about this notion as science (or hubris), one should not overlook the implications of the mind-sets it trains.

I accept Orr's good faith and take him at his word. I also think he is going to die. But by stating the incredible so matter-of-factly he presages a more credible possibility: one can transform a habit of neurosis and presumption of misery through a breathing and affirmation technique and make oneself into a healer. After all, if we tell ourselves (while breathing *prana*) that death is a mirage, what is depression or AIDS?

Esoteric rebirthing trains a new attitude toward the relationship between body and spirit—an attitude expressed in enhanced breathing and new thought patterns. Immortality is the password for that relationship; it does not have to be also a guarantee of everlasting life.

Ideas about transfusion of body into spirit (matter into energy) are not in themselves shocking. They are part of everyday Christianity. They permeate science, holography, telecommunications, and cybernetics. But we do not usually take such ideas personally. Not only do we not live them, we do not know how to live them. In fact, most people believe that we cannot live them. They are meant for the transdimensional universe or some future evolved race, not for us as individuals. "Think again" is, in essence, what Orr says. "Everything is here. We *are* the evolved race."

A conventional version of his thesis might be: We are assemblages of elemental substances based in energy fields. Our minds are also energy fields. If we cleanse and renew these fields in the manner taught by ancient yogis and avatars, then we can travel at will between matter and energy, body and spirit. We can redirect negative thought patterns and deter their replications in the flesh. We might also be able to change the basic catabolic "thought pattern" that leads to our dying. We have no idea what might be possible eventually through human consciousness. After all, if mind and body are both energy, then if we become skillful we should be able to prescribe any pattern for them we want, including new bodies (like the Kriya master Bhartriji who "can have two bodies if he wishes [and] . . . can adjust the age of his body as easily as we adjust the dial on our TV"[46]).

Orr is not saying it is easy to become that skillful. I do not even think he is saying that it is possible, though he would surely dispute me on this point. Trickster that he is, Orr states everything with the same casual certainty, so it is not possible to know what he truly believes. I am not sure it is even important. The real issue is: does rebirthing work? Does it heal neurosis and physical disease? If it does, then affirmations are legitimate medical tools.

If rebirthing is a viable therapy, then the rhetoric is merely another affirmation, a means of invoking the correct mind state for personal growth.

Of course we know that, despite the legends of Babaji and Bhartriji and Orr's confident assertions, average people cannot simply turn immortal. I wonder, however, what *can* they accomplish by simply breathing and taking responsibility for healing themselves *as if they might live forever?* What might occur after many centuries or even millennia of such practices? How would an Earth populated by full-breathing beings change? If we don't ask such questions and entertain such possibilities, we will never unlock the potential of humanity. Even beginning this process may be generations away from us, but that is no excuse for failing to take the first step, for not defying scientific authority and finding out what is possible.

"Not your average American lifestyle,"[47] Orr wistfully concludes.

Faith Healing and Karma

WITH SO MUCH potential in laying on of hands, channeling dis-incarnate spirits, shooting energy out of palms, conducting Reiki, and breathing immortal bodies, why do people get sick at all and die? Why is spirit healing at best sporadic? Why can results not be replicated and taught to the masses? Drunvalo Melchizedek offers one explanation:

> We live in a school, and so diseases actually do serve a function. There is a learning process in it. A lot of times when I ask permission of someone if I can heal them—not me, but if I can be involved in that process—their Higher Self will come in and say, "No, uh-uh, get away." And I have to back away from it. In fact, I find this about fifty percent of the time because that person's learning something. They're learning compassion; they're learning patience; they're learning humility. . . . On the other hand, sometimes the person has learned the lesson but has become attached to the pain or the situation and doesn't know how to break that—in which case the Higher Self will usually say, "Yeah, if you can do something, go ahead." I had to learn a hard lesson on that one time when I had a very good friend who was almost dying in the hospital—she had a baby who had died in her and been dead about a month, and the infection went through her whole body. And they didn't think that she would live for another two or three days. My inclination was, "I want to help you." And when I went to her Higher Self, it said, "No, stay away!" In fact it was very energetic about it. It really did not even want me to get near her. I backed away and said, "Okay." But I felt in myself that she would probably die—which is okay too. I mean there's nothing wrong with dying; it's part of life. But what happened was—and I saw the wisdom in the whole thing afterwards—she healed herself all by herself, and in the process became a much stronger and better person. . . . My interference could have really harmed her.[48]

Spiritual healing may propose to embrace and trump every kind of medicine, drug, and technique, but it can do so only in the context of the sick person's karma and position on the path of life and death. Potentially the spirit healer can accomplish anything, but if he routinely tapped that power, then there would be no place for the complexity of life experience. Everyone would become healthy and complete and behave only in behalf of all sentient beings. We do not have a healer on the planet capable of this, so we can hardly hope to cure the populace of its malaises and lesions in progress. Instead, we are being asked—and this is certainly explicit in the present global quandary—to heal ourselves as best we can.

Agency

T HIS SECTION OF the book is a shot in the dark.
None of the following scenarios could be true; yet each one expresses an aspect of who we are.

Sometimes I imagine that the fabric of reality is cohesive enough that we can trace cause and effect in most esoteric cures; other times I believe we are fooling ourselves with a coverlet that is coming unravelled at every possible margin, as we pretend to foretell the birth and death of the universe itself. The cosmos is likely far murkier than we allow, and what we call truth may be better characterized as the "truth mystery."

The "stories" I am about to tell reflect a verity we cannot intuit any other way. In fact, it may be that our most significant truths are hidden so far beneath the surface that their nature can be intimated only by extraordinary statements of myth and hyperbole.

Scenario One: Spirits or Intelligence in Other Dimensions

The universe is not as we perceive it. Although scientists propose to characterize all events, they like the rest of us are operating with five senses that record a meager portion of the *known* spectrum of radiation (and they are relying as well on only a few aspects of those five senses).

Psychics who dissent in the particulars of their descriptions of other dimensions all agree that Earth is but one possible zone in which to be alive and aware. Other dimensions and realms impinge on this one—and perhaps even have a hierarchical relationship to it such that spirits (many of them once incarnate here) can assist those on this plane.

Scenario Two: Aliens and Spirits Confused

Extraterrestrials are presumably the outcome of molecular chemistry and natural selection on their own planets and have had to travel here over vast distances in ships (by a method of propulsion unknown to us, thus suggesting access to more powerful energies). Spirits, whatever planet was their origin, are not presently embodied on this plane at all. If they "traveled" here, it was across nonmaterial dimensions. The two sets of outsiders overlap in our interpretations of them. As long as channels and contactees do not know the nature or source of an encountered humanoid or leprechaun (and these visitors either do not tell them or they prevaricate), we could assign any beings either to the myriad unknowns of other dimensions or journeys across the vast physical distance between us and other solar systems. Even this distinction may not clarify the matter. After all, the supertechnologies of more advanced planets may allow multidimensional travel, resembling spirit visitation.

In the late twentieth century people—almost randomly with respect to regions of the world, educational levels, and walks of life—reported contact with intelligent creatures who were seemingly not human and claimed that they came from other planets. These beings, not unlike those from exotic races portrayed in the "Star Trek" TV series, invariably had developed remarkable techniques for psychokinetic healing and/or machinery that allowed microsurgery and reengineering far beyond our level of expertise.

Once we admit a plethora of outside entities and divine forces, there is no end to what is possible. All manner of disincarnate intelligences and transdimensional energies—for cursing or for curing—can be summoned by a magician or healer.

More materialistic and scientifically advanced beings from other worlds and dimensions can contribute psychotronic tools and medical technologies still removed from us by billions and billions of years at our developmental pace, including machines that beam instant orgone, alchemical elixirs, and microdose potencies. By such a time, argue some enthusiasts, anything will be possible, including intervention in our world across time.

One popular rumor is that the ancestors of one of these races cloned our species hundreds of thousands of years ago from a fusion of their own tissues and the tissues of native terrestrial primates. They now amputate cattle and collect dead birds for continuing biotechnological research.

So we are confronted with the contradiction of aliens (or spirits) who either wound and hypnotize or heal and empower and who resemble or masquerade as each other. Any of these extraterrestrial creatures might behave identically to the postulated hidden intelligences of cells and coronas of the body, so their hypothetical presences become other ways of explaining the same things. We can blame our misfortunes or credit our healings to extraterrestrials and humanoid intelligences much in the way aboriginal peoples assigned agency to pagan spirits and ancestors. By this argument the agency of faith healing is always a spirit guide or trickster. He, she, or it needn't even visit our planet or dimension.

Electronics engineer L. George Lawrence, in experiments conducted in 1971 in the middle of the Mojave Desert (in Southern California) with cacti, wild oak, yucca, electrodes, and a telescope pointed at the heavens, seemed to pick up messages from planets in Ursa Major, or rather he claimed to detect them in the living vegetal tissue of terrestrial plants. There are no visiting ETs in this scenario, merely a holograph of them lasered so powerfully onto the Earth that it can be tracked in every flower, the cells of every wasp, and in the lattices of our collective unconscious minds.[49] We imagine their presence—and even their activities and accoutrements—only because they are transmitting a subliminal mandala of their world into our minds, holding us collectively in a psychotronic trance.

Even if proposed extraterrestrials could not visit the Earth (too far or too inconvenient!), they could hypothetically communicate the same energy to us telepathically across galaxies (like Reiki masters), intrabiologically through plants, or even as messages in nucleic acid from which they seed the Earth (or once did). This primal substance would then have spawned not only our bodies but our collective unconscious minds. At such a point, the occult rituals of the Egyptians, enacted by Aleister Crowley in the cult of the Golden Dawn, become etiologically synonymous with the wisdom of a Hathor race on the fourth overtone of Venus or "dolphins" on a planet of Sirius.

Scenario Three: Internal Energy

Our whole technology is a kind of rinky-dink imitation of the real internal science the higher races of the cosmos have mastered. We have cars and planes and computers and use rockets to penetrate the most meager spans of space. We treat our diseases mainly from without. Meanwhile, the real "technology" of most of the beings in the universe is a science of healing (and creating) through mind and breath. Spiritual medicine is an attempt to get Earth in touch with a cosmic order of physicians.

Yet as long we build and rely on machines, we lose in ourselves the precise equivalents of each power those machines tender. We cannot cross galaxies because we have restricted ourselves to mere, highly polluting local travel. We cannot redirect cells or heal directly, except sporadically, because we have manufactured robots to work in our stead. By externalizing science, we lost our own natural powers.

Scenario Four: Consciousness

Newtonian-Darwinian science proposes a universe of matter in which

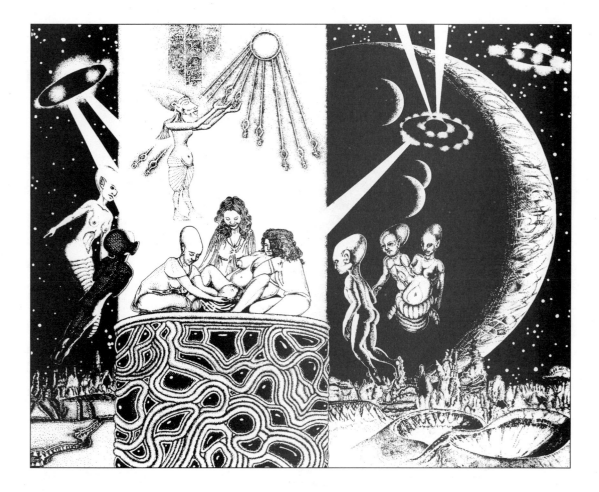

mind arises randomly as an epiphenomenon of complex molecular systems. However, consciousness may come first; it may precede atoms, molecules, and cells, and fashion them from its own proclivities, its tendencies toward form and expression. All consciousness in the universe would thus be one, a singularity from which life forms on myriad worlds draw their breaths and minds. Sentient beings everywhere would be in touch and in latent collaboration. We would then have the possibility (at any time) of returning to pure consciousness and redirecting matter—atoms, molecules, cells—which are actually epiphenomena of it.

Spirit Healing

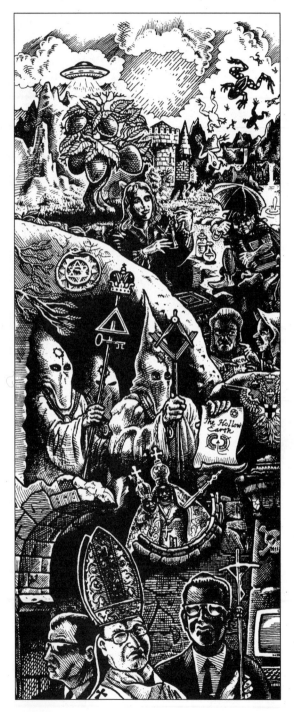

This is not an easily accessible undertaking, for mind is deeply entangled by local matter and is subject to its colossal thermochemical energy and dense, binary infrastructure.

Scenario Five: Love

Transit across the cosmos and healing have *absolutely nothing* to do with metal ships, jet propulsion, and surgery, but leapfrog in vehicles from one whole region to another through the centers of stars and beam the equivalent of *chakra* stem cells. Entry into our sun, for instance—a foolhardy act which would occasion instantaneous incineration in our primitive form of spacecraft—in an appropriate vehicle sets one on a swift issuance out through double-star Sirius. In vehicles composed of feelings as well as matter, the propellant (and the medicines and life-support systems of their occupants) is the transmission of pure love![50] *Merkabas* (translated from the Semitic as "chariots") are vehicles. In a primitive form, they can be simply cars or planes. In a more sophisticated context, they are devices used for passage between star systems and galaxies, time travel, and transdimensional relocation. We build external metal *merkabas,* fuelled by chemicals without love or spirit, and run them like taxis, while real spaceships

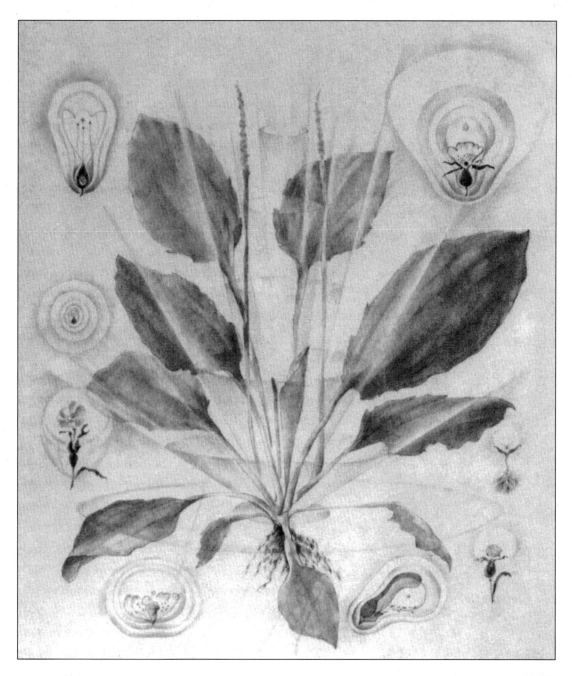

use pure love to move among starfields.

An internal *merkaba* is literally a spaceship created by a spiraling sequence of sixteen or seventeen breaths, each fused with (and thus ostensibly energized by) a projection of love and an image of three star tetrahedrons—in essence, gigantic supersonic Cho-Ku-Reis and Dai-Ko-Myos.

This is not romantic love or anything resembling Valentine's Day conceits. It is molecular-telepathic love, divine love as an actual force, like gravity, which Christ consciousness once drew on in its Divine Incarnation on Earth but which we are now having difficulty manifesting even in trifles because of our obsession with machines. This force is the major factor in the cohesion of substance and gives rise to romantic love and all creatures born from syzygy. It is the purest and most resonant energy in the universe and the only one that can propel mind and matter at speeds faster than light. It is the basic universal fuel and medicine.

SOME INVESTIGATORS IN the early 1990s purported to have discovered a universal series of shapes behind all alphabets and languaging code systems, so that a sacred morphology (representable in its most basic form as a series of two-dimensional projections of a torus inscribed in a three-dimensional tetrahedron) can give rise to all Hebrew, Greek, Arabic, and perhaps even Roman, Chinese, and Cyrillic letters. An alphabet that speaks in the rudiments of creationary geometry and Divine Intelligence is telling us, no matter what we say otherwise, that we are constructed—body and mind as well as speech—from a sacred binary sequence of syntaxes. Hence, while the text of Genesis narrates the myth of the Creation in one voice, it lays out the precise mathematics of it in an anagram of its Hebrew letters. In this interpretation, there would *always* be two simultaneous writings: one in contemporary vernacular code and the other in the esoteric code of the root iconography. Curative power might thus come from the potentization

of a latent alphabet that translates the seed forms of sounds and shapes

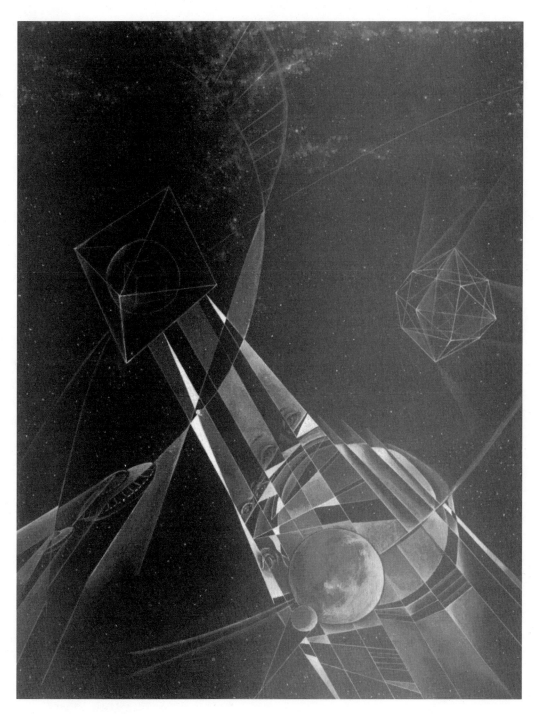

75

into sequences which are potentiated in objective psyche and soma, including the transcription of DNA into amino acids and protein configurations. The Qabbala purports to depict the genesis of all matter and shape from an alphabet of Yahweh's speech.[51]

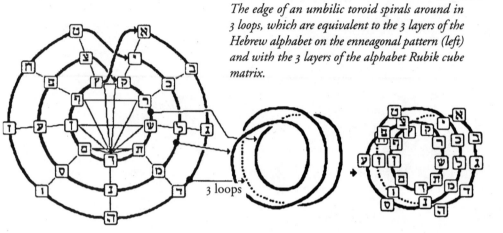

The edge of an umbilic toroid spirals around in 3 loops, which are equivalent to the 3 layers of the Hebrew alphabet on the enneagonal pattern (left) and with the 3 layers of the alphabet Rubik cube matrix.

3 loops

© Stan N. Tenen/Meru Foundation, San Anselmo, California

Umbilic toroids

To make one's own internal *merkaba* one must breathe these primordial alphabets through deep geometrical properties and simultaneous affirmations. Pyramids, star tetrahedrons, isocahedrons, dodecahedrons, spheres, and the interplay between binary sequence and the Fibonacci Series are the underlying matrices of creation; they brought stars, time and space, worlds and their life forms, and our own mode of consciousness into being once upon a time. They provide a wellspring of energy immeasurably greater than nuclear fission, inexhaustible, healing, and nonpolluting—the hidden source (agency) of all spontaneous healing.[52]

Scenario Six: Sacred Geometry in the Hands of Aliens, Ancient Astronauts, or Spirits, or Implanted by Higher Intelligence

This universe is seen as a grand experiment in geometry, a play of forms in which we are the original mathematicians who have located ourselves experientially in an event we continue to improvise. Here on the cutting edge we make reality as we go. And we are alone. Or we are "them."

All power extends from the internalization of numerical ratios and primes of numerology (34/21, 46 mitoses to generate the cells in the human body, universal constants such as pi, etc.) in the context of simultaneously opening our heart *chakras*. This is how love in the universe is translated into energy and vehicles of transit, originally by compassion (as in Buddhism) and by direct *prana* breathing (rebirthing), or by a combination of these while building *merkabas* through progressions of ratios and primes.

I WILL LEAVE THESE scenarios and their arguments because they go on forever. The hypothetical healing agency is always going to be more complicated than its cover stories. Finally, our relationship to natural healing power is compromised by all our belief systems, whether those systems be ones of utter skepticism or naive acceptance, whether they be conscious or unconscious. Any time we assert that "this is what spirit healing and vital energy are" or "this is where they reside," there is someone else with a different allegiance and just as good a story. So, in the end, we are doomed to practice and cultivate something which is inscrutable and unknown, in the context of a greater mystery.

Notes

1. Edward Bach, *Heal Thyself* (London: C. W. Daniel, 1931).

2. David G. Jarrell, *Reiki Plus: Professional Practitioner's Manual for Second Degree* (Celina, Tennessee: Hibernia West, 1992), p. 11.

3. Drunvalo Melchizedek, "Flower of Life Workshop," Dallas, Texas, February 14–17, 1992 (video recording).

4. Bodo J. Baginski and Shalila Sharamon, *Reiki: Universal Life Energy. A Holistic Method of Treatment for the Professional Practice/Absentee Healing and Self-Treatment of Mind, Body and Soul* (Mendocino, California: Life Rhythm, 1988), p. 67.

5. Jarrell, *Reiki Plus,* pp. 12–14.

6. Paris Flammonde, *The Mystic Healers* (New York: Stein & Day, 1974).

7. Edward Whitmont, personal communication, 1986.

8. Anonymous (by request), personal communication, 1987.

9. Edward Whitmont, *The Alchemy of Healing: Psyche and Soma* (Berkeley, California: North Atlantic Books, 1993), p. 66.

10. Ibid., p. 67.

11. Dana Ullman in the preface to Richard Grossinger, *Homeopathy: The Great Riddle* (Berkeley, California: North Atlantic Books, 1998), p. ix.

12. See also Norman Cousins, "The Mysterious Placebo," *Saturday Review,* October 1977.

13. Thelma Moss, "Kirlian Photograph and the Aura," interview with Roy L. Walford, in *Io #19, Mind Memory Psyche,* Plainfield, Vermont, 1974, p. 174.

14. Brian Inglis, *The Case for Unorthodox Medicine* (New York: Putnam, 1965), pp. 109–112.

15. Paris Flammonde, *The Mystic Healers,* p. 71.

16. Ibid., pp. 165–66.

17. Ibid., pp. 153–54.

18. Ibid., pp. 143–44.

19. John G. Fuller, *Arigo: Surgeon of the Rusty Knife* (New York: Crowell, 1974); reprinted by Pocket Books, New York, 1975, p. 20.

20. Ibid., p. 234.

21. Ibid., pp. 196–200 et seq.

22. Lee Pujols and Gary Richman, *Miracles & Other Realities* (San Francisco: Omega Press, 1990), pp. 169–70, 215.

23. Fuller, *Arigo,* p. 121.

24. Ibid., pp. 119–21 (quotes rearranged for emphasis).

25. Barbara Emerson, *Self-Healing Reiki: Freeing the Symbols, Attunements, and Techniques* (Berkeley, California: North Atlantic Books, 2001).

26. Barbara Thomas, personal communication, 2001.

27. Baginski and Sharamon, *Reiki: Universal Life Energy,* pp. 22–23.

28. Emerson, *Self-Healing Reiki,* p. 7.

29. Ibid., p. 16.

30. Ibid., p. 71.

31. Jarrell, *Reiki Plus,* pp. 14–15.

32. Ibid., p. 15.

33. Ibid.

34. Ibid., p. 11.

35. "The Best Things in Life are Free," words by B. G. DeSylva and Lew Brown, music by Ray Henderson, from the musical *Good News* by Mary Lawlor and John Price Jones, 1927.

36. Emerson, *Self-Healing Reiki,* cover.

37. Ibid., p. 19.

38. Leonard Orr, *Bhartriji: Immortal Yogi of 2000 Years* (Chico, California: Inspiration University, 1992), p. 22.

39. Bob Frissell, *Nothing in This Book Is True, But It's Exactly How Things Are* (Berkeley, California: Frog, Ltd., 1994), pp. 178–79.

40. Ibid., p. 176.

41. Ibid., pp. 203–204.

42. Leonard Orr, *Physical Immortality: The Science of Everlasting Life* (Sierraville, California: Inspiration University, 1980), p. 11. The material from this and other books by Leonard Orr has since been collected in Leonard Orr: *Breaking the Death Habit: The Science of Everlasting Life* (Berkeley, California: Frog, Ltd., 1998).

43. Orr, *Bhartriji,* p. 18.

44. Orr, *Physical Immortality,* p. 9.

45. Orr, *Bhartriji,* p. 22.

46. Ibid., p. 25.

47. Ibid., p. 29.

48. Melchizedek, "Flower of Life Workshop."

49. Peter Tompkins and Christopher Bird, *The Secret Life of Plants* (New York: Harper & Row, 1973), pp. 46–49.

50. Melchizedek, "Flower of Life Workshop."

51. Stan Tenen, *The Matrix of Meaning for Sacred Alphabets* (San Anselmo, California: Meru Foundation, 1991), VHS videocassette.

52. Melchizedek, "Flower of Life Workshop."

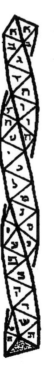

CHAPTER TWO

Healing, Language, and Sexuality

The Healing Dialogue

NO MATTER WHAT energy or information is transmitted from a healing source, nothing will improve unless the sick person can receive and assimilate the message. The receptivity of the patient is ultimately more activating than the power of the physician. Somehow, through the nervous system and viscera, the various energy fields hypothesized around the body, and/or the "Intelligence" associated with the cells themselves, a meaning called "cure" is transposed from a medicine or healer into flesh. However little or much we think we know about its ontology, the cure must not only communicate to the essential nature of the organism but communicate convincingly *one tiny thing*. An acupuncture needle, a microdose of arsenic, or a surgical excision are equally subject to this condition. All healing rests on the potentiation of a curative message.

As much as psychic surgery, conventional medicine begets a subtextual "dialogue" that conveys systemic meanings. The actual curative message may travel not only apart from but *despite* the express methodology of the healer. The best surgeons, for instance, communicate an *essence* of healing while, at the same time, making appropriate physiological repairs.

The "worst" doctors, by contrast, are the ones who simply cannot be "spoken to" and—despite their words—say nothing. They continue

to talk in the deceptively neutral language of technology and business.
They prefer to abstract the patient and to be abstracted. They may be
"nice" to a fault, but that niceness is mostly affect—an unintentional
parody of the concerned healer. Their expressions of concern mask a
lack of real concern. However modern their tools and skillful their techniques, they cannot help but transfuse the persona of the uncaring
robot they aloofly mime. They can deliver the benefits of technology,
but they can never heal in addition.

LAYERS OF CODES denominate the various veils and deep structures
of our world. Behind every known language is an unconscious one—
not only associative codes of the psyche, but buried strings of atavistic
forms and unremembered memories. Margaret MacKenzie reports that
shamans in the Cook Islands lapse into ancient languages only they and
the sick understand, and then only during actual treatment.[1]

In reality, it is all "language," from cell formation to texts of mathematics describing those cells. We are located in bottomless subtexts
of chromosomes, tissue fields, histories, common law, belief systems,
jurisdictions, "technologemes," etc. Even our claims to locale in time
and space (individually and collectively) are more diagnostic than historical. "Past" and "present," "mind" and "symptom," are conventions.
The writing of the world on its own body approaches us as intimately
as any disease, so each disease and each cure writes us again as a text.

ACCORDING TO CHIROPRACTIC THEORY, "signaling errors" are transmitted from the articulations of the bones, from the nervous system, and within the viscera and settle in both the skeleton and personality.
Curative snaps of spinal vertebrae arouse signaling mechanisms that
either have lapsed into repetitively tracking or are totally numbed. In
the simplest, most mechanical sense, an adjustment of the subluxated
vertebra merely eliminates an impingement, but a chiropractic recoil
also releases "energy" and information in a discrete burst. Feldenkrais
and Alexander Techniques alter patterning errors by "reinstructing" and

recoding stress cycles. Osteopathic unwinding follows tissue grain to a stuck point and shows it both where it is and where it still has freedom; it adds a few grams to tissue resistance, then reads the new tissue state and elicits another motility. Homeopathic microdoses supply resonant disease images and reflections in order to give the system an alias in which to read itself at a different vibration. An Ayurvedic physician takes a patient's pulse and then attempts to select an herb or other remedy vibrating at the same frequency as the homeostasis or disease pattern he feels. All of these are language systems, not in the formal or diplomatic sense but insofar as they transduce one form of structured code into another. Organ recovery is literally recovery of morphogenic memory.

Faith healers likewise cure by *addressing* disease, making words and prayers into instruments of power and summoning in "divine" voices (which also have a cellular basis). Shock of inner recognition is far more effective than mere insight or repair. Oral Roberts doesn't even have to attend seminary (if a school is needed, he can start his own). His so-called Christian bias is after the fact. The patients he treats are Sooners like him in some fundamental way. He touches the objective part of them, which recognizes him as their medicine. Then something profound, something underlying structure, changes.

Deepak Chopra posits a field in nature woven of vibrating Intelligence and permeated by waves of cosmic sound. The billions upon billions of threads that represent the *sutras* of Vedic science, Chopra says, are the "superstrings" of physics—and perhaps the runes of Reiki. Even as subatomic particles assemble reality where there was nothing and cells organize in tissues, symbolic "messages" alter illness grids at their core. Cure resides in the potency of a hieroglyph, symbol, molecule, or sound unit, individually or linked together in sequences, compressing "mind, body, DNA, and bliss into one undivided whole":[2]

Ayurveda would say that many diseases begin where there is ... a break—bliss slips out of its groove, so to speak, throwing off the cell's intelligence. To repair the break, a specific signal needs to be inserted back into the circle—a primordial sound. In this way, a vibration is used to cure a vibration....[3]

Potentized *Sepia,* Dai-Ko-Myo, *prana,* a mantra, a Navaho lighting stroke in colored sand.... But remediation is not always possible:

Both cancer and AIDS seem to be cases where the proper sequence of *sutras* must be unraveling at the deepest level. In other words, they are failures of intelligence, like "black holes" where bliss gets distorted out of its normal pattern. What makes both diseases so intractable is that the distortion runs so deep—it is locked inside the DNA's own structure. This causes the cell's self-repair mechanism either to break down or turn against itself.[4]

In immune diseases such as lupus and multiple sclerosis, as well as neurological disorders such as strokes and epilepsies, the sickness mimics signaling errors in ways that suggest a reversal of morphogenetic code—a cellular speaking in tongues that, rephrased in "bliss," might restore the *sutra* of the failed biological transmission.

"Consciousness would be curing people today," Chopra is convinced, "except that we diagnose disease too late, after years of stress have hardened the physiology and made it difficult for bliss to penetrate. But the gate is always open, even if only by a crack."[5]

Holism and Coherence

HOLISTIC PRACTITIONERS GO from whole picture to whole picture. They seek to grasp the coherence of a person, his or her *essential nature,* even when they know little of a complex disease process. They seek the "signal," the character of the illness.

In orthodox medicine, symptoms are separated into quantitative events with explicit phases. Doctors attempt to cure diseases in the ways they have named them. They follow Ariadne's thread through labyrinths of diagnosis: they can stop at any point, effect a partial repair, pick up, and follow their thread on, to further partial cures—each one a predesignated category. Murphy's Law is the ruling axiom, for the body is a fallible machine.

A holistic healer has established that he will not be working by abstraction or in parts, so he does not need different remedies for different aspects of diseases or stronger pharmaceuticals to penetrate the stubborn mass of the body. Instead he tries to capture the character of the pathology and shatter it so that it will form a new pattern like ripples in water. If a thing is a one, it can be altered by altering, even to an infinitesimal degree, any facet of that one. The succussed, dematerialized nanodoses administered by homeopaths are like subatomic bullets aimed at disease patterns. This transcends Murphy's Law, and even reverses it: anything which can heal *does*.

Legend has it that Babaji, pestered repeatedly by a yogi who said he could not practice because of a pain in his knee, finally declared, "I will fix your sick knee." He spat on his hand and flung his spit toward it. Suddenly the knee no longer hurt.

I believe the issue here is not the holiness of the spit but the gesture of disinterest, "spoken" so precisely it cut into the obscurity of the other's life. It used the subliminal senses and their codes to awaken the body to the vibration of its own defect and stubbornness. It addressed the deeper distortion, of which the knee was only a warning. Zen koans lead to sudden transformations in much the same fashion.

Where holistic practitioners fail, by their own definition, is when they miss the whole, or when the patient cannot receive or assimilate it. No partial virtuoso solution can catch disease at its roots. If a healer goes to the wrong whole, he has simply missed the case. But his errors provide a path toward future interpretations: he may well arrive at the correct whole by successive instructive mistakes, as long as he doesn't capitulate to palliating individual symptoms. Homeopaths do this as a matter of course; a wrong remedy can throw everything into perspective and show why something masquerading convincingly as symptomology is not the operant disease. Then a new remedy is given, not for the dominant symptom but for the next whole picture.

Distortions are transposed through tissues, and ailments often arise far from sites of initial compromise. A severe stomach inflammation may be less deep-seated than a speech impediment, especially if the latter goes back further historically and attaches more tightly to systemic roots. If breath is restricted and an eye twitches years after because of the toxic effects of a childhood vaccination settling in the liver, no amount of attention to eye muscles or the chest is going to get at the real disease.

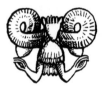

The body unerringly directs attention to its strain lines; the doctor has to learn how to see or feel it: a limp or stutter might deflect the organism many degrees from center, with flaring up in the stomach one symptom of this tilt.

Healing is finally a dynamic interaction between the character of the disease and the character of the medicine, no matter how these are framed.

Addressing the Practice of Self-Cure

Students of *t'ai chi ch'uan* remark how their form changes over the years even though they were ostensibly always doing "the form." One practitioner told me he was startled to realize only after some five hundred classes "That's what the teacher means by 'move from the center.' He doesn't mean, 'Get an image of the center and sort of shift that way.' He means—there really is a center to the body." There is also a center to health, a different center to each disease.

Peter Ralston, a proficient martial artist, recalled that for many years he tried to "sink" his body in every imaginable mechanical and mental way, using different exercises and images, and suddenly one day

he let go of an unexamined postural belief on which he was relying

without realizing it; then his entire being sank as though on its own.
A correct cure sinks the body likewise.

Ralston adds: "You know you're there when a car whips around the corner and there's no time to think. Instead of jumping up, which is perhaps the first instinct, you go right to the ground and just stride past low down. It's faster than thought. You don't think, 'Oh car! I better do what my teacher says and sink!' You find yourself having sunk because you know it at the deepest level."[6]

T HE SELF ACTS only on the basis of what it knows for certain. The unconscious, unarticulated animal never visits the physician, or at least never declares itself when the social persona brings it there. The most intransigent diseases lurk in its shadow, but also the most miraculous cures. They exist on the primordial level of a crocodile or wild mouse, which do not even address their existence ontologically, let alone their ailments and dying.

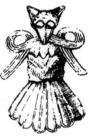

The intellect, no matter how placating and convincing, cannot sell the animal self anything that threatens it. In fact, the self already knows the tricks the intellect has for convincing it, so it cannot be convinced. That is the role of the healer. He or she must contact the animal inside the person, the creature on whose needs the fate of everything rests and who can die and take the body with it, without the mind ever suspecting the disease originated in internal conflict and symbolic distortion rather than in germs or genes.

So tricky is the personality that it will take any lesson it learns from the self and exaggerate it in order not to have to learn any more. The success of realignment depends on getting around this, on *not* replacing one inflated gesture with another—that is, it depends on curing cleanly with a stroke of a sword rather than slapping aside a disease like a punching bag only to have it come swinging back later with more force.

One physician writes of an alliance that must be negotiated with "the patient's *practice of self-cure*, which is rigidly established by the time he reaches us. To treat this *practice of self-cure* merely as resistance is to fail to acknowledge its true value for the person of the patient. It is my belief from my clinical practice that very few illnesses in a person are difficult to handle and cure. What, however, is most difficult to resolve and cure is the patient's practice of self-cure."[7] (italics are the author's) Only when the patient lets go of this habit of sham cure at a deep enough level is her system open to a real cure.

"When I was very young," Manocher Movlai, the founder of Breema bodywork, told a practitioner, "they brought somebody who had a back problem to my great-grandfather. My great-grandfather asked me, 'Manocher, what do you say about this person?' I said, 'He is sick, he has a back problem.' Then my great-grandfather said, 'That's what you don't understand about Breema! This man is a complete man, a healthy man, nothing wrong with him, and he's playing being sick, he's playing having a back problem!' "[8]

In other words, a patient's practice of self-cure has probably been successful for him *until* this present disease. If he is resisting treatment, it is not because he wants to be sick but because he is unconsciously trying to participate in a "cure" in the one way he knows how. The physician must convince him to abandon his over-collaboration at the level at which it interferes—that is, abandon its negative aspects without abandoning its raw energy. Once again, it is not a matter of literal dialogue between doctor and patient, but one of the doctor seducing the patient's latent resistance in order to aid a cure rather than have it be hampered by some ambivalent inner state. This seduction can be in the form of a needle at the correct point on the correct meridian, a chiropractic torque, an herbal formula consisting of just the right combination of tonifying and sedating elements, an allopathic pill reducing blood pressure, a sudden insight, or a tincture of rosemary.

Medicine will remain obscure to the degree that our lives are obscure. A system of healing must finally reach within and touch real imperatives, as the Yellow Emperor of China reached within the lives of his "subjects." It simply doesn't work to give up all to science and technology and to the verdict of Western history and ask them to solve it—and then only when it is manifested as disease and discomfort. We are more in the battle than this.

Character

We will now move from the arena of disease and cure as such to the ritual domain of medicine described in Volume One. Here we explore the origin of social and totemic categories of healing—the symbolic universe in which ailments are indistinguishable from supernatural beings and in which cultural poses reflect the invisible edges and patternings of psychophysiological disorders.

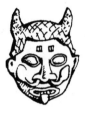

Indigenous society is made up of fusions of character states, spirit embodiments, and ritual projections of disease states. Of course, things have not changed in the modern world, though we seem also to have many so-called *bona fide* concrete pathologies as well as X-ray and ultrasound images of them and other standard categories, devices, and techniques of health, death, autopsy, and burial to distract us from the actual complexity and idiosyncrasy of diseases in individuals. What gets named is what is known and treated, but it is hardly all that is there.

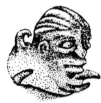

In the present HMO era in which medicine is overseen by actuaries and bureaucrats, doctors have become so involved in identifying familiar categories and flagging authorized problems that they are not only unresponsive to disease somatics and subtexts, but no longer even outcome-oriented. The first priorities are not correctly diagnosing and curing diseases and making patients healthier; they are filling out forms, processing cases quickly and cost-effectively, and not getting sued. Mysterious disease patterns and inexplicable pain and dysfunction simply get overlooked.

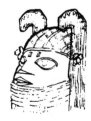

What is missed is the disease totem.

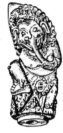

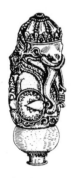

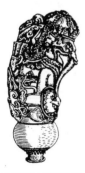

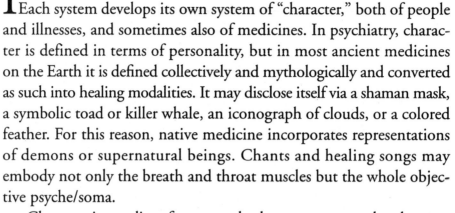

Indigenous medicines are invariably based on reading character. Each system develops its own system of "character," both of people and illnesses, and sometimes also of medicines. In psychiatry, character is defined in terms of personality, but in most ancient medicines on the Earth it is defined collectively and mythologically and converted as such into healing modalities. It may disclose itself via a shaman mask, a symbolic toad or killer whale, an iconograph of clouds, or a colored feather. For this reason, native medicine incorporates representations of demons or supernatural beings. Chants and healing songs may embody not only the breath and throat muscles but the whole objective psyche/soma.

Character is a replica of energy—both energy expressed and energy denied. Life literally takes its "character" from a person's energetic and unconscious state. Energy in the context of resistance is also character. Culture shapes character profoundly. How different is any Comanche, Dinka, or Aussie from any Turk, Ainu, or Tibetan despite similarities of personality! Just look at their postures, their masks, their degrees and tilts of repression, their relative projections of machismo and empathy, their overall ambiances. Compare an African-American baseball pitcher to a Sri Lankan guerrilla fighter hurling a grenade. Something is similar, but the stances represent radically different intentions, belief systems, and energetic bundles. Psychoanalyst John P. Conger defines this in contemporary language:

> Character provides a meeting place for psyche and soma. Character as a defense structure gathers us when we are scattered and organizes us into an identifiable pattern of rigidity and energetic withdrawal, binding our anxiety, rage, sadness and longing. Character is what keeps us separate, exempt and special, and what holds us back from surrender to our energetic nature. Character represents a practice of self-cure, an ongoing, hasty, rigid solution imposed over our instability to maintain an intact sense of self. Daily our anxiety persuades us not to relinquish our protections.

Typically, when character establishes itself in a growing organism, it disrupts and inhibits the scheduled somatic function, so that muscle remains flaccid and unresponsive. With our diaphragm contracted and the ribs gripped with fear, we may never establish a pattern of full breathing. We may never develop coordinated movement between the left and right side. We may never stand up and walk in a natural easy way. Character is the shell that energy leaves behind, and as such it provides a house; but the shell, as we grow, becomes too small.[9]

African, native American, and Aboriginal Australian character exists always with respect to gods, ancestral forces, and systems of totemism, even as our character manifests in respect to our own social, cultural, and technological activities. A poor doctor in any culture fails to grasp the relationship of the levels on which psyche and soma reconstellate and thus treats the wrong chronic and emotional diseases.

Wilhelm Reich's *Character Analysis* is a basic Western text for reading disease. It would serve equally for an acupuncturist, a homeopath, or a psychiatrist. Sigmund Freud laid down the first rule in reading character: Pay attention to *exactly* what the patient tells you. Reich took it a notch further: It is not what he tells you but how he tells it—his mode of description, his breathing and movement and disposition of energy while he talks, the eye contact he makes or fails to make, his precise choice of words and rhythm of speech, the general sense he has of who is doing the talking. This character knows far more than either the doctor or patient about the ailment. It may be part man, part god; part woman, part ancestor; part human, part beast, part hungry ghost. That is why the Yellow Emperor of Chinese traditional medicine puts forth what to us looks like a massive diversion constituting a whole system of relationships among earth, fire, water, air, and metal. It is also a formal medicine, though the surface formality increases ambiguity and negative capability instead of purging and sterilizing it, as does allopathy. This makes it a double-edged healing system.

In ancient Africa, Amerindia, and Australia, although they are not documented as such in the ethnographic literature, we can find thousands of mind-body ceremonies with a character-emotional import. Consider the following two from Australia and Bali, respectively. We do not know the inside of them, but it is clear they have profound physiological and emotional impacts. Even their mythologies, i.e., their inner voices and drama, have subtle physiological effects transcending our conventional notions of mind and body.

The first account is a physician initiation in Australia:

> . . . a very old doctor threw some of his crystalline stones and killed the novice. Some of the stones went through the latter's head from car to ear. He then cut out all his insides, intestines, lungs, liver, heart, in fact, everything, and left him till next morning, when he placed more of these stones in his body, arms and legs, and covered his face with leaves. After "singing" over him until the body was swollen up, he put more stones in him. He then patted him on the head, causing him to "jump up alive," and made him drink water and eat meat containing magic stones. When he awoke, he had forgotten who he was, and all the past.[10]

The second describes the finale of a healing ceremony in Bali:

> By the spell, the krisses in the hands of the men turned against them, but the magic of the Barong hardened their flesh so that, although they pushed the sharp points of the daggers with all their might against their naked chests, they were not even hurt. . . . Some leaped wildly or rolled in the dust, pressing the krisses against their breasts and crying like children, tears streaming from their eyes. Most showed dark marks where the point of the dagger bruised the skin without cutting it, but blood began to flow from the breast of one, the signal for the watchmen to disarm him by force.[11]

With intimations of acupuncture, bioenergetics, and *Chi Gung,* these ceremonies leave little doubt about their symbolic significations of self and other. These are the raw material of curative systems.

I cannot emphasize enough how subtle and inextricable character is and how central to accessing the core of personality, disease, and

health. Paul Radin says that Maori character "is very complex and unusually profound. According to them, man and every sentient being ... consists of an eternal element, an Ego which disappears after death, a ghost-shadow, and a body."[12]

The eternal element is called *toiora*. It is a spark of the vast divine force materializing mortally. The pure Ego comprises three elements. Its *mauri* arises as its active life principle and also as the symbol for that principle. A material *mauri* might be a tree planted at the birth of the child and an immaterial *mauri* might be the totem of that tree. The Ego also includes the life-essence *(hau)* and the physiological manifestation *(manawa ora)*. No standard Freudian (or even Reichian) character analysis will work in a Maori context without addressing these elements of psyche and soma. It may well be that a specific tree (or the symbol of that tree) must be treated at the same time as the person.

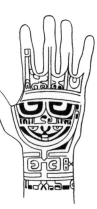

> In the ghost shadow, the *wairua*, we are dealing with the soul, strictly speaking. It is partially visible but does not properly possess a material form until it appears in the underworld. *Wairua* is the ingredient which mediates us to the external world; we would be lifeless and decay without it. We might possess the life principle and form but we could not be seen. In the same way it is the *wairua* that enables us to give form to things, to actually accomplish them. A Maori remarked to [Elsdon] Best, "My *wairua* is very intent on this work that it may be well done." It is well to remember this, to realize that it is not simply with our senses that we see and touch and think. "Be of good cheer," a woman was told, "although we are afar off, yet our *wairua* are ever with you." And it is in the same strain that an old Maori wrote to Best, "We have long been parted and may not meet again in the world of life. We can no longer see each other with our eyes, only our *wairua* see each other, as also our friendship."[13]

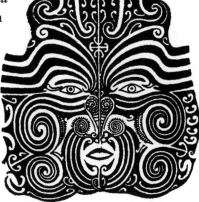

Healing in a Maori context must incorporate, even as an unstated presence, the role and condition of the *wairua*. Whether it is "real" or not in a anatomical sense, it is absolutely real in a "character" sense. It

is the glue of Maori life. It lives and dies in the bodies of the culture, along with the flesh and ego. It can be affected positively by charms and mantras, negatively by voodoo and "evil eyes."

> Although the *wairua* could not be destroyed, a person could be killed through his *wairua*. It was easily affected by magical spells. It was the *wairua* also that was affected when a man found himself afflicted with fear of becoming evil, with a dream of impending danger, or if he had polluted his *tapu*.[14]

The Maori recognize the physiological body of stomach, intestines, and liver too, but it is integrated with the *toiora, wairua, mauri,* and *manawa ora*. We have *"wairuas"* too, but we either don't recognize them or give them other, provisional names. After all, elements of personality reside simultaneously in organs (feelings and desires in the heart and stomach, the seat of thought and the mind in the viscera, memory in the stomach, etc.) and in the immaterial aspects of the self.

> Looked upon as a material entity [the body] may have an immaterial form, and regarded as an immaterial entity it may possess a material form. In other words, it possesses, as an integrated unit, both form and substance. The first the Maori call *ahua* and the second, *aria*. . . . Best quotes a Maori as follows: "I saw clearly his bodily form *(ahua);* it is not the case that I saw distinctly *(aria)*."[15]

To heal, one must first see.

Wᴴᴇɴ ᴛʜᴇ ꜱʜᴀᴍᴀɴ calls out the illness, he *is*, in that moment, the illness externalized. "I am the crocodile," he chants. "I am lightning. I am a lion. I am a shooting star." Of course, he can externalize the illness only to the degree that his supplicant can internalize *him*. When his performance resonates along a vector of power and

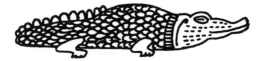

pathology in native vernacular, he merges with the disease and becomes a force which can dislodge it. "My psychic power is strong enough to cause others to believe in themselves,"[16] explained an Australian indigenous healer.

All medicine men and doctors address the precise coda in which character is written in their cultures. The Yellow Emperor spoke as the master physician of his time, mixing medicinal advice with curative tropes:

> Beginning and creation come from the East. Fish and salt are the products of water and ocean and of the shores near the water. The people of the regions of the East eat fish and crave salt; their living is tranquil and their food delicious. Fish causes people to burn within (thirst), and the eating of salt injures (defeats) the blood. Therefore the people of these regions are all of dark complexion and careless and lax in their principles. Their diseases are ulcers, which are most properly treated with acupuncture by means of a needle of flint....
>
> Precious metals and jade come from the regions of the West. The dwellings in the West are built of pebbles and sandstone. Nature (Heaven and Earth) exerts itself to bring a good harvest. The people of these regions live on hills, and, because of the great amount of wind, water, and soil, become robust and energetic. The people of these regions wear no clothes other than those of coarse woolen stuff or coarse matting. They eat good and variegated food and therefore they are flourishing and fertile. Hence evil cannot injure their external bodies, and if they get diseases they strike at the inner body. These diseases are most successfully cured with poison medicines....
>
> In the North is the region of storing and laying by. The country is hilly and mountainous, there are biting cold winds, frost and ice. The people of these regions find pleasure in living in this wilderness, and they live on milk products. The extreme cold causes many diseases....[17]

This means precisely what it says and, on the other hand, is so latent and anonymous it means nothing. It bears a relationship to reality not unlike that of a dream. Its text is literal, but only when we have penetrated its other, surface literality. It substantiates a closed system of diagnosis and health maintenance—a complex which works prior to any application of needles or ingestion of herbs. Its unknown originators have not chosen their images because they are picturesque and suggest Oriental painting. They have chosen them because they were already imbedded in the world, hence in personalities.

The homeopathic materia medica is a compendium of character statements posing as symptom complexes. The doctor must routinely match the image of an individual with the image of a disease and a medicine; it is not sufficient simply to add up a patchwork of parallel symptoms in both. For instance, *Nux vomica,* the poison-nut remedy, is used for a diverse range of ailments, but always on the basis of collective synergistic traits of the medicine, never of singular or isoalted symptoms. The *Nux* person is husky, strong, ambitious, hard-driving, even over-ambitious to the point of working all night. He is self-destructively competitive, fastidious, and lacks perspective, preferring to drive himself. This symptom complex is also prone to stimulants and compulsive sex. Yet these are just *our* words, and a patient needing *Nux* may have none of these characteristics, at least on a perceptible level. The *Nux* meaning may be condensed, synopsized at an organ level, or even reversed. The successful physician reads it anyway.

We must also emphasize that these character traits lie beneath any actual pathology yet sustain even life-threatening malignancies. In homeopathy they are "derived" from potentized substances in provings (that is, from the characterological effects that these substances have on healthy people), and medicines made from them are prescribed only on the basis of the Law of Similars. By homeopathic precept, the Simillimum in the minimum dose is the unique message that potentiates character rigidity into vital energy.

Acupuncture would seem to rest primarily on the subcutaneous transmission of energy from the insertion of a needle, opening internal channels for the circulation of *chi* energy. The acupuncturist, however, starts by taking the patient's pulse. Each wrist has three pulses, and any pulse can be diagnosed at two different levels; in these twelve pulses there are twenty-eight common readings, every one a distinct persona. The pulse may be empty, disappearing on pressure. It may be too urgent, too sunken; it can float on the surface of the skin from the Wind Evil. It may slip and slide; it may overflow from Fire floating and Water dried up. It may bounce like a fiddle string; it may be inflating but leathery from the cold; it may be blurred; it may be shaped like an onion skin, hollow from great loss of blood. It may be overquick and halting or soft and fine; it may be shaped like a bean from fright. The vibration of this pulse must then be replicated in a remedy. The match can be somatic, pharmaceutical, energetic, or symbolic.

According to *The Yellow Emperor:*

The feeling of the pulse should be done according to method: for when it is slow and quiet it acts as protector and guardian. In the days of Spring the pulse is superficial, like wood floating on water or like a fish that glides through the waves. In Summer days the pulse within the skin is drifting and light, and everywhere there is an excess of creation. In Fall days the torpid insects underneath the skin are about to come out. In Winter the torpid insects are all around the bone, quiet and delicate like the nobleman residing in his mansion.[18]

We couldn't ask for a more sensitive rendering of the layers of characters and disease. The landscapes are incredibly subtle vibrations, impeccably rendered.

Of course, any self-respecting allopath explores beneath the surface, too. His training is to investigate beyond the description and to pay attention to actual physical occurrences *in* the patient rather than to what the patient says. Yet, to be successful, he has to read the patient absolutely. He cannot fall back on gross diagnosis as an excuse to single out those things that are heavily stated; he cannot rely solely on his tests and X-rays. Otherwise he may cure a layer which is inflamed or psychosomaticized but not truly the source, and not only leave the disease to fester but cut off one of its avenues of expression and dissipation.

Healing,
Language,
and
Sexuality

The radiologist or surgeon has to first "see" the disease too—the characterological aspects of lab tests and radiation images.

Codes

A N OBSCURE HEALING SYSTEM which dramatically accentuates the
characterological components of cure is "Curative Eurhythmy,"
a treatment arising from Rudolf Steiner's anthroposophy. Eurhythmy
is simultaneously a para-linguistic code of indeterminate depth and a
literal morphophonemic symbology. Each medicine is "taught" to the
patient as a motion-sequence made up of the letters of a "word" the
therapist has chosen as a cure. He demonstrates the word over and over,
and the patient imitates him until he picks it up. The stages of imper-
fection and correction *are* the healing process. Each successively less
imperfect spelling communicates a layer of compensation to the character—the faulty template of self-cure—but, as the spelling becomes
truer and truer, a cure is transmitted.[19] The body is addressed in letters on the unexplored assumption that the etiology of disease and the
etiology of language-making share a chrysalis deep in some archetypal
code.

The Steiner "alphabet" is made up of Germanic calligraphy acted
out as body postures and movements. Each letter has a gesture, the
enactment of which can occur on a number of different planes or scales.
A "U" for instance can be written close to the ground or high in the
air. It can be suspended vertically or extended horizontally. Like a Reiki
symbol, it can be drawn with the toes or fingers or with the whole body.
The underlying goal is to communicate essence.[20]

Although vowels and consonants seem to be semi-arbitrary
graphemic units of sound, Steiner considered their representations a
fixed aspect of their meanings. While a mere semantic "meaning" is
communicated to the conscious self, the inner self receives the discrete
primacy of a sound or shape. The relationship of semaphors to actual
words and meanings is considered basic and ontological on some level.

The sound "M," where it occurs, from "mother" to "hum" to "rhythm," is a Eurhythmic seed, empowered by its relationship to other seeds in clusters. "S" in "sun" and "sleep" and "asthma" is the same "S," so a remedy with many "S's" might be given to someone with asthma, or those "S's" might be mixed with other seeds in making up different medicines. A person with heart disease might well be given "H's" and "R's" to enact. He might also be fed "L's," which would not be surprising, since "L" is "love" and "light" and "life"—emotional properties assigned to the heart and its circulatory system.

A prose song (abridged below) was composed by a lupus patient working eurhythmically with the internal "L" which represented her own name Laura as well as the name of her disease:

> To summon inside—The brave shining warrior, glittering hero of the skies, with flaming sword, astride a horse so white you *know* you are ready, to meet and overpower the dreadful. I've got my firm together now, my word drawn up, to hold and to swing into warning. Big "L's" begin lifting, for lightness and levity, raising the sediments Up in the body. L is for *lucia,* I said with my slipper, for all of the liquid that rises and falls into falls to further the flowing to keep us in motion.... The globe itself hovers there before you. Yes, you can touch it, give it a little "L."[21]

For people to engage in complexity and rhythm is transformative in a primal, even cellular sense.

It may be idealistic to think that we can cure the crab of cancer with microdoses of poison nut or drive out the wolf of lupus by acting letters, but it *is* apparently possible in some manner to confront and tame diseases as characters in masks even as Haitian voodoo performers and Kwakiutl totem dancers do. There is a long tradition on the Earth of chanting and making icons and talismans to banish diseases. These modalities may well persist in medicines because the deepest biological and totemic codes respond to them.

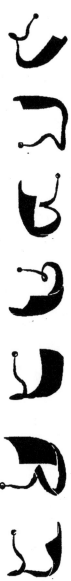

© Stan N. Tenen/
Meru Foundation,
San Anselmo,
California

Martial Medicines

While the seeds of Eurhythmy are basic units of human language, those of *t'ai chi ch'uan, ba gua,* and *hsing-i* were once movements of animals—snakes, birds, fish, monkeys—observed by martial artists in medieval China. There is no strategy or compensation in the escape of the fish or deer, no considered persona behind the attack of the rhinoceros or tiger. Animals exist purely in the expression of their bodies, as signatures prior to language. They cast objective expressions of their total beings, so it is objective being that we learn from them. Animal postures are stances for confronting internal blocks.

How one engages an *external* opponent is translated into a healing process through an internalization of combative movements. Whereas psychotherapy proposes to locate trauma in a primal event and then to expiate it through cathexis, martial arts provide sets of energetic moves—aggressions and their neutralizations, punches and their feints, uproots and their evasions. These forms integrate *Chi Gung* breathing modes, subtle responses to pressure, sensation of fields around the body and beneath the feet, and fundamental principles of mobility and energy, all of which have possible morphogenetic effects. The activities learned through practicing sets (martial alphabets) are then integrated into sequences of blending, using partners.

Martial practice allows one's self to bottom out in the expression of one's body/mind. Recruits must fight their way out of their own fears and stuck points. Where the self bottoms out, the shadow is no longer a memory of damage done or a fear of danger colored by past trauma; it is a present and actual inability to strike and defend oneself. An opponent, even in a practice situation, is a representation of one's disease tendencies, hence his attack provides ceaseless opportunities to practice movements which are simultaneously martial strikes and feints and psychosomatic seeds.

Fighting arts are directly associated with healing modalities in Taoist tradition. As the opponent is repelled, a medicinal meaning is communicated inwardly (Eurhythmy). If the opponent is not overwhelmed, his body/mind receives a blow or jolt that breaks its apathy (chiropractic).

A SO-CALLED TRAUMA or pathology is re-energized again and again as a rigidified character state *and* the attack of the opponent. One must blend each time anew, and, despite exhaustion or distraction, summon up resources to engage this "other." The roots of impediments are not evident. The difficulty in learning *t'ai chi ch'uan* or capoeira is not the complexities of techniques but a prior difficulty in one's own body/mind. In fact, one discovers not only one's obvious armoring but limitations one did not know existed, discovers them simply by breaking through (via a rollback, cartwheel, throw, or yield) into unrestricted territory beyond. The impalpable moment just before the breakthrough is the impediment, the moment of the flinch, the flinch that is unconscious and unexperienced.

The martial-arts practitioner (like the healer) must stay "real" because he or she responds to and accommodates an actual opponent rather than a fictive or intellectual one. She must neutralize not only the imagined threat of "bad guys" but a litany of misleading internal psychobabble and empty reassurances. Potential victims of violence are as much the prey of their own minds as of criminals and their weapons.

Without an attack, there is no impetus to remedy this or attempt accute, effective movements. Without the crisis of the external opponent, the inner necessity is unregarded and unclaimed. In some *aikido* workshops, students stand in the path of strikes, stepping aside only at the last moment. This demonstrates poignantly the nature of emotional energy in relation to force and its deflection.

It is possible that certain healing aspects of this activity could be accomplished by pure exercise—and no doubt are—but the internal martial arts provide techniques and their execution in a concrete system of self-cure; they enforce clear discrimination between pretenses of effectiveness (negative character projections and congested organs) on the one hand and unimpeded actions (health) on the other. Speed and power in isolation are as ineffective in real cures as in combat; brawn and agility (drugs and surgery) *per se* are only superficially transformative of one's actual position and situation, the actual situation that is always unknown despite the most thorough diagnoses. Groundedness, attention, and timing are required, which means going deeper in oneself. A curative "alphabet" must be trained.

Wendy Palmer, who teaches students intuition and blending under the title "Aikido as a Clairsentient Practice," explains:

> In body-oriented situations like aikido or sports, we do not have time to ask a mental question. By the time we have asked the question, it is too late. In fact, we want to keep the intellect out of it altogether and allow our energy field to respond automatically. In order to suspend thinking, we occupy our attention with basic practice. We concentrate on the movement of our breath, the balance and perimeter of our field, and gravity and our receptivity to the earth. When we focus in this way, our system responds automatically, sometimes brilliantly.[22]

During the 1980s and 1990s, unknowing pedestrians on Telegraph Avenue in Oakland often did a double-take upon spotting the sign proclaiming Peter Ralston's School of Martial Arts and Ontology. Yet who could question that dealing with other creatures through conflict and battle is a fundamental rubric of existence. "'I am here and you are there' is a profound statement,"[23] Ralston reminds his students. It is a premise equally of healer and warrior. In case the students listen without really hearing, he repeats it, often more than twice: "I am here and you are there." This is also the situation between healer and healee. How that distance is mediated energetically and characterologically is the basis of any cure.

In an ideal training (or healing), the linear confrontation of foes (or predator and prey) is replaced by two people in a sealed energy bubble, each—whether they know it or not—trying to fill every hole in the field between them as it arises. The battle becomes their collaboration, their healing. They are each other's doctor. Palmer writes:

> In aikido the blend is what dissolves the conflict. When we blend we go *with* the energy or direction of the attack. From a mental standpoint, the head center, we "see the world from the attacker's point of view." The heart center tends to feel what our partner is feeling. The *hara,* or belly, knows how and where the body will move. When all three centers make contact with those of our partner, we have the sense that we have disappeared. We become so like the person who has attacked us that there is no one to attack.[24]

If a student respects these levels of feeling in himself—along with sensations from the energy field of his opponent, the "signaling errors" of his own tension, and the constant of gravity—a somatic transformation occurs. Traumas and energetic blocks are reexperienced, cathected, and shifted. Whereas in psychotherapy such a process is mediated by words and symbols, in shamanism by masks and chants, in allopathy by concrete vectors inside the body, in martial arts it is processed by ritualized battles.

D ISEASE IS A MOST SUBTLE and grievous opponent, but at what point do you distinguish armed teenagers in a dysfunctional society from industrial toxins in the same society? A disease is simply a stage of a physical manifestation relative to the organismic field in which it occurs. A meteorite, a prison uprising, or a suicide bomber is a disease too. The boundary of internal and external effects finds only the self, reflecting both ways that the ultimate enemy is always one's own imbalance and tension.

As Don Juan Matus taught Carlos Castaneda, one is a potential victim of spirit forces that can take any form—thug, vandal, wild beast, or disease. If a person moves in balance, her internal organs are in balance and resist disease. Likewise, her outer body is resilient enough that an attacker has a more difficult time targeting, injuring, or killing her (and may even harm himself trying to do so).

A mugger is an imbalance, like a disease; he provides too much energy before one is ready for it. If one were ready, one would deflect the attack and thereby heal the attacker. Paul Pitchford, *t'ai chi* practitioner and healer, recounts returning from seeing an herbalist in San Francisco's Chinatown in 1975:

> Suddenly these two men came up to me. They wanted to give me energy. I tried to tell them that that was quite generous of them, but it was more than I needed. I told them I couldn't use so much energy. But they were real insistent on giving it. So I had no choice but to return it to them.

This is a charming tale of a street skirmish, but things have deteriorated in the last quarter century beyond the possibility of such graceful heroism. One is rarely ready these days, and the diseases of urban civilization, intensified by domestic abuse, drugs, and guns, are hardly curable by anything less than a legion of Taoist masters. In the imaginary cities of some utopian world, street samurai might be the police, healing "criminals" on the spot by converting their energy of rage to medicines. Not here, not now—but "planet medicine," if it is anything at all, transcends conventional therapeutic boundaries.

The world is a much more complex place than one in which attackers do only bad and healers only good. In the *dojo, nage* and *uke* become doctor and patient, each in their respective roles, trading potential blows.

Too much energy harms, maims, or kills; less energy more discretely

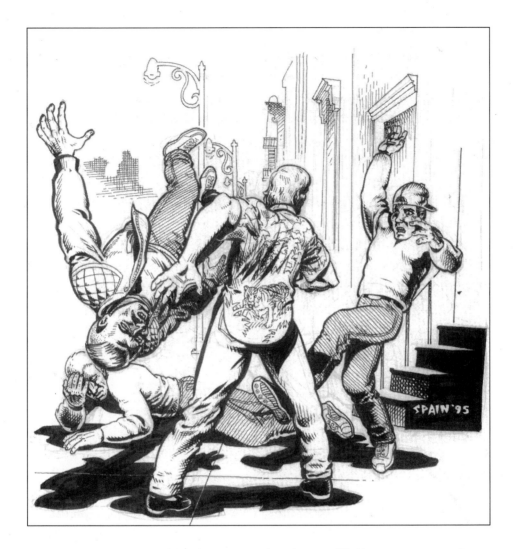

applied stimulates and heals (Ayurvedic charts of kill points on an elephant are also guides to treating sick elephants with acupuncture). Adhering movements done even more softly and with erotic intent become seductive. "Shoot Tiger," a *t'ai chi* move for immobilizing an opponent by twisting his arm upward and back and delivering a blow to his shoulder blade, may also be enacted with gradual pressure to heal tensions at that same point as well as to treat diseases forming along its meridian.

Healing,
Language,
and
Sexuality

When a proficient martial artist learns massage therapy, he or she can utilize the attributes of *chi*, blending, and organ sensitivity to function directly as a healer. Forms of *shiatsu* and osteopathy which effect cures from palpations utilize the reciprocal and transferring relationships among muscles, nerves, skeleton, and organs in a curative rather than pugilistic context. The engagement of internal organ leads to myofascial redistribution of subtle impulses.

JAPANESE SHIATSU REQUIRES the practitioner's firm contact along acupuncture meridians. *Nuad bo-rarn,* traditional Thai massage, employs slow full-body stretches and joint releases with conscious breath. There are parallels among these, yoga, and various *san shou* and *ta lu* sets in *t'ai chi ch'uan.* Vulnerable zones of the opponent's body, with a revision in attitude, become energetic points of the patient's body. In principle, the two-person sets of *t'ai chi ch'uan* done with a different emphasis are therapeutic massages. The black belt or *sensei* conducting force at their precise vectors also transmits *chi* and startles the viscera into activity, even during battle.

Kumar Frantzis explores the vast domain of martial medicine:

All of the Ba Gua techniques and movements as well as the techniques of Taoist meditation have a direct cognition of the way in which you move your energy for healing. These techniques also have direct applications for healing. The hands-on healing technologies of Tai Chi, Hsing I, and Ba Gua are all derived from Chi Gung. They are collectively called Tui Na, or more specifically, Chi Gung Tui Na. Chi Gung can be considered a healing method that uses your energy to heal your body. Once you become proficient in Chi Gung it is a logical progression to apply your sensitivity and energy to heal someone else's body using Chi Gung Tui Na. . . .

Chi Gung Tui Na has hundreds of basic hand techniques that include tissue work like massage, deep tissue work with the fascia, muscles, tendons, and ligaments, and balancing the energies of the body by working with the energies of the internal organs. These last methods are typically used on people suffering with extreme diseases. Other techniques include joint manipulation, bone-setting, working specific points of the body as in Shiatsu, and shooting your energy through the energy lines of the patient, including work with the spinal and cerebrospinal systems and glands.

More sophisticated techniques include raising the vibratory levels within a person's body. The Ba Gua system has a particular method of using vibratory sounds to effect the energies of eight energy bodies. . . .

The author's experience of working for more than ten years as a Chi Gung Tui Na doctor in clinics and hospitals in China is that while the three systems of Hsing I, Tai Chi, and Ba Gua share many techniques, each has its own particular specialty areas of medical bodywork. Hsing I people are well known for their bone-setting skills and deep tissue work. They are also skilled at repairing heavy traumatic damage to the body, called Die Da in Chinese. Tai Chi people are very sophisticated in working with the yin aspects of Chi and are particularly skilled at treating diseases of the internal organs and cancers. Ba Gua people are proficient in all of these areas, with very specialized skills in working with the central nervous system and nerve damage.[25]

Once cultural categories are relaxed, healer and warrior blend into each other; Bear and samurai doctors embrace.

Sexuality and Medicine

A NY CONTACT BETWEEN humans is potentially pathological or therapeutic. Healing occurs from touch when resonance is processed and transferred positively through character. For a moment of fusion, healer and healing agency are identified with each other and understood as one: "I am here and you are there." The spectrum from martial to medicinal to sexual clarifies that healing is not so much a categorizable act as a focus and an intention in relation to energy.

Affinity between healer and lover is implicit. In our American vernacular, we speak of love as a "medicine." Popular music is filled with such references: "You heal me," "I was sick until you came along," "I'll die without you," and so on. *Witch Doctor* and *The Voodoo Man* are love songs.

Yet these lyrics disguise in their comic riffs the vulnerability of our situation as lovers and healers. The real healing implications of lovemaking remain unacknowledged. In the West, men and women prefer sex to be explicitly erotic; media images are jive, stylish, and dissociative. Pathology and eros work close to each other; witness such tropes as the virgin whore, the nasty boy, the g-string diva, the now-antiquated Marlboro man. A playboy/playgirl version of sex insinuates itself through the culture in subtexts of artifice and conquest. Lovemaking turns into a game of power, and power can manifest in any number of guises; in fact, play, seduction, and power are significant components of shamanic healing, too. That lovemaking *is* medicine is an equation Wilhelm Reich institutionalized in his medicalization of sexual intercourse, prescribing it for a variety of diseases, few of them explicitly emotional (see Volume One). Reich was hardly the first scion of sexual medicine. Tantric yoga for millennia has taught a *prana*-based form of sexual activity resembling *Chi Gung,* in which charge generated between partners and channeled through their body/minds is converted into curative energy—orgasm without discharge. Tantric postures are not only sexual but more profoundly so than most so-called erotic acts, combining (as they do) two-person yoga stances with genital *chakra* activation. Here lovemaking and healing are mature and committed, and partners, while opening the meridians of their own bodies, provide each other with vital energy.

I N AN ODDITY of our present civilization, sex has been isolated in a category all its own (a null set containing only itself and displayed in lights). As sociologists, psychologists, and philosophers, began to deconstruct this glitzy cipher in the 1990s, it became evident that people were carrying out an exotic array of activities under the pretense of having sex (or fantasizing about sex), only a portion of which were sexual. Some of our most obsessive acts of sexuality are in fact projections of healing

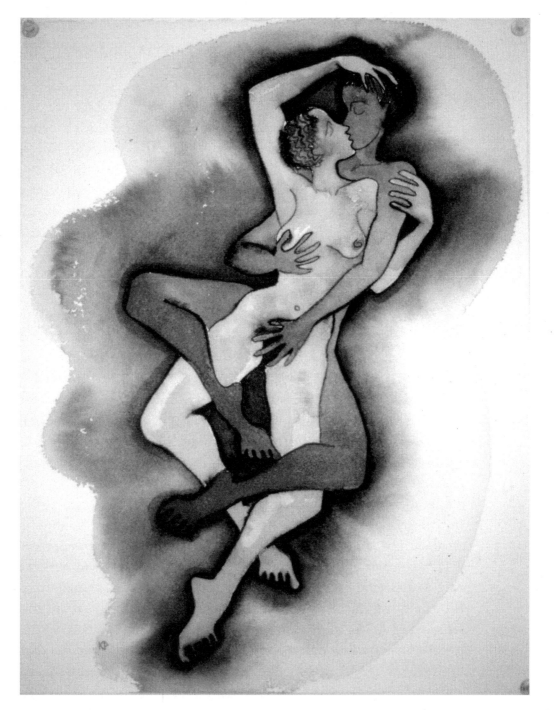

(and love). Others, of course, are projections of alienation, depersonalization, dominance, self-abnegation, and rage. And, trying to transcend of all this, is the ritualized motto that healing somehow *is* love.

In a culture that eroticizes to the point of idol worship and floods itself with fantasies of sexuality as nirvana, the main "curative" outcome a person is conditioned to seek is explicitly genital. Sex becomes

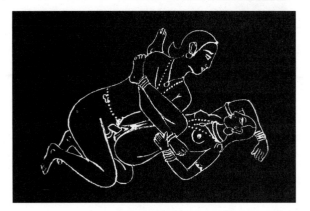

its own existential solution—a sole reason for living. But this is not explored to a level that will release what it actually means: that eros is energy operating subliminally and ontogenetically.

In a classic confusion of medicine and sex, psychotherapists (and, likely, other doctors) have been sleeping with patients at an alarming rate, a phenomenon discussed as an ethics issue as early as the 1976 meeting of the American Psychiatric Association.[26] Although most speakers tried to blame this event on the ethical failings of specific doctors, it speaks also to a breakdown in the therapeutic model. Desperation reflects not only the inability of the psychiatrists to produce positive change in their patients but the lack of self-esteem and boundary on both sides that results from that failure. There *are* therapies of sexual relations, but they do not arise improvisationally from insight analysis.

Moshe Feldenkrais describes "how many mistake the longing for affection or the need for social power for sexual tension, and proceed with the sexual act to satisfy these cravings.... [P]eople who proceed with sexual action when there is [only] the tension of habitual extraneous motivations that were mixed up with sex ... rarely relieve that tension. They just mitigate it and they find themselves changing one partner after another in the hope of finding one who will do the trick for them."[27] Others, he adds, supplement actual sex with aphrodisiacs and vitamins in search of lost potency.

The main impediment to erotic healing is perhaps even less a shallow view of sexuality than an epidemic denial of healing as a nonmedical modality in any form. We tend to confine the doctor to an office, though diseases, of course, follow their own rules. They also work on Sunday.

Those holding to conventional sexual roles and unexamined views of "fun" may reject the notion of deep erotic conversion because self-awareness is not an issue for them in *any* part of their lives. They are buttressed against it. Even among "New Age" men and women who honor healing rhetorically, there is often a failure to understand the depth and danger of real acts of intimacy and sexuality.

Just as there is no healing machine, there is no lovemaking machine. Energy exchange between people is erratic and variable, and sexual healing is no more universally accessible than any other kind of medicine. Lovemaking becomes healing only when emotional and psychic shadows are integrated and actual empathic contact is extended between partners.

THERE IS NO LANGUAGE for therapeutic touch. Most people are not even clear on the difference between the overly eroticized imagery churned out by the desire mill of Madison Avenue and their own sexuality. Titillated relentlessly, they cannot tolerate the complex feelings that arise from attraction or contact in any form. Muddles on this point lead us to misidentify some of the more intimate forms of healing touch as seduction because so much human contact has been interpreted only in terms of its potential flirtatious nuances. Bioenergetic therapist Stanley Keleman writes:

> The deprivation of actual physical contact is so enormous in our culture that anything that touches us has such an enormous impact, and anyone practicing touch becomes a guru.[28]

This is not just a Western problem. In many Islamic cultures women must hood their faces to avoid even the scintilla of attraction. In some

African societies, clitorises are castrated in primitive surgeries. The potential damage being guarded against must be fearsome indeed to require as prophylaxis such a brutal disfigurement. In some tribal cultures the fear of menstruation is so great as to lead shamans to disavow and disclaim the healing power of blood.

O UR SOCIETY HAS defined such an enormous repertoire of ostensibly seductive behavior (and misbehavior) that we have virtually no repertoire at all for any *other* forms of touch and exchanges of energy, especially between the sexes. While we wildly overestimate both our appetite and capacity for genital activity, we virtually ignore our hunger for sheer contact. As the former becomes more virulent in the frustrations and abuses it generates, the latter becomes depleted, and the combined effect is a neurosis of touch and human contact that gives rise to exotic pathologies in both somatic and psychological realms. If the line between massage and seduction is blurred, it is no wonder that the line between healing and loving is blurred.

Behind each of our catchwords ("erotic," "seductive," "adore") lies such a host of cultural habits and prejudices that we hardly know what they each mean. How do we distinguish sexual energy from other forms of healing energy? Do we have any real notion of the role eros plays in the energetics of therapeutic touch? Could suppression of eros (in either party) hinder healing? Might not all healing touch require some erotic component? When does mere contact become erotic? Can there be touch that is energetically erotic but does not have seduction as its goal?

Of course, there can. Sexual energy is a form of cosmic energy, an aspect of *prana:*

> The healing potential of shiatsu might well originate in creative or sexual energy. At its very best shiatsu contact is very nurturing, loving and a great turn-on. As Reuho [Yamada] professes, "Human energy is sexual in essence, but in shiatsu that energy melts into a more general ecstatic feeling. Ooooo, feels good. That's all. Sometimes I call my shiatsu Tantric Zen."[29]

Yet this is also shifting ground. At a gut level we suspect that if an interaction begins as therapeutic touch and changes into seduction, there has been a violation of boundaries and ethics.

This is because Western culture is particularly depleted in providing stages one goes through to transmute energies. Many powerful forms of healing touch die in impulse because their impulse seems to arouse inappropriate erotic feelings. The heart within healing is stifled as it passes through the lower *chakras*. If the practitioner could contain and blend with its feeling rather than either act rashly upon it or suppress it, then he or she might find energetic attraction suddenly converted into an effective therapeutic tingling resembling the flow of *tantra*. This would be an initial step toward healing as a form of love.

Breema, a bodywork which includes embraces, belly-to-belly contact, and periods of holding partners in cradle-like positions, is so frequently misinterpreted that American master Manocher Movlai has stated during trainings that he believes vigilance about sex corrupts our ability to make physical contact with each other to such a degree that it threatens the existence of our species.

In reaction to one student's complaint that some of his postures were exploitative of women, this giant Kurdish man paced the room making astonishingly and fierce faces while roaring that he was a bear; then pranced like a horse. "The bear is so cute," he growled. "The horsey we think is cute. But people, no! What? If I want to make love, I don't need this [imitates the intimate posture in question]. I can make love to a single hair on her head."[30]

Sexual and Healing Massage

IT IS NOT ENTIRELY happenstance that the term "massage" has become a euphemism in our own culture not only for a hedonistic, hands-on treatment but for prostitution itself. So-called massage parlors are businesses where sexual pleasure is marketed under the guise of muscle relaxation, or, in some cases, not even under a guise at all. This has

at least two implications: that sex is more merchandisable than healing, and that sensual pleasure and sex are irretrievably confused with
each other.

The body does not make intellectual or semantic discriminations;
it just responds. Men visiting erotic-massage parlors are (in terms of
their latent hungers) going to the "doctor." Even a symptomatic relief
of their fever translates through the body as a real medicine. Though
few of the prostitutes are intentionally involved in healing, as long as
there is seductive touch (or even a charade of making a client feel good),
the healing archetype is inescapable. Sex workers are unskilled nurse-
physicians practicing a rough medicine the body recognizes without
the mind. That doesn't mean that the experience is always positive, but
its touch does fall within a therapeutic context.

In a number of documentaries, interviews with lap dancers, strip-
pers, and prostitutes reveal how these women are not only sensitive to
the complexes and erotic compulsions of their customers but sympathetic and anxious to meet them and relieve frustrations. They *are* massage therapists, even if unbalanced in their approach.

Whereas a deep craniosacral treatment or a skilled *shiatsu*
massage can be an effective treatment for someone with
capacity for translation of sensual energy
to their organs, a person without that
subtle capacity may be seeking an
approximation of the same sensations by genitalization. Although it
is often not sex which such people
seek in sex, ironically only sexual contact will get it for them. Lust so overrides natural hunger that satiation, while symptomatic, becomes
the only means of breaking the stasis and allowing the
mind, if it is receptive, to reclaim the body's actual needs.

Women are natural healers insofar as they bring life into the world
and then nurture it. Even women who never give birth gestate ener-

gies and organs receptive to healing. Men may seek sex more ardently partly because they lack (i.e., have not developed) their own intrinsic healing functions. They are dependent on others to supply these aspects because their biology and their culturally prescribed personae and roles combine to prevent them from developing it in themselves.

In this context sex surrogates (participatory sexual teachers and healers) function as healers, initially on the level of treating specific genital dysfunctions but secondarily on the level of literally transmitting erotic energy. These professionals are often hired by disabled people or others considered so unattractive by society that sexual (or even physical) contact otherwise is a virtual impossibility.

IT IS DIFFICULT enough for most people in our culture to accept a relationship of lovers as fundamentally one of healers. But once that is established (as it sometimes is in free-love circles), it becomes difficult (anew) to explain why, if loving is healing, often sex is so pathological and destructive. Yet it should be no surprise if, during impassioned and emotionally charged episodes of physical contact, a person's compulsions around sexuality instead of its healing aspects are reinforced. A seductively forced opening can lead to a deeper closing later. A good general rule is that defenses exist for a reason and should not be recreationally or idly removed, especially without cognizance of what is being protected. By letting too much charge flow into one plexus of the body (one *chakra*), sexual activity may somaticize biases and blocks which are ultimately quite degenerative. It may also reinforce habits of somatic rigidity. No matter how pleasurable the experience may seem, people do not truly open themselves until they are ready. Thus, the extra energy has no place to go. Exploitation of sexuality often generates inability to tolerate it at all, so people go from promiscuity to abstinence. Incest is also a taboo for psychological as well as sociological reasons.

Healing,
Language,
and
Sexuality

In the absence of healing contact and recognition of each other, we exist in stupors of unacknowledged desires and projections of lust, frustrated violations of each other's boundaries, misappropriations of freedom, and dysfunctionalizing sexual taboos that mask actual sexual expression in a host of bizarre sex-image customs and rigid erotic dances. It is no wonder that abuses of core energy lead to serious sexual pathologies, including pedophilia, necrophilia, and sadism.

Beneath the surface of desire is often a more fundamental holding back. If a therapist is lucid and clear on his or her own feelings of attraction toward a patient, the patient experiences without seduction any energy projected and both move through it. The massage practitioner thereby deepens his or her quality of touch. Always beneath titillation and fantasy is a deeper sexuality that is slow and serious and has no compulsive quality; it is the fundamental arrangement the self makes with its male or female personality, and from it alone do authentic sexual feelings and healing energies emerge.

Basic Hexing

LOVERS ARE A SUBSET of basic human dyadic interaction. Between any two people, a quality of energy arises. It can include parts of empathy, condolence, anger, repulsion, fear, contempt, attraction, attachment. It is the basis for the common arrangements people have, including marriage, games, governments, communities. Psychoanalytic and shamanic transference derive from this quality.

"Male" and "female" are social categories at the same time as they are biological distinctions. In each society genders are fixed at birth (with the exception of transsexual operations), but what is manly or womanly ("macho" or "feminine") is an outcome of layers of cultural history and modes of social development which define gender roles. Behavioral sex is yet another realm and does not require any of the above distinctions. Two organisms can participate in an erotic relationship without one being male, the other female. There are innumerable variations on the theme of the standard heterosexual pair.

Individuals born these days with at least the rudiments of both male and female genitals (intersexuals) have one set have surgically amputated at birth according to the recommendation of an endocrinologist. Usually arbitrarily selected, the "ambiguous" genitalia is removed not for health reasons, but because gender is considered an absolute in Western civilization; you are not allowed to be both male and female. As adults, many intersexuals experience a sense of having been robbed of their identity. Perhaps intersexuals also have unique healing abilities, which ablated with their ostensibly superfluous organs.

Sex is multiform in nature. Reich's requirement of male-female genital embrace for orgastic exchange and health was a culturally provincial interpretation of sexual energy and biological capacity. Shared age, race, culture, gender, even species are neither anatomical nor emotional prerequisites for sex, though violation of any of them brooks many societal taboos (depending on the culture). Science fiction has even probed the possibilities of sexual relationships between creatures from different worlds. This is all part of the unresolved question of biological identity.

Gay men have developed their own systems of *tantra* based on males participating genitally with each other in exciting charge and withholding sperm. There may be many other *tantras* and diverse genres of orgone embrace, including lesbian and auto-erotic ones.

More University, a commune based in Lafayette, California, offers a series of courses on Enhanced Sexual Performance (ESP in their playful terminology) in which women (in particular) learn to expand their orgasms—to lengths ranging from an hour to fourteen hours and even longer. Although heterosexual contact may be involved (and usually is), genital intercourse is considered incidental. Instead, sequential mutual masturbation is practiced, with an emphasis on each partner aiding the other in enhanced sensation (sequences and rhythms are developed to prolong tumescence and extend the experience). The contact is viewed mainly as an aid —it is more "pleasurable" to be acted upon than to act

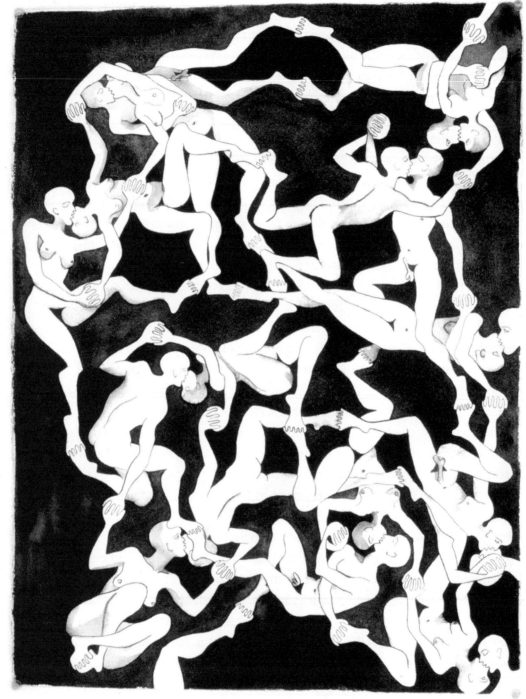

upon oneself. But the orgasm itself is sexual medicine.

In the overall More philosophy, full orgasm— individual capacity for feeling and erotic pleasure— is a prerequisite to the expression of human generosity and consequently to community harmony. It is also a means of preventing disease.

From years of research at the commune, members have come to believe in distinct human estrus cycles less explicit than in other primates but no less powerful or dominating. In fact, because human hormonal arousal is not strictly cyclical like simian "heat," it is more at play potentially in every situation, with oft-disastrous results (given the roles assigned by society and what is considered appropriate behavior). Females (mostly 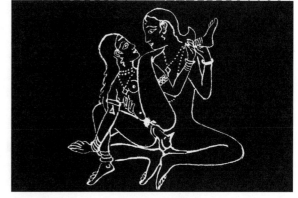 unconsciously) arouse males and control male sexual behavior. This unacknowledged biological event, constantly and subliminally experienced, leads to a variety of mating rituals but also a much larger variety of diversions, secondary sublimations, and other rituals of denial. More studies and exposes these with an aim toward neutralizing their danger. In evening community sessions (called Mark Groups) people talk about their lives, relationships, and desires, and other members query them about what they mean, trying to root out jealousies, self-deceptions, and disingenuousness. Sexual projections and fantasies are named, acknowledged, and neutralized by being shared.

While More activities reveal women's fake innocence and constant estrological seduction of men, everywhere, of all ages and statuses, they place even more weight on exposing men's abuse of their power. Men, they argue, dominate the sexual act with their own more limited orgastic capacities, devaluing the exponentially broader range of female orgasm and creating the entire social and professional pecking order by their own unconscious (or at best semi-conscious) act of rating women according to desirability—a rating they make little sexual use of except to fulfill their own minimal needs. Their less generous uses have defined the workplace and general social environment. "All women are judged by all men according to their fuckability," one More teacher proclaims. "No matter whether these women are their mothers, daughters, or sisters; no matter their age, from children to great-grandmothers;

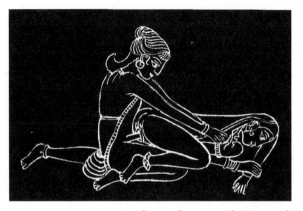

no matter how feminist and socially conscious the male—women are rated and given status by how fuckable men consider them, and are denied status on the same basis. All women. Equal-rights laws notwithstanding." Another More instructor warns, "Watch out especially for those men who claim they are above this or don't do it, for these are the ones who do it most covertly and cover their tracks most skillfully. In fact, they use their claims of being advocates of women to disguise their more devious and desperate appropriations of them."[31]

The More goal is to make men and women aware of these habits: women repressing their awareness of unconscious flirtation and seduction, feigning innocence of how men get turned on and pretending it is all nuance and charm, men denying the role of sexism in how they treat women and kidding themselves that their attraction for *some* women gives them the moral authority and impartiality to assign social domains to *all* women. Only then can each begin to be real with the other.

No doubt there are abuses of authority and sexuality at More too (some apostates have made very specific claims), but More's relative success at the practice of sensual joy for social well-being, health, and sanity is an indication that planetary justice and innate contact between people are based on erotic ritual and recognition of sexual danger to a greater degree than allowed by our belief systems and religious prejudices.

Although denigrated in the press as a "sex commune" and belittled in both holistic-health and left-wing circles, More has survived since 1968 and produced a service-oriented community most traditional spiritual and political egalitarian groups would envy. Many Buddhist, Catholic, yogic, Marxist, and other guru-led or New Age communities have been torn apart by abuses of power and sexual exploitation (or distortions of their basic practice arising from avoidance of the issue)—and also have difficulty finding time amidst their tasks and rituals for more than sporadic or rote charity. The main occupations of More's home-based commune and various regional communities are teaching courses on sensuality and man-woman relations under such titles as "Money, Sex, and

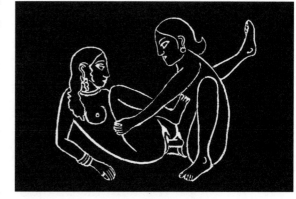

Jealousy," "Estrology," "Basic Hexing," and "Love for Sale," and feeding the poor. In fact, quite anonymously, they run one of the largest ground-roots charities in the United States. Every member of every More house and most of their students throughout the year collect groceries, produce, and other surplus goods and distribute them in inner-city neighborhoods, often at personal risk. More has mastered logistics for how to give away subsistence goods in places where poverty, drugs, dealers, gangs, and guns abound. They also set aside a large portion of their Lafayette commune for the homeless to camp. They feed and provide shelter for these "guests" and fight a daily battle with zoning agencies to maintain and expand this activity.

This is not altruistic or strategic generosity; it is not even an attempt at social action or piety. For generosity is more than just a More credo. It is a functional basis of sexual identity, community, and charity. Men and women "give" to one another not because they think it is right or expect something in return but because gifts open to them their own unlimited bounty.

This philosophy is the diametric opposite of the ritual victimhood practiced not only by most therapy groups but as a political tactic throughout American society. All too many people seek to be victims because they plan to exact a legal or emotional claim on someone else or on a social institution. Also, victimization legitimizes their sorrow and failures.

More treats such martyrdom as the abnegation and squandering of a vast personal wealth. To indulge in wretchedness is what makes us wretched. To be bounteous liberates our own richness to ourselves. A More member told me, "Our philosophy is, when you wake in the morning, ask yourself, 'What is it today which I have to give?' If it is nothing but grief, then ask, 'To whom may I make a gift of my grief?'"

The Pathogenic Healer

IN THE WEST there is the illusion that methods are what cure disease. As Carl Jung observed, we honor "... the 'right' method irrespective of the man who applies it." But this, he pointed out, overlooks an ancient Taoist law: "'... if the wrong man uses the right means, right means work in the wrong way.'"[32] By this measure, it is not the method but the physician who determines the success of the remedy.

What binds preachers, oncologists, shamans, homeopaths, tantric healers, psychologists, Reiki masters, massage therapists, and surgeons is that, in reading the "character" of their patients according to the systems in which they work, they stand as mirrors in which sick persons "see" themselves—not photographically of course but in an almost imperceptible shimmer or warble. The mirrors are there before any medicine is administered. They are the medium *through* which the medicine is administered (much like the water into which mirrors melt in Jean Cocteau's *Orphée*). In seeming to discover psychoanalysis (character transference) as medicine, Freud and Reich may have actually discovered the mask behind which all medicine men and women hide.

Transference, inculcated by the resonance of mutual discovery, is what cures people in psychotherapy. The therapist reenacts the patient's emotional states, thus accelerates them into new orbits. In the discussion of a dream it may not matter what symbolic referents therapist and patient assign as long as in the process they experience a curative dialogue between themselves, as long as their empathic interaction sows new elements in the psyche. After all, cultures survive not because their beliefs and ideologies are rational or accountable but because people adhering to them respond to one another in satisfying ways. No laws can enforce this; yet a functional community, from its feelings of connection alone, arrives at appropriate institutions. More prisons cannot protect a community nor can harsher laws restrict criminal activity. One might as well argue with diseases.

To the degree that a doctor is comfortable with his or her own life and role as a physician, he or she will practice medicine at an appropriate level without medically hexing or projecting disease complications. Yet, any confusion a doctor has, conscious or unconscious (but particularly unconscious), will be transfused onto the patient along with the cure.

Projection is inevitable as long as there are two breathing animals. This is more obvious in dyadic abreactive therapies like shamanic healing and psychoanalysis, but it is *always* the case, along the entire gamut from Reiki to surgery. Sometimes projections may get minimized or deflected, but, despite all attempts at neutral clinical environments, they roam unchastened and unimpeded. They are the great howling silence in every hospital and medical office in the West—the unacknowledged and uncompensated-for madness behind the antiseptic act of spiritless cure.

The more technological healing facilities become, the darker the shadows they will cast, the more heinous the monsters that arise from those shadows to dominate the very furniture of waiting rooms and officious facial expressions of those operating the bureaucracy. Doctors are mere secretaries themselves, agents for steel-silicon giants girded with artificial intelligence. *Their* motives are projections of something unknown and unprobed in us (what about those science-fiction tales in which machines develop personalities and become restless "wannabes" or "terminators"?).

For all we *see* in a hospital, the absolute reality staring us in the face is virtually invisible.

In fact, we are purposely hypnotized not to see what is happening: a great disease factory, a repressed horror movie in self-parody of its own darkly comedic genre.

Set aside the vast ritual of institutional health care and janitorial disposal of bodies for a moment. Edward Whitmont points out that, on even the personal level, the field between doctor and patient routinely includes not only "the patient's wounds and complexes, his or her pain, anger and yearning for healing . . ." but the doctor's "empathically tuned resonance that arises from his own wounds and his more or less consciously realized anger at the limitations of the human situation as it affects himself as well as the patient, as well as his urge to assert his capacities for helpful intervention. . . . [These are] mobilized when the pathogenic impasse is activated in the encounter."[33] The implication here is not so much that there are neurotic doctors but that the very profession of objective medicine, its epistemological shallowness and disregard of the shadow in the midst of horrific diseases, tumors, corpses, etc., is generative of sociopathology and archetypal disease.

"Most—yes, *most*—physicians are suffering from Post-Traumatic Stress Disorder," writes Bernie Siegel, the renowned M.D. author. "They have a classical exposure to traumatic events and no place to appropriately express them. Many are ashamed to show their pain, and cry in hidden places."[34] This emotional suppression projects disquieting fantasies through the doctor's professional persona, smiles and good will pasted on over them. A patient instinctively fears such a persona but can find no rational justification for her unease.

Suppression also leads to an increasingly more mechanistic practice of all aspects of medicine. If one is trying to conceal deep and disturbing feelings, these manifest rampantly both as ghosts and hexes.

Whitmont again:

A great healer once remarked that "a physician never enters the sick room alone, but is always accompanied by a host of angels or demons." Whether the healer comes with angels or demons will be determined by the degree of the healer's conscious awareness of his own wounds and impulses toward wounding and by his ability to process them, to potentize them to their symbolic essence and hence not to be carried away by them nor to project (and projectively induce) them in his patients.[35]

Potentization is what converts most of the nonallopathic modalities in this volume into medicines. It is not just a homeopathic modality. By thermodynamic, alchemical, and semeiological dynamics they transduce one type of energy and manifestation into another. They penetrate character. But potentization in the service of drugs and machines can be secondarily pathological. What looks terrifying (more like a morgue than a healing temple) *is* terrifying, for good reason.

The illusion that the doctor is an efficient automaton—or that he feigns neutrality successfully—overlooks the fact that his or her own "illness potential" is activated by not only the patient's symptomatic pathology but the particular complexes in the patient's personality that resonate with that potential: "When the healer unconsciously acts out those complexes, they operate like poison and add to the patient's disturbance."[36]

Later, Whitmont adds:

The surgeon scrubs to free himself of infectious material he might introduce into the patient. Yet "infection" is not merely a physical, bacterial or viral phenomenon. It is a field dynamic that occurs in every human interaction and deserves special attention in the healing dyad because of its potential to confuse the process and even inject iatrogenic pathology.[37]

Perhaps the most dangerous aspect of the healer is his adoption of medical authority. This mantle, conferred on him by his role and stature within the clinic and community, is reinforced by his warrior stance confronting disease. Whitmont insists that who become our doctors is no accident, for "... to the degree that [a] doctor's unconscious obsession and fear of death, the urge to control illness and death for his or her own preservation, happen to motivate the choice of profession, he or she will fight illness and death as such."[38] Again, I emphasize, this is true on an unconscious level no matter what talents a physician cultivates outwardly and no matter how neutral and technologically proficient his or her manner of healing. Often the more technically skilled a doctor the more virulently he activates a patient's resentment of false authority. Those attitudes determine how the patient unconsciously receives and assimilates the medicine.

On the surface, the doctor may be carrying out his hero-physician role to a tee and the patient may be playing the model recipient. Underneath, though, they are evoking a more tortured mythology in which the patient resists the doctor's authority and becomes sicker in order to confound it, while the doctor projects onto the patient unresolved conflicts from his own life. As latent complexes arouse one another, both attract the shadows that give each of them the greatest difficulty and thus present the most compelling challenges. The patient's disease and doctor's training collaborate to form a virtual arena in which the unlived fantasies of both parties play themselves out. When the doctor views himself as a hero and the disease as his adversary, it is not far from there to the patient becoming the adversary, especially if he or she does not respond appropriately.

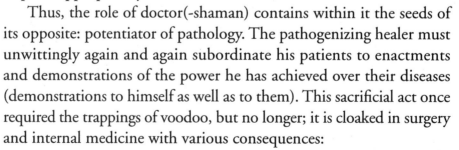

Thus, the role of doctor(-shaman) contains within it the seeds of its opposite: potentiator of pathology. The pathogenizing healer must unwittingly again and again subordinate his patients to enactments and demonstrations of the power he has achieved over their diseases (demonstrations to himself as well as to them). This sacrificial act once required the trappings of voodoo, but no longer; it is cloaked in surgery and internal medicine with various consequences:

MODALITIES

- The patient is reduced to an object.

- The empathy the doctor attempts to project rings false, so an intimation of deceit replaces that of presumed good will.

- The doctor aggressively takes on himself the role of dispelling the illness and deprives the patient of his or her own healing power (in fact, the doctor may unconsciously resent any healing that cannot be attributed to him).

- Identifying with his own falsely inflated role thereby erodes the doctor's real skill in whatever modality he practices.

- The patient, depersonalized—perhaps even infantilized—becomes so passive (again, usually unconsciously—there may be collateral assertions of activity and participation in getting well) that he or she does not draw on natural healing powers or fails to perceive the profound level on which transduction is needed in order to be cured.

- The doctor may diagnose on the basis of superficial signs because he is unconsciously always seeking the same adversaries or reflecting his own conflicts (this explains the tendency of certain doctors to find the identical conditions over and over in patients bearing different etiologies).

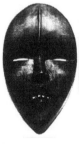

- He may also get carried away with his image of what the disease is and practice outside the realm of his competence, attempting to heal something that isn't present or subtly transforming the actual disease into his imagined disease. He may iatrogenically worsen the disease or impart a new disease.

- He also may literally transpose his misrepresentation or exaggeration of pathology onto the patient, who will unconsciously pick it up and become sicker (thus the doctor will become not the specialist diagnosing a complex but, transpersonally, the source of disease).[39]

Because we are neophytes in understanding the role of mind in transmuting matter or the relationship of psychological meanings to cell morphing, we do not know the degree to which a doctor's projections can cause neuroses, attachments to already-existent diseases, and resistance to self-cure in patients. Maybe such transmutations occur purely on the psychological level and become somaticized only over long periods of time and only when other negative co-factors also exist—thus, they do not constitute a sole iatrogenic factor in the causation of tumors *et al.* Maybe, on the other hand, patients can walk into a doctor's office with relatively minor diseases and leave with far more trenchant ones grafted spontaneously during the examination. What happens is that the physician actually projects a malaise he later diagnoses as present. The patient's fear of what the doctor will uncover, merges with the doctor's unconscious guilt from his wrongfully seized power: all he did to earn his status was complete medical school and an internship; he was never broken by crystals like the Aboriginal doctor or otherwise initiated and cleansed. Thus, he is continually subject to his own fear of what he might reveal to both of them. These become self-fulfilling prophecies.

Every society faces this terrifying and imponderable crisis when it looks squarely in the eye of voodoo and sorcery. Bad will causes accidents and transmits infection as surely as the firing of guns. I am not suggesting that doctors unwittingly fling diseases into patients like pins into proxy dolls. I am merely indicating that as long we do not know all the parameters of either negative or positive projection, we should be careful about whom we choose to treat us.

All of the above is of course not just limited to doctors and patients; it is the vibration of life, seen dramatically in the relationships of spouses and secondarily in boss-worker, teacher-student, pilot-passenger dyads. In doctor-patient realms it contacts pathology directly and thus becomes entangled in the language and sociology of disease and cure.

It is worth summarizing this plot: Doctors may not intentionally abuse their roles or the power bequeathed them, but underlying confusions about power and shamanic identity will *always* lead to the projection of pathologizing distortions. It is not possible for human beings not to abuse it. Whitmont notes, "[Power] is a pathological aspect of ego functioning and cannot be dealt with in a simple way by ego-will and good intentions. An attempt by the ego to renounce power is as unhelpful as ego hubris and the misuse of power for self-gratification. Both extremes equally arouse the wrath of the transpersonal elements."[40] That is, both ring false in a situation where rectitude is crucial—authenticity is required by the literality of the disease and the trial by fire that pathology exacts. This is why medicine is so difficult to practice. A doctor attempting to get around the power issue by asserting his all-abiding good-will actually invokes it in the arrogance of his very attempt. Thus, in pretending to be more than a doctor he becomes less than a doctor. What he lacks in actual compassion is transformed into his hex.

Drunvalo Melchizedek offers a view of this same ego dynamic in faith healing:

> You've got to get your ego out of the way and not [presume] that just because you think someone should be healed they really should be....
>
> Healing someone else means taking on the responsibility for that person. It might not just be a five-minute little thing or something you do. It might mean you have to spend a year with them. If you're not willing to totally stay with that until it's done, maybe you should go fix cars or something.[41]

This is why the lack of shamanic initiation and transference in the training of modern physicians is so insidious. It is no wonder we are either fast approaching or have already arrived at a system which is as generative of disease, despair, and alienation on one level as it is technologically adept at excising or suppressing symptoms and dread malignancies on another.

CHANGING THE WHOLE medical system is impossible. The arch-diocese that confronted William Clinton in 1995 was more deep-seated than the Vatican. It is now well beyond that stage, functioning as a giant megacorporate conduit for the abstract materialization and quantification of bodies, minds, genes, and spirits. Who we think we are stares back at us in X-ray and other radiation images as little more than a puppet-activated corpse. Yet, in individual cases (where alone healing is manageable), therapeutic impasses and negative projection cycles are broken magically as they occur. The doctor subconsciously undergoes the transmutation of a shaman (who himself experiences an illness, at least in symbolic form, in order to serve as the vehicle of its cure). Whitmont explains:

"The fact that the healer's propensity to his own illness is activated in a mutually containing field with the patient makes it possible to have his own 'illness' become the 'simillimum' that is offered for the healing process."[42] The same illness potentials, "when 'potentized' into symbolic awareness by the healer ... help the healing process."[43] A transpersonal event paralleling the mysterious alchemization of homeo-pathic microdoses from toxic substances transforms pathogenic atti-tudes into beneficent waves. The debilitating factor in the physician is itself potentiated into the cure. Likewise, an unacknowledged "micro-dose" can originate either metachemically or cognitively in any thera-peutic situation, even within the framework of allopathy. As pure shamanism enters each medicine in a set of its own archetypes, the doctor's personality becomes the vehicle of the cure rather than its impediment:

Often this activation of the simillimum is brought about as the result of the pain of having to renounce one's desire for intimate personal relationship with the patient and the acceptance of the ensuing lone-liness, should this be the case. It also may be the effect of the doc-tor's training or personal experience in which he passed experientially through the illness-healing process himself.... It helps him or her to partner the patient's individuality on an inner quest, by feeling, perceiving and resonating with him or her, and hence also perceiving the nature of the ailment and its appropriate therapeutic modality and curative similarity . . . such as a proper potentized substance, the meridians or points to be activated, and even his or her own relational influence.[44]

This is why the novice must be killed with "crystalline stones" or their symbolic equivalent.

The archetypal function of the healer includes the function of the sacrificial *pharmakos,* the scapegoat who offers himself and his sensitivities and ability to suffer pain as a sacrifice. He chooses to carry and metabolize his patient's ills, and shares his patient's imprisonment in the incubatory container. . . .

He allows himself to know that he is meant to carry and suffer the "evil," the pathology of others. Hence, in order to avoid "infecting" others (his own infection he cannot avoid), he . . . undergo[es] a constant "purification," that is, [he] must maintain a perpetual scrutiny of the nature and appropriateness of his reactions (and/or overreactions) that may be similar to the patient's state.[45]

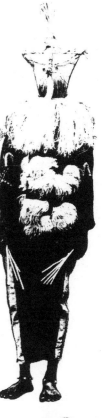

When the physician steps back and accepts his or her role as the true healer, letting the patient's systemic wisdom cure illness within its own domain, then the patient gains access to the archetypal healer and all his/her powers, as mediated by an actual physician. A mutation takes place that transcends and transforms both.

The Archetypal Healer

THE TRUE HEALER and inner physician is the hologram of independent cells orchestrated as tissues and organs that formed embryogenically from the seeds of the zygote and continues to rebuild and restore its template. Transit across a lifetime is itself a passage into the innermost chambers of a genome-*wairua*—and this process is unique in each person. It cannot be generalized or socialized accord-

131

ing to formulas of demography or even genetics, and it cannot be dealt out in mass medicine. It can either be catalyzed or impeded by doctors, but not manufactured.

If all disease is etiologically karmic and psychospiritual, then the truest modality of a healer is his or her ability to activate archetypal and cosmic factors. The practice of a particular craft, with its skills and paraphernalia (which may comprise synthesized drugs, movements and palpations, sophisticated surgeries, or symbolic transference), ideally awakens an unconscious impetus to modes of healing that succeed beyond any actual mechanical act of medicine. By this definition all healing is, to a certain degree, archetypal, and all feats of medicine are likewise sleights of hand. The techniques, temporally functional, do not themselves effect embryogenic tissue transformations. The great variety of healing systems is necessary not because of the variety of diseases but the multiplicity of routes of access to individuals and blocks in which these are character-bound.

THE SIGNAL OF LIFE is uniform like a wave, but the body often does not perceive it singly or take its own existence seriously. If nostalgia and fantasy dominate, and sensation is always in the past as sweetness of memory or in the future as daydream, then the wave of life will be fragmentary and remote. "Tired of livin' an' skeered of dyin'," the lament of the dockworker Joe in "Ol' Man River," is the chorus now for all of modern habitants. When the resiliency of biological existence rigidifies, one also shuns the final singleness imposed by death. If an organism cannot express its whole nature, it seems to need all of time in which to accumulate and express its partial natures, so it is greedy for experience. Living and dying are both violations of its hoard of fragments.

The successful healer presents an "other" that enables the core of the "sick" person to "perceive" his own health. This proprioception may be conscious or unconscious, biochemical or psychospiritual, highly cathected and painful, or silent and brief as a breeze over a field of clover. The same mystery that marks daily autonomous self-healing arises from the twaining of healer and patient.

Healing is a vibration between a doctor (or modality) and a patient on whatever plane we choose to reify it. A message is sent to the wholeness of the body, either emotionally, vitally, by meridians, by herbal or pharmaceutical blends, by muscles and nerves, structurally, or by language and other linguistic codes. The integrity of the system interprets the message and organizes around it anew.

Every medicine has an amplitude and a periodicity. Even a curative experience, which is a shock or tilt, expresses itself finally as a wave. The cure may originate in a snap or ping, but the ripples it sends forth are perfect wholes.

Healing occurs at a frequency or vibration present in the patient and tuned to a medicine. Whatever ensues subsequently may not matter—even a lapse in the treatment. After all, adjusting the frequency or the stimulus does the same thing to a cure that it does to a wave; it changes its amplitude without changing its nature. The shape may be different, but its congruence remains.

The patient also experiences the wave before the treatment, *is* the wave, but in a fragmentary sense or without sufficient energy to mobilize or expand it. He does not feel his life as a unity. Thoughts are scattered and depressed; purposes are at cross-purposes; physical movement is uncoordinated; organs are restricted; systemic responsiveness is uncommitted and interrupted. The wave is discordant or intermittent.

A good healer does not do too many things or too much. He tries to do the one necessary thing. The person who is being healed cannot judge the result according to a standard of symptomatic relief. The goal is to assert the wave, to end an outgrown practice of self-cure.

Bone cracking is "silly," but the bones that are cracked do not laugh. Their pulse rides into the body like a horse throwing back its head in midflight, the *hsing-i* horse which delivers a powerful blow in *shiatsu*. New spasms may interrupt unity, but eventually the wave completes itself because it is already there.

Disease also has a singleness of expression, and it will reimpose itself if there is no wave to release, or transmute it.

A WHOLENESS COMES ON GRADUALLY. A person first feels better, has fewer symptoms, is less depressed, more energetic. Then she experiences greater coordination, unjustified optimism, unexpected freedom. Relapses may be resting periods before greater expansion. Later on, the person is springy and responsive. She mocks herself less in interactions with people. If she laughs or cries, these are also coordinated and part of her expression as a living creature. Eventually the wave will transpose itself in social situations; she will make better decisions and friends, have more coherent thoughts, experience more poignant and grounded desires. Unity is irresistible.

Her death is now a single thing too, and she can face it, as part of the wave, with poignancy that is no longer restless yearning.

T HE PROCESS CALLED "bodywork" gets that name not because it is physical rather than mental, but because it honors our incarnation in a physical universe as an irrevocable condition of therapeutics. It little matters whether we believe that spirit has arisen in matter or matter itself is possessed of remarkable attributes: disease and cure prove that we have manifested here in bodies alone. We cannot out-think or exogenously spiritualize our anatomical destiny; we must think *in* it, find mind through it. In this sense, bodywork (and healing in general) is a restatement of the condition of birth. We come into being through the body of another who came into being likewise, back to the beginning of a universe. The doctor must replicate, in some manner, the act of gestation. She has to be a maternal force because her cure cannot evade the root of biology and cellular continuity. She must impose herself into the biological message with the same seriousness with which the mother *is* the biological message.

Christ's dying for our sins archetypally empowers healers to "save" sick persons through their own bodies. Psychoanalytic transference reenacts the Crucifixion symbolically, not because the doctor is sacrificed but because the patient accepts the intercession of an archetypal being in his own cure. The Crucifixion and transference are different faces of the same creed.

When doctor and patient begin to work together, a breathing together is established, and everything in both individuals is represented in that breathing somewhere. The two bodies reclaim the ancient message—or, as Johnny Cash sings: "Flesh and blood needs flesh and blood, and you are what I need."

He means loving not healing, but the meaning could not be clearer.

Notes

1. Margaret MacKenzie, personal communication, 1978.

2. Deepak Chopra, *Quantum Healing: Exploring the Frontiers of Mind/Body Medicine* (New York: Bantam Books, 1989), p. 247.

3. Ibid., pp. 248–49.

4. Ibid., p. 250.

5. Ibid., pp. 251–52.

6. Peter Ralston, dialogue during a class, Oakland, California, 1990.

7. M. Masud R. Khan, "Toward an Epistemology of Cure," quoted in John P. Conger, *The Body in Recovery: Somatic Psychotherapy and the Self* (Berkeley, California: Frog, Ltd., 1994), p. 95.

8. Cybèle Tomlinson, "Breema Bodywork," *Yoga Journal,* November/December, 1994, p. 94.

9. Conger, *The Body in Recovery*, pp. 95–96.

10. A. P. Elkin, *Aboriginal Men of High Degree* (Sydney: Australasian Publishing, 1944), p. 125.

11. Miguel Covarrubias, *Island of Bali* (New York: Alfred A. Knopf, 1938), p. 334.

12. Paul Radin, *The World of Primitive Man* (New York: Grove Press, 1953; Revised Edition, 1960), p. 58.

13. Ibid., pp. 58-59.

14. Ibid., p. 59.

15. Ibid., p. 60.

16. Robert Lawlor, *Voices of the First Day: Awakening in the Aboriginal Dreamtime* (Rochester, Vermont: Inner Traditions, 1971), p. 370.

17. *Huang Ti Nei Ching Su Wên*, trans. by Ilza Veith as *The Yellow Emperor's Classic of Internal Medicine* (Berkeley, California: University of California Press, 1966), pp. 147–48.

18. Ibid., p. 163.

19. A. Veronica Reif, "Eurhythmy and Curative Eurhythmy," Berkeley Anthroposophical Society, 1978.

20. Ibid.

21. Laura Chester, "In a Motion," unpublished manuscript, 1978.

22. Wendy Palmer, *The Intuitive Body: Aikido as a Clairsentient Practice* (Berkeley, California: North Atlantic Books, 1994), p. 72.

23. Peter Ralston, statement during a class, Oakland, California, 1991.

24. Palmer, *The Intuitive Body*, p. 94.

25. Kumar Frantzis, *The Tao in Action: The Personal Practice of the I Ching and Taoism in Daily Life*, unpublished manuscript at the time of publication (Berkeley, California: North Atlantic Books, 1996).

26. "Sex Between Therapist and Patient," transcript of a meeting of the APA, June 21, 1976, *Psychiatry*, Vol. 5, No. 22.

27. Moshe Feldenkrais, *The Potent Self: A Guide to Spontaneity* (New York: Harper & Row, 1985), p. 26.

28. Stanley Keleman, "Professional Colloquium, October 29, 1977" in Grossinger (ed.), *Ecology and Consciousness: Traditional Wisdom on the Environment* (Berkeley, California: North Atlantic Books, 1992), p. 25.

29. Barbara L. Schultz, "New Age Shiatsu" in Berkeley Holistic Health Center, *The Holistic Health Handbook* (Berkeley, California: And/Or Press, 1978), p. 195.

30. Manocher Movlai, in a class at the Breema Institute, Oakland, California, 1991.

31. These quotations are informally recalled from a lecture entitled "Love for Sale" at More University in 1993.

32. C. G. Jung, *Psychological Reflections*, edited by Jolande Jacobi (New York: Harper & Row, 1953), p. 71.

33. Edward C. Whitmont, *The Alchemy of Healing: Psyche and Soma* (Berkeley, California: North Atlantic Books, 1993), p. 188.

34. Bernie Siegel, "Letter to the Editor," *Common Boundary* (September/October, 1994), p. 9.

35. Whitmont, *The Alchemy of Healing,* p. 200.

36. Ibid., p. 189.

37. Ibid., p. 198.

38. Ibid., p. 208.

39. More complete descriptions of some of these may be found in Chapter Nine, "The Healer," in Whitmont's *The Alchemy of Healing,* pp. 187–212.

40. Whitmont, *The Alchemy of Healing,* p. 203.

41. Drunvalo Melchizedek, "Flower of Life Workshop," Dallas, Texas, February 14–17, 1992 (video recording).

42. Whitmont, *The Alchemy of Healing,* p. 197.

43. Ibid., p. 189.

44. Ibid., p. 198.

45. Ibid., pp. 208–209.

Healing,
Language,
and
Sexuality

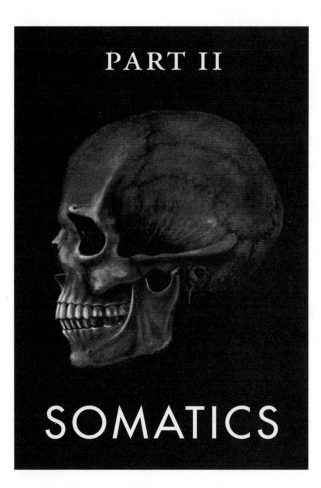

PART II

SOMATICS

Background to Somatics

Roots of Somatics

DEFINING SOMATICS IN the context of medicine is at once deceptively easy and extraordinarily complicated. The easy part is simply to note that, throughout the habitation of our species on Earth, body therapists have restored or enhanced health by massage, adjustment, hands-on energetic changes, and (more recently) guided exercises. The osteopath reinvented the jack-of-all-trades Pleistocene doctor.

The complicated part is that somatics deals with not only well-being but meaning that originates in a distinction between straightforward modes of touch and exercise and inner proprioception of embodiment. It has more to do with the body experienced from within than the body manipulated from without. Somatics can never be just massage or palpation, no matter how skilled or inventive these may be. It requires layers of sensation and integration that are not recognized in most physical therapies. One can be a resourceful and talented cranial worker, Rolfer,

---

This chapter could be placed at either the beginning of the "Somatics" section or the end—or, for that matter, at any other point along the way. Readers encountering Somatics as a concept for the first time might prefer to postpone it until learning about individual systems. Similarly, the order of Chapters Four and Five is interchangeable; the information in them is presented so that either could be read first.

Feldenkrais practitioner, etc., simply by carrying out diagrammatic postures and manipulations. What distinguishes somatotherapy is a conversion to viewing the body—in particular, one's own body—as a medium of inquiry into the nature of existence. Thus, a dedicated student of *t'ai chi ch'uan* can be a more authentic somaticist than a veteran bioenergetic therapist.

Somatic methods arise from the epistemology, phenomenology, and kinesiology of a body and reach beyond the body itself to a body image, an inner body realm, to social communication and space itself.

In describing her modality years later, somatic elder Gerda Alexander wrote:

> In touching we do not reach beyond the surface. In eutonic "contact" we move consciously beyond the visible boundaries of the body. Through this "contact" we can include also the surrounding space in our awareness. Thus, without touching, we are able to make real contact with other human beings, animals, plants and objects, passing through external boundaries.
>
> This conscious "contact" has greater influence than "touch" with regard to changes in the tonus and the circulation.[1]

The distinguishing features of the field of somatics (as defined at a 1992 San Francisco conference) are "focus on body image, anatomy, sensory and kinesthetic education, and nonverbal language."[2] I take this to mean the *simultaneous* priority of all five domains.

Perhaps more than any other present field of investigation, somatics portends the emergence of a phenomenological, self-organizing paradigm of reality, one that shares aspects with chaos theory, superstrings, structuralism, and deconstruction. In fact, somatics implicitly throws open the question (in daily life) of who is the observer, who is the subject.

The mainstream of medicine is somatic to the extreme—doggedly and literally so—without any phenomenology or philosophy beyond its linear rationalism. From this perspective, somatics *is* medicine. If we had to choose one modality whereby to treat everything, its ontology would be somatic: surgery would be its acute branch and pharmacy would provide a proximal method of penetrating and altering viscera.

More sophisticated somatic philosophies do not treat the body as a concordance of independently functioning viscera or as a separate entity in dialogue with an abstraction of mind. Somaticists address not the body *per se* but the mind in the body and the neural, corporeal aspect of the epiphenomenal mind. This is what defines the profession.

Some hijacked versions of somatics may seem to be less phenomenology or even manual medicine than a blend of pop philosophy and positive thinking. Their techniques and trainings suggest ritual exercises and mind-bending more than real cures for concrete diseases.

The EST of Werner Erhard is not somatics, nor are similar "positive thinking" and empowerment practices and seminars. These are secular religious rites not dissimilar from corporate sales meetings. Guided visualization, hypnotherapies, and instructional change by imperative from biofeedback machines are also not somatics in the pure sense. They are systems of behavioral modification. They impose an external authority inculcating a particular pattern of behavior or lifestyle. They borrow techniques, terminologies, and rationales from somatic systems, but they are linear and proscriptive. By contrast, true somatics teaches people how to listen to themselves and awaken their own inner life impulses. It does not have authoritarian agendas or patriotic ideologies.

S OMATIC THERAPIES ARE spiritual processes. The cranial osteopath follows her touch inward to a fluttering that seems to lie at the "soul" of the organs. Ilse Middendorf's breathwork not only enhances physical health, it leads a person into the meanings of her own untouched profundity. Eutony cultivates phenomenology through rhythm. Polarity massage is guided to karmic levels within the self where the destiny of the organism lies. Just as indigenous peoples entered their sweat lodges with a prayer to have their spirits soar like eagles, so somaticists bring the parameters of the sweat lodge with them and impose the functional equivalent of such heat and prayer on their clients.

Touch

IN OUR CROWDED CIVILIZATION, we have become dislocated from a sense of mutuality and connection with one another. In earlier times physical contact melded a richer and more diverse set of experiences, both spontaneous and ritualized. The pure kinesthesia of love and hate was somaticized instead of being sublimated and commoditized in the way it is today. Although this included acts we presently define as violent and cruel, the overall framework of human contact was tactile and embodied.

Stanley Keleman notes:

I am seeking a language of the basic metabolism of being, a matter-of-fact language arising out of the process of our biological existence.

One doesn't need ritualized methods to practice contact. We need to understand the organism and how it lives, and not develop methods.

What I practice comes from my understanding; it is not a method.

For example, in loving, we participate in a whole series of events at different levels; there are cellular and blood components; there are interpersonal actions and symbols. Loving ... is arousal, it is memory, it is pulsation, it is attraction, boundary-ending, connection, image-making. How these are shared is what contact is.[3]

The modern rebirth of contact and "touch" has come about, at one pole, from disciplines of physical and psychological therapy and medicine seeking a manual avenue of access and, on the other, from a suppressed and depreciated function of mutuality seeking new and acceptable modes of expression. It is what our overly abstracted and medicalized civilization most craves. Now that the intellect and concept rule, touch is the shadow, the depreciated function seeking to reclaim us. Whether in extreme sports (X Games *et al.*), exotic sex toys and erotic play (dildos, lap dancing, etc.), devotion to domesticated pets, or acts of deadly violence, the need is to touch each other and feel our own and other bodies.

Somatics as a separate discipline has roots in art, philosophy, naturopathy, and folk healing. In fact, it was once a branch of humanities and medicine, later overshadowed by the formalization of physical therapy, the medicalization of healing, and the triumph of aesthetics over expression in art and philosophy. The somatic synthesis vanished or at least went underground for the better part of a century.

> [Somatics] dates back to the mid- and late nineteenth-century Gymnastik movement in Northern Europe and the Eastern United States. At a time when physicians were still engaged in the crudest forms of surgery and medication, and when psychotherapy was just beginning, the practitioners of various branches of Gymnastik were already doing sophisticated healing work using expressive movement, sensory awareness, sound, music and touch.[4]

The founders of this movement included Frederick Matthias Alexander in Australia, Leo Kofler in New York, and Gerda Alexander, Ilse Middendorf, and Elsa Gindler in Germany. They wrote very little, transmitting their systems mainly through participants in their workshops, so most of their innovations went undocumented.

> World War I broke up the early interdisciplinary Somatics community, leaving individual schools intact but isolated and fragmented. World War II further dispersed the pioneers, forcing many of them to put aside the more visionary aspects of their work, and to eke out a living as refugees, marketing their work under the more acceptable forms of physical rehabilitation or psychotherapy.[5]

This certainly describes the journey of Gindler disciple Marion Rosen who, upon escaping Hitler's Germany in the 1930s, came to the United States and, not finding any public receptivity for somatics *per se,* began doing rehabilitative therapy. Out of this practice she eventually developed her own Rosen system of movement awareness.

A NEW SOMATICS HAS EMERGED simultaneously from the old nineteenth-century Gymnastik tradition; from modern arts, dance, and experimental theater; from the previously underestimated realm of the exercise class: Pilates, aerobics, kick-boxing, weight-lifting (of course, true "exercise" also includes yoga, *tai chi,* and *Chi Gung*); and from engaged forms of manual medicine and physical therapy.

Somatics is no less than the health-oriented aspect of the rebirth of touch. No longer confined to systems of adjustment and massage, modes of palpation and proprioception extend into science, art, spiritual practice, recreation, self-improvement. Bodywork, massage, myofascial touch, musculoskeletal palpation, breath, and autonomous movement have launched a medicinal avant-garde tradition following poetics and jazz in the late twentieth century, conferring (in palpation modes) the generosity and personal energy that once characterized communities of writers and musicians. Even business leaders and soldiers and their brass take workshops in how to know themselves and act effectively. Personal trainers restore a sense of physical groundedness and bodily purpose to people who can afford to pay them. Our modern situation has become so desperate that we must turn to professional guides for how to love, how to express anger, how to begin and end relationships.

People experimenting with somatics have improvised variants out of every imaginable component—meditation, guerrilla warfare, theater, puppetry, equestrianship, tennis, wildlife management, Gurdjieffian exercises, kayaking, African drumming, eroticism, sailing, skiing, sweat-lodge rituals, movement improvisation, hallucinogenic plants—or like somatic pioneer Frederick Matthias Alexander, they stand in front of a mirror and ask how (and where) the human mind/body begins to move.

Body/Mind

The somatic definition of "body" is such that it means just about everything the familiar use of the word "body" contradicts. Nothing more centrally expresses the body's creative power than the sheer fact of its physical existence. Our organisms arise and continue to sustain themselves and grow from cell division and differentiation through a lifetime, even as they retain the ability to make seeds for other living systems. Cells bearing Golgi bodies and mitochondria are truly alchemical in their transmutation not only of metabolic substance but their own intrinsic nature. Sex cells turn into stem cells, then into raw undetermined tissue, layers of flesh moving in unison that can become banks of cones focusing light or goblets absorbing nutritional material.

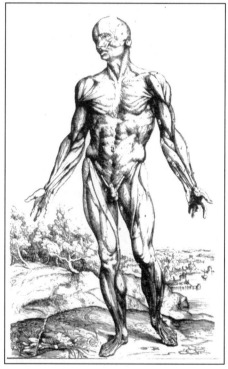

This process contains mysteries, mysteries that do not have to be solved for us to embody them, and, by embodying them, to think them without thinking them, to express them in our analysis of everything else, every moment we live. The development of a living creature-form from a germ cell requires coherence and complexity far more resembling metaphors of mind than of body. Beside this deeper body/mind, the mind of psychology and philosophy is a brief flash in an abyss.

Those who deal professionally with the body—doctors, athletic coaches, and physical therapists included—tend to see a functioning unity of organs and systems, of which one, the nervous system, connects mind to the rest of the material network. By this formula, health is assigned to body and medical etiology to mind, but a description of physical processes hardly covers the range and multiformity of the former; likewise, body can be intuitive and imaginative with resources of creativity rivaling mind at its most sublime.

Body and mind in every way are levels of the same manifestation. Can we speak of coordination separate from a mind? Can music exist without a body? Is telekinesis only the brain pulling? How does the mind even know it exists in order to pull? Is the heart only a pump or also the seat of emotions? Is yoga an act of mind or of body? Is healing mindwork or bodywork? For the traditional Apache of the Western Hemisphere and the Aborigine of Australia these questions do not exist. Their science intersects the life forms that make up the world, human and otherwise, in a different plane.

Things which are neither and both are things not in our system. Yet the young Jívaro initiate and Pomo Bear shaman stake their lives on a fact that is both mind and body and neither mind nor body, assignable to neither, even by component, as we might assign the impulse behind a dance step to mind or the breathing of meditation to body.

THE SO-CALLED mind-body split that we work holistically to unify is probably better described as a split between the mind of the body and the mind of the mind. As long as we are incarnate, we are separated from the vast unconscious archetypal body. The problem is that we are often dissociated from the mind of the body as well. Meditation, some schools of psychoanalysis, and even more "physical" therapies like osteopathy and herbs clearly address the mind as body (or the body as mind), that is, open a channel through our moment-to-moment proprioception into the patterns of energy and substance in our tissues. If the process is successful, physical and mental change are simultaneous.

By somatics I do not mean "physical therapy." Somatotherapy is a psychotherapy of the body. Somatotherapy also comprises skeletal, neuromuscular, and visceral medicines for treating actual physical lesions. Admittedly in this form somatotherapy has a conventional medicinal (osteopathic, neurological, even surgical) component, but this indi-

cates the subtlety and complexity of the mind-body nexus rather than an independent medical domain. Psychotherapy and somatotherapy are *both* psychosomatic medicines that explore the mysterious borderlands of the mind-body axis.

This dynamic might be made clearer by our distinguishing between the intellectual mind, which objectifies itself from the phenomena it experiences (in one of its most sophisticated forms, it is the scientific mind), and the mind of the body, which uses its subjective experiences to develop an internal language of sensations and functional connections. When we speak abstractly of the heart in relation to love for instance, we are not attributing characteristics to the physical aorta; we are identifying the charge we feel from the pumping of blood and the deep oxygenation of the organs *and* our capacity to contain and integrate that charge, to translate it into feelings about another person and acts of emotional exchange. The *aikido* master identifies the same "love" with the harmony of spirals between *uke* and *nage*. When one puts his or her heart into an act, the projection is far more complex than either the semantic metaphor or the life-giving actions of the circulatory system.

Certainly a major failing of Western culture, and industrial civilization in general, is that it cuts off everyone—capitalists as well as workers—from the mind of the heart, i.e., cuts them off not only from healing but the acts of compassion that arise from healing.

Breath

CONSCIOUS BREATH—nothing more than the act of internal breathing—is a crucial modality in holistic medicine. It is an active element in meditation, *Chi Gung*, rebirthing, Continuum, and various other therapies, including the famous nineteenth-century German breathing schools of which the last remaining *in situ* is Ilse Middendorf's "perceptible breath" (still taught by the founder herself in Berlin at the turn of the twenty-first century). Breath (integrated with movement and internalization) supports yoga and the Taoist martial arts. In all somatic therapies, including Reichian work, Feldenkrais, Rolfing,

Polarity, chiropractic, craniosacral touch, and visceral manipulation, breath is an integral and indispensable axis.

The differences between somatic systems and so-called direct "breath" forms like rebirthing are merely those of emphasis. The universal goal is to achieve deeper, more aware breathing, usually breathing that can be distributed from the lungs and belly to the organs and limbs, to the cells. A more subtle tenet is that the breathing of the practitioner is no less critical than that of the patient; in fact, the practitioner's fullness (or shallowness) of breath is communicated to the patient, thus can unconsciously cue his or her breathing (or rigidity). This is as true for an M.D. as a bodyworker.

Where a specific breathing technique is not taught, guided breath is often encouraged—sometimes by explicit exhortation, sometimes through exercises, sometimes by the energetic exchange of the treatment itself. The gasp of bones being adjusted, the root-seeking charge of acupuncture needles, and the tissue-molding of Rolfing automatically summon deeper, fuller, and subtler tissue and cellular breathing which then energizes the whole mind/body.

Polarity, rebirthing, and many massage-breath forms have a moment in them where one feels that one simply cannot go on breathing fully. This is exactly the point at which one *must* go on, for it is anxiety, not physical limitation, that holds one back, though there is also a weariness and a sense of not being able to push any further or maintain concentration. Once one travels past this point, breathing begins to free itself. The body is transformed by its unity of muscles, emotions, organs, and fluids (for which breath becomes the catalyst and agent). Instead of continuing to resist, the flesh softens and trembles to a visceral level; concentration becomes suspended; attention hangs in an alert but relaxed state; cells change.

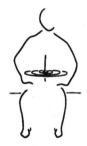

Horizontal breathing—forming a center

Let the middle area gyrate

Lower area with rising breath

IN ILSE MIDDENDORF'S CLASSES, students learn the minute differences between cadences and levels of breath, how to perceive these ever more subtly, and to deepen them by following their paths and expanding their range. One places his hands successively on different parts of his own body and takes time to allow each natural breath and its sensation to arise and take shape there. This may be as subtle as touching the outside of the nose and feeling the nostrils saturate with air or chanting a vowel and sensing the shape it transmits through viscera. The breath, once aroused, grows in unexpected ways, becomes embodied at deepening levels. It trickles, glides, chants, dilates, rebounds, pirouettes, excites, and expands. As the breath—or the projection of the breath's metaphors through mind—contacts the periphery of the body, it vitalizes digestion, circulation, immunity, and makes the spinal column more flexible. Repetition of variations of these exercises increases the range of perceptible breath and vitality of the organs.

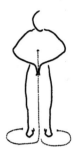

Straightening up with rising breath

Middendorf's assumption is that if "natural" breath comes into resonance throughout the whole body and subsumes more isolated, artificial breaths, well-being will naturally follow. The center gathers strength and disperses it to the periphery. She writes:

> The breathing coming out of your own conscious and unconscious meanings, freed from the control of your ego, shows itself to you through the movement you allow yourself, resulting in a pleasant feeling of release, and directs itself to your creative forces which, once released, express themselves full of joy....
>
> The perceptible breath always needs patience, especially as every new start of the movement growing out of breathing extracts material from one's depths, new, and unknown....[6]

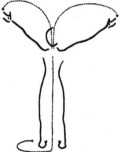

Inhalation in the upper area

Bodywork Psychotherapy

SPEECH OCCURS ON two levels—one as words, shaped by the mind into meaning; the other as sound, shaped by the breath and muscles into expression. Chanting and conscious breathing are clearly somatic, but so are gossip and chatter. How a person talks is part of how she also moves and breathes, how her body talks to her and how she talks to her body.

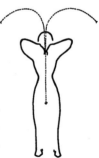

Bending down again as you exhale

Interpretation of the psychosomatic basis of language has given rise to many of the so-called "direct" and "gestalt" psychotherapies that use a combination of speech, action, gesture, tonation, etc., as collective inroads to character. These are transmitted as movement and voice exercises. Not all of them are strenuous. Some are as simple as tightening and loosening the throat or trying to experience sensation in a certain organ. In Gestalt therapy, for instance, narrative is used not for a recovery of primal events in language nor purely energetically in the Reichian mode, but as the medium for a psychodramatic reenactment of a historical conflict. The therapist does not deny a legacy of traumatizing incidents, but she wants to encounter their contemporary form, and this cannot be a gamble of truth-telling or a day's mood. She must elicit a somatic interaction in the context of transference. In bioenergetic therapy this interaction is even more physical and includes exercises, registers of voice, and even direct confrontations between therapist and patient.

The laws of holism demand that everything be present at every moment in some form. So even the most verbal holistic therapies emphasize physiology and character. In fact, modalities that are at once herbal, somatic, and energetic (like Polarity, Ayurveda, or Body Electronics) are vintage "alternative medicine," for holism is precisely the *nondistinctions* among treating with an herbal remedy, with palpation, and with words or prayers.

F ULL HEALTH IS dependent upon breath circulating, skeletal harmony, cerebrospinal range, and metabolic rhythm. Violations in the coherence of an organism include shallow breath, nervous speech rhythm, uncoordinated posture, limited range of flexion and extension, reduced motility of organs, and tight control of diction; these are symptoms not just of emotional disturbances (as is most commonly assumed) but also of skeletal, muscular, and visceral diseases. They can be viewed as psychosomatic waves locked in errant patterns. After all, the heart and the liver have no other way to express themselves. As

Stanley Keleman tells us in the title of one of his books, the "body [also] speaks *its* mind." The muttering of the mind manifests as small talk or philosophy, but the expression of the body is not athletics or hunting or sex. It is the body's version of conversation and philosophy—just as intricate, subtle, and metaphorical. The kidneys and lungs have their own distinct personalities, but we rarely acknowledge them.

Practitioners working with postural and functional integration have come to understand that rigid body stances (including systemic pathologies) reflect customs of etiquette and professional or militaristic discipline more than underlying somatic requirements. Emotional traumas and lesions get built into static poses. Thus people *become* their personal histories, their niches in society, their jobs, rather than *their* humanity or flowingness. Uncompromising patterns lead to psychostructural diseases. Eutony, Alexander Technique, Feldenkrais Method, and Rolfing are all modes of realignment and body balancing that are intended to affect simultaneously the personality and dynamic physiological state of the organism. They address (almost exclusively among medicines) the dysfunctional habits of poor "self-cure."

Without skeletal, massage, and visceral traditions, there would be no holistic medicine as we understand it, for there would be no emotional, energetic link between pure physical exercise on the one hand and vitalistic pharmacies and shamanic rituals on the other. Potentized minerals, organic vegetables, and vision quests in and of themselves do not restore deep physical health for many people. Most Westerners cannot jump into symbolic transformation or *Chi Gung* without guidance in gradual stages. The body has learned its habits too well to "think" its way out of them. Bodywork provides support for unaccustomed uses of breath, sensation, and neuromusculature. The viscera need "osteopathic instruction," Rolfing, or even, in some instances, allopathic drugs or surgery before they are strong enough to sustain a different lifestyle. One of the weaknesses of many of the "New Age" adaptations of traditional herbal and homeopathic medicines is that they overlook the multi-layered energetic basis of anatomy and character in their enthusiasm for the vital components of their pills, aroma essences, and runes. Bodywork fills that gap.

I N HOLISTIC MEDICINE, definitions of health are based upon the organs' relationships to one another. If personal behavior or organic function are aberrant, then the organs are usually also out of position. It does not matter which came first, which initiated the drift; it is "neither and both" and functionally the same. The chiropractor believes that by adjusting bones he reorients muscles; by reorienting muscles, he changes tissue qualities. The changing tissue qualities cause the body to reorganize itself and, as the body reorganizes, the intellect begins to recognize its neuroses, transcend them, and deepen the expression of its life.

For most people, as *t'ai chi* master Benjamin Lo notes, simply to stand symmetrically at their natural height is a major undertaking. The strain from this task is not because it is punishing—or even necessarily because of physical frailty; it is because the person is organized away from normal functions, usually out of fear and protection. He is avoiding the feelings that go with past failure and discomfort or that represent these in the economy of the psyche.

As sensations rush up during a bioenergetic session or exercise, a deep rhythm from the system tries to impose itself and, since the rhythm is more fluent, more coherent than the personality, it runs into blocks posing as attitudes (character). The person will tighten and resist, and this will be felt both as pain and the wish not to continue the exercise. Although the discomfort is immediate, it is also vestigial. It hurts now because something else hurt back then, and the body numbed itself away from that in protection or hardened against it in defense. The present resistance is what hurts, not the actual mechanics of the task.

Moshe Feldenkrais' exercises are used to engender the practice of gradual sensual pathways toward restoring function. The person replaces awkward or painful mechanics with new movements that support daily activity. The movements are not gymnastic feats. They are learned in tiny increments, restoring sensation, for instance, in slight orbits of the pelvis or ankles.

Since defended feelings are perceived as pain, there may be apprehension that to persist in such exercises will cause injury or disease. The irony is that a disease feared, such as a back going out or heart failure, is more likely to be caused by the *absence* of the exercise than by following it through—by decades of stiffness, shallow breathing, and withholding. Fear of disease, in this case, is fear of self; and from fear of self, malignancy arises. Reich left little doubt that he considered cancer and heart disease literally diseases of the personality, the breath, and suppressed sensations. If such is the case, somatic character exercises keep the body from cellularizing emotions as pathologies.

A student's complaint that Lo's *chi* exercises were only very difficult calisthenics was more a confirmation than a dismissal. In a sense, prior to *chi*, they *are* merely calisthenics, but not calisthenics in which one pushes oneself past the point of feeling or numbs oneself to sensation in order to achieve some victory. They are calisthenics in which one tries to regain a natural, pre-armored structure and mobility, a sense of ease with simply standing in gravity in the world, metabolizing oxygen. This process itself causes feelings to bubble up and spread patterns that were suppressed or ignored. An athlete may sometimes be able to use such surges of memory and visceral texture to spur performance; other times he must override them as distractions.

In somatic disciplines (unlike sports), one *must* accept and integrate the feelings aroused by the use of the body exactly as they come up and in the way in which they come up—first in the exercise, subsequently in life itself. There are no extraneous meanings, no goals, no finish-lines; the meaning is simply: this is what's happening; this is who I am.

We see this graphically in a practice from Keleman:

> ... [K]icking can ... help us understand, experientially, the notion of self-forming. Kicking encourages the use of the voice as well as moving the whole body into action, either as protest or an expression of joy. Kids kick with glee. Tickle a child, and watch its legs

Background to Somatics

start bouncing around. When a child is angry, he screams and his legs want to move. Then finally, it ends with jumping for joy, or stomping in a tantrum and walking away.

Lie down on your back with your shoes off. Make sure you can move and breathe easily. Now begin to kick the bed. Start with raising your legs to right angles to your body so that they go straight up in the air toward the ceiling. Then bring them straight down, hitting the bed with your heels. Keep kicking, always lifting your legs at right angles to your body. Begin to feel what the emotional experience is as well as the action.[7]

Deep into a bioenergetic episode a patient may become the animal she is, wailing in creature sounds, doing creature movements. The inner being is brought into alignment with the surface personality and shares a moment of coherence with it. This coherence is so sweet and medicinal that its superficially unattractive traits are a price worth paying.

In experiencing these things, the personality understands that there is another life it has not been living. It comes to a point, past exhaustion and past the driven expression of emotion, where the self begins to express its own being. This pours through the flesh as an elixir, a homecoming, a recognition. Suddenly anger or passion no longer needs a situation; it is one of the core things in the body. The voice now speaks for the organs too.

A physiological change takes place—muscles are stretched, the skin changes color and temperature, liquids and breath move through cells. Molecular changes may also take place; after all, oxygen is molecular in its activity.

Fake psychodrama perhaps, but then no one protests that a pill or an operation isn't real because one is prescribed in language, the other performed in a clinical setting. As mind and body flow together and achieve their nondifference, tension momentarily lightens. The sky outside the window becomes as luminescently blue as Reich, in his vision of orgone bliss, would have had us believe it is. The blossoms on the trees hang as globes of fuzzy light, expanding eternally without weight and made of tenderness more than of matter. Memories that seemed to have been lost forever flood back in layers. Life becomes so large and expanded in their return that it is itself sufficient and ample; there is enough to drink forever, but there is not so much that one would drown. One's size changes, the sense of being cramped in a body softens. The torso expands to hold a figure which is at once more muscular and firm and more angelic and graceful. For the duration of the feeling, lost functions flicker back and are sometimes even recovered.

A single such experience may not dissolve chronic internal illness. It is the accretion of such moments and their chains of perceptions that ultimately penetrate pathology or immobility at the core.

Fields of Somatics

B ECAUSE OF THE profusion of somatic systems, it is impossible to deal adequately with many of them in this book. In order to map the variety and complexity, I will approach the various disciplines in terms of their shared lineages and themes, comparable techniques, fusions, and divergences, and also in terms of an emerging somatic field.

Though major osteopathic, bioenergetic, constitutional, cognitive, and *chi*-based methods have for the most part developed independently of one another, the combining of elements has become so prevalent that many lineages now overlap and give rise to hybrids. In fact, it is reaching the point that almost every practitioner has his or her own unique modality. As the specific manual and palpation techniques that define any one tradition become components of universal somatic modes, they also move beyond the contexts of their own systems.

Individual somatic modalities may be viewed as either tools of different sizes, shapes, and fulcral points or different protocols and ontologies to deal with the ragged and often disjunctive interzone between semantics and tissue (language and embodiment). Usually practitioners of separate modalities acknowledge the virtues of others and redirect clients whose conditions or temperaments predispose them elsewhere, even to treatment by herbs, diet, homeopathy, psychoanalysis, etc. However, to the more ideological adherents of any one system, theirs is the premier and purest therapy. Reich, Alexander, Rolf, Feldenkrais, Movlai, Upledger, etc., are revered as saints and gurus by their followers. Worshippers and xenophobes will always deny that the work of their system is improved by the techniques of another or that some people are better served by a rival practice. They proselytize and strive to keep their own rosters growing rather than participate in developing a pan-somatic modality. But these purists are important to us too, for the logic and rigor of an old system may be lost in the modernistic *carte blanche* and ease of switching among frames of reference. They themselves would argue that the techniques only work in the context of their development and systemization, whereas others override such purism on the basis that manual mechanics are nonsectarian and can be learned and applied in a limitless range of contexts.

When a Rolfer stops his deep tissue integration to respond to the craniosacral pulse, does that enhance or detract from the cohesiveness of the structural integration, and is his craniosacral work as productive as it would be in the context of its own system? It is quite possible that neither sustained pressure nor stillpoints are as effective in hybrid treatments as either would be alone, but that the combination of them still contributes new elements to individual treatments by initiating responsiveness at more than one level. Amalgamating systems provides somatic information and tissue vectors not available in any one lineage. The different modalities then resonate with each other in practice. The success of a treatment depends finally upon the skill and sensitivity of the practitioner rather than any explicit checklist of techniques. New modalities spring up empirically, as traditional methods emanate new applications and meanings.

Since everything cannot be done, the selection of what *is* done during the limited time of the treatment is paramount. Any technique is

at the expense, potentially, of another. A skilled practitioner, well trained in more than one method, can cross boundaries therapeutically as long as she is aware of her patient's changing capacity to respond to what she is doing and as long as she brings the application of each technique to its natural terminus. Problems may never be solved when the context is always changing. When a condition is constantly being redefined and recontacted, there is no therapeutic outcome. The danger of switching from one set of techniques to another is that the organism being worked on will be confused (or overloaded) and respond to neither. For a new combination to be completely counterproductive, however, it would have to induce confusion and loss of cohesion in the organism receiving it.

Each set of techniques is uniquely valuable in its own right, and the integrity of its developmental stages is critical for the effective meanings of a system. Each modality was organized in terms of serial signals and feedback loops that might be distorted by improvised segues or discrepant messages. Conversely, practitioners develop their own skill (sense of touch) by feeling their way out from systemic considerations. Some therapists are totally eclectic and improvisational as to what modality they choose at any one session, moving seamlessly from one core technique to another.

New inquiries into tissue structure, character, resistance, somatic layering, energetic reciprocity, and transmission of palpative pressure lead therapists through many of the same realms of discovery that the innovators of somatic systems travelled. There is no limit to the varieties and levels of therapeutic touch and no requirement of purism except for a given practitioner to keep his treatments cohesive and integrative, as the addition of new procedures inevitably means the deemphasizing of former ones and a change in the meaning and effect of the trajectory being applied. Ultimately, unified somatics is a method of entering into a dialogue with cells, tissues, skeletal and visceral structure, psyche, and life energy and resonating with their immediate motifs.

IF THIS ARGUMENT SEEMS TO BE going in circles, it is because there are nothing but circles here. They are circles which exist everywhere in the somatic field. They support traditional trainings and disciplines, and they work toward producing idiosyncratic and hybrid systems. If any electic mode becomes unique and distinctive enough and with a complicated enough training (like Zero Balancing, Trager Approach, or Integrated Manual Therapy), then new subfields and courses within somatics are born. When previously sectarian techniques are redistributed among fields, then they change their meanings and uses. If, over time, a technique becomes more universal than sectarian, its separate discipline may disappear.

In areas where techniques are similar, compatible, parallel, or even, in some cases, provide different paths to the same structure (including formerly related techniques that have diverged from one another), synthesis is presently occurring despite purism and professional sanction, and practitioners are learning one another's methods. Some of the newer somatic forms (such as Zero Balancing and Body-Mind Centering) and many traditional disciplines (chiropractic, bioenergetics, Ayurvedic massage, and cranial osteopathy) are practiced now both as narrow formal systems and general somatics.

Applied Kinesiology has been adapted to the meridians of traditional Chinese medicine. Chiropractic has been redefined in a more proprioceptive mode by Feldenkrais "Awareness Through Movement" practitioners and craniosacrally oriented therapists. Craniosacral Therapy, visceral manipulation, lymphatic drainage, and myofascial release have been blended together in diverse practices, sometimes with acupuncture and shamanic work as well.

A chiropractor, if so educated, can select moments at which to apply visceral work instead of adjustments in order to realign specific organs, or she may even choose to lead her patient in a series of Feldenkrais or Alexander exercises, or recommend yoga.

Randy Cherner recalls that in the early days of his practice he relied heavily on a straightforward use of "chiropractic-like" adjustments.

Patients would come in; he'd look them over, spot their distortions, and correct them with swift, direct motions. The patients would feel relief, thank him (often profusely), and he thought, "This sure is easy work."[8]

His first warning that it wasn't going to be so easy came when patients began showing up at their next appointments not only with their prior ailments recurrent but often more severe versions. Gradually he came to realize that it wasn't enough just to adjust their shapes; one had to engender a fresh attitude beneath the shape, to address the forms of being in the personality/organism from which the shapes were originating, and to give the person a means of experiencing his or her own process on an ongoing basis.

As his practice developed, Cherner began searching less for effective modes of immediate correction and more for an elegance of function. He prioritized overall coordination and a freedom to move (especially in the presence of formidable mental impediments—what he called "scoliosis of the brain"). In classic osteopathic fashion, he began emphasizing indirect work, always *away* from the area of the problem. Instead of grappling with the jaw of the lion, he would pick an arm or a leg, find the line of tension in it to the core, and begin working it inward, reaching its "jaw" only at the end of the session or in a subsequent session. The goal was to demonstrate somatically to the patient how she was the source of her own trap and thus its most likely remediator. This was best accomplished by giving her the broadest field of proprioceptive experience. The transmission was mostly palpation, with a few carefully chosen words in a Feldenkrais educational context.

Ida Rolf set as one of her prerequisites for improving structural alignment an ability to work with reciprocal relationships of organs and neuromusculature. If there is a "problem" someplace, that is never the source but the place where the organism is holding out in order to protect a deeper dysfunction or sense of incapacity and emptiness, which invariably manifests many other places as well and is rooted in some core structural dilemma. Attacking a problem directly does not solve the problem; it merely gives the organism a new dilemma—to find another place to hold out. Working on reciprocal sites (for instance, the hamstrings instead of the muscles of the neck to deal with restriction at the neck) allows the organism to experience its own biodynamics and adjust accordingly across a great breadth. It restores its capacity to fill in its own space.

Body-Mind Centering teaches its own independent method of following energy and strain patterns, resembling, to some degree, traditional cranial osteopathic techniques but having a separate origin. Thus, a "bilingual" practitioner can alter the intention of her touch to convey subtle differences between the two modes, following and holding a bit more in the craniosacral pattern and leading and developing spirals in the Body-Mind Centering mode. If also trained in *Chi Gung*, she may interpose Taoist methods of transmitting vital energy. If a Reiki master, she can work off the body for a part of the treatment, channeling direct energy. Ideally, the different vibrations harmonize and enhance one another.

Rolfer Michael Salveson reads the craniosacral pulse (in a mode taught him by John Upledger) while doing his structural integration; he also applies *Chi Gung Tui Na* energetic techniques (acquired from Kumar Frantzis) to areas that have deep-seated blocks. His practice of Rolfing is now one dialect of Ida Rolf's original system. At Esalen, Rolfing was differently combined with Gestalt psychology and a Reichian etiology to form a broader-spectrum Human Potential therapy.

Joseph Heller, an aerospace engineer at the Jet Propulsion Laboratories in Pasadena, became interested in human development, bioenergetics, and Gestalt psychology and, like A. T. Still and Moshe Feldenkrais before him, applied insights from physics to physiology, particularly in interpreting tissue mechanisms and stress. After studying with Ida Rolf for six years, he became the first president of the Rolf Institute. However, he was not satisfied with her "ten session" program of structural reintegration. Because he did not believe that altering fascia could ingrain long-term psychological changes, he enlarged the Rolfing model to include elements of Reichian and bioenergetic bodywork, Feldenkrais Method, and Aston-Patterning. Under the name Hellerwork, he developed a system that combined deep tissue integration with movement awareness and cultivation of emotions. In bioenergetic fashion, while carrying out the basic Rolfing protocol, he elicited a fuller verbal exploration of the feelings that inevitably arose from fascial engagement, seeking their historical and developmental sources while leading the client to new somatic outlets for them. At the same time, he retrained key sensory-motor activities. In his own words:

> As Hellerwork highlights psychological issues and patterns embodied by physical structure, it also explores energy, starting with gravity and including the sense of connection people can discover between themselves and the universe beyond them. . . .
>
> Release of the rigidified musculature is, itself, a teaching aid through which the practitioner enables the client to see what her body has done in the past, what effect its doing so has had in the present, and what choice she has about realigning her relationship with her own mechanical, psychological, and energetic components, as well as with those of other people.[9]

Lomi Work is a somatic therapy grounded in the Esalen hybrid of Rolfing, bioenergetics, and Gestalt, with an emphasis on breath. Polarity Therapy was subsequently integrated within Lomi as a derivation of a set of exercises taught to founders Richard Heckler and Robert Hall by Randolph Stone, who provided some of his techniques by invitation in a series of seminars in Northern California during the mid 1970s. Later, elements of Feldenkrais Method, *aikido,* craniosacral therapy, and Vipassana Meditation were added to the Lomi repertoire by individual practitioners.

Today, Lomi exists less as a separate modality than as a general somatic training curriculum. Heckler has gone on to develop a leadership program founded on Lomi principles and offered to corporate executives and military personnel. (See Resource Guide.)

Meanwhile, Polarity Therapy is practiced in an opposite mode at

Northern California's Heartwood Institute, where it is combined with alchemical hypnotherapy, Taoist dietary practices, and psychotherapeutic massage. Additionally, Heartwood founder Bruce Burger has developed a specific shamanic version of Polarity, merging aspects of Stone's methods with spiritual modalities from his own Hindu and Plains Indian teachers.

P**RIOR TO ANY UNIFIED** somatic field theory, the different systems balance one another in terms of directness versus indirectness, passivity versus activity, subtlety of vector, and depth of palpation. For someone with heavily bound musculature, the impressing of new tissue memory by a Rolfer into muscles, ligaments, and epithelia provides a necessary first step for reorganizing structure to reduce strain, but then, without Feldenkrais or Alexander work to reeducate the "uses of self," the person may unconsciously resculpt many of the strain patterns. On the other hand, someone else's neuromusculature may be trenchantly resistant to Rolfing, their system hypersensitive to the degree that deep-tissue work overwhelms its delicate homeostasis, so Feldenkrais exercises may suitably come first, with Rolfing never used or broached only later after the tissue texture and sense of "body" has deepened. Or chiropractic may be utilized in place of Rolfing—bones and joints emphasized instead of muscles and fascia (of course, Rolfing also works on bones and chiropractic on muscles). Some people respond better to less mechanical and less behaviorally directive techniques and are far more able to assimilate and enact change subliminally suggested by craniosacral or Breema touch.

Functional transitions between somatic systems operating at different musculoskeletal and neurovisceral levels may also be incremental. A person with a stress pattern encompassing diverse physiological symptoms is first treated craniosacrally through his mandible and the temporal bones of his skull. This relieves an outer layer of constriction and dysfunction. A year later the person does a series of lessons with a Feldenkrais practitioner. She leads him through a sequence of head, eye, and pelvic movements while his thoracic torso torques at different angles respectively in relation to his sacral torso and legs. This layer-by-layer investigation of habitual movement locates another zone of obstruction so that it can be gradually "taken off" in daily life. Success makes the person receptive to educational somatics. An Alexander practitioner teaches him how to inhibit a habitual series of gestures that always arises concurrent with certain daily activities (talking on the phone, answering email, sitting at staff meetings) that seemed to exacerbate the remaining layers of the syndrome. Practicing that conscious change of orientation during his work life, he experiences the dissolution of another layer of difficulty along with some of its painful symptoms. The syndrome is now situated more on an emotional plane with fewer physical outcroppings. During a session a month later a Lomi practitioner asks him if he can locate and amplify the neuromuscular pattern at the base of his effective inhibition. Since the signal to inhibit was initiated at such a subtle level, the client cannot initially discriminate it and does so only after a number of exercises conducted in front of a mirror. However, once he "finds" his point of activation in tiny, almost imperceptible facial movements he is able to make these more palpable and express the rivulets trailing from their impulses. He taps into a network of emotional blocks and unexpressed feelings going back to early childhood. These become his next layer of work. After that he is able to approach the purely ocular aspects of the condition by the Bates Method.

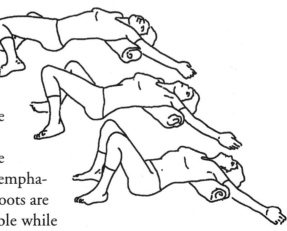

I have oversimplified and optimized the sequence described here; what I mean to emphasize is that symptoms themselves at their roots are biological, psychospiritual, and incalculable while somatic systems are always syntactic and paradigmatic. The match of any system to any real condition is temporal and approximate. The above sequence might have equally gone from Body-Mind Centering to Eutony to Continuum to Hellerwork. There are limitless modes and progressions of access to core. While one system may accomplish a quicker, deeper, or more lasting cure, that does not disqualify any other system from working at its own level toward a sound resolution. If it is the "wrong" system (i.e., if there is a more essential, less peripheral approach), the "wrong" system may prepare the client for the transition to a more appropriate modality. It may also accomplish similar goals but over a longer period of time. Or the person may never get to the core in this way. She still lives a rich and satisfying life with many episodes of autonomous self-care.

None of us is ever "fully treated." We travel from missed opportunity to fortuity to ever new possibility. Between formal treatments (if they even occur) our inner physician treats us and we are "adjusted" by the culture and environment. There is no programmatic outcome to any of these sequences. In somatics more than in general medicine, existential and mechanical issues overlap and entangle each other. Remember, somatics goes back to folk art, self-inquiry, Stone-Age medicine, and the natural movements of animals. Life itself is bodywork and spiritual practice. It impresses its own malignant and curative seams in tissue.

The truth of somatics, at the most subtle and sophisticated level, is that the intrinsic strength of a deep-seated function, especially once it is somaticized, overwhelms the relatively linear and simple effect of an adjustment. Bodywork itself—and medicine in general as a technological refinement of bodywork—cannot establish lasting change unless it activates the one thing more powerful than the mechanics of a dysfunction, and that is the prior cohesiveness and elegance of natural function. This is true even in the case of people born with disabilities. Life itself is an elegant solution to entropy. The bodyworker

who palpates and adjusts merely mechanically is like someone trying to affect the ripple pattern in a lake by stirring the surface of ripples. Whereas a lake is too vast to be altered, at least by noncataclysmic means, an organism has a mind, a consciousness, which directs levels of intention and reorganizes posture and alignment down to the subtlest fascial—and perhaps even cellular—integer. Thus, the right combination of touch, energy, and sometimes language can create a whole new moiré out of the source. It must be wooed, not wrenched, though that does not exclude some very powerful direct techniques.

Somatic Philosophy

IN MAPPING THE evolution of somatic systems during the last century, we might consider as baseline disciplines: visceral and myofascial palpation, musculoskeletal adjustment, various movement systems, traditional massage, *Chi Gung*, Ayurvedic exercises, yoga, and the physical components of a variety of shamanic and spiritual practices. In addition, psychotherapy and characterological bodywork contribute their own dimension to the practice of all somatics by reifying relationships between experiences and tissue structure.

To the pure somaticists we may also add innovative martial artists like Bruce Lee, Derek Jones, and Peter Ralston and a whole range of improvisational choreographers (Yvonne Rainer, Nancy Stark Smith, Anna Halpern) and multimedia artists all involved with redefining the uses of the body and the relation of mind and intention to action.

Most contemporary somatic systems may be characterized as syntheses, built up from the raw material of baseline practices in some combination or other. For instance, Rolfing has roots in osteopathic adjustment, Gurdjieffian work, and yoga. Feldenkrais drew material from yoga, Alexander Technique, movement rituals, and judo as well as Western science. Polarity syncretizes Ayurveda, cranial osteopathy, and shamanism.

The sets of relationships among the elements of multidimensional, hybrid systems can be extremely complex, operating both consciously and unconsciously. A new Rolfer may pick up variants of traditional aspects of cranial adjustment and bone-setting indirectly through their historical role in Rolfing, or learn them in their more pure and palpative form from an osteopath and then reapply them to Rolfing at a different level of treatment. Thus, it is not unusual for aspects of osteopathy, traditional massage, or bioenergetics to manifest at more than one level of Rolfing (or of Feldenkrais work, Alexander Technique, etc.).

Innovations within somatic areas have now become more common than orthodoxies. Look at the business card or shingle or website of most practitioners, and you will more often see a list of techniques than a single specialty. In fact, I would propose that just about every system currently coming into existence under a new name (or subsequent to the publication of this book) will be a third- or fourth-generation somatic synthesis rather than an entirely novel method. It will also be a new method insofar as its elements will be fused in a novel way.

In one syncretic system Judith Aston, a student of Ida Rolf, has put together elements of Alexander Technique, Feldenkrais Method, and osteopathy in an idiosyncratic amalgam. Aston employs three very different kinds of hands-on manipulation, one similar to Feldenkrais' mode of light touch, a second using manipulation to make the joints more mobile, and the third a subtle palpation of the connective tissues of the body. Together these represent her own spectrum of intuitive touch.

Aston diverged from Rolf particularly on the issue of a symmetrical bodily line:

> Unlike more traditional body mechanics of symmetry and alignment of the body perpendicular to the ground, I found that all movement is naturally asymmetrical and that everybody develops slight asymmetries through the intrinsic structure of having one heart, one liver, etc., as well as through adaptation to all the kinds of injuries, sports, and daily habit patterns....
>
> Around 1975–77, I made two discoveries that were critical to the development of Aston-Patterning: (1) That movement came from

asymmetry and (2) That I was seeing a very different model for body mechanics than the one based on accepted medical and human factors that designers model.[10]

Aston then took her innovation into the artifacts of our culture's technology. The health implications of a mechanical world-view, after all, are not limited to the explicit practice of technologized medicine; they extend to patterns imposed by all structures arising from a mechanistic world-view and a rigid, arbitrary artificial environment. Most products we use are not human or even organic, and they contribute in their own ways to somatic dysfunction.

While Matthias Alexander began by having his clients practice sitting in a chair and then standing, Judith Aston decided to redesign chairs themselves. She closely examined and then reformulated a variety of furniture, clothing, vehicle interiors, and tools:

> My paradigm participates in [the] general realization that linear causality doesn't properly explain the way things work.... Since 1975 I have been working with a very specific aspect of a paradigm shift. This unique aspect has to do with the understanding of assumptions about the body's best posture and mechanics for motion and the body in relationship to any object that it touches such as utensils, a chair, a keyboard, golf club, steering wheel, and so on.[11]

After all, a golfer or basketball player, as well as a truck driver or plumber, is regularly adjusting his or her body kinesthetically to the rituals and artifacts of a trade. These unintentional manipulations have far-reaching consequences:

> The idea of ergonomics was the final piece in this body-sense puzzle. For once you have changed, you may need assistance to use these changes in your normal everyday environment. I found that no matter how long I worked with people and no matter how great the changes seemed, if they climbed right back into the same car seat or old shoes, for example, old patterns would be immediately reinforced. I started using duct tape, foam and towels to modify people's

car seats, office furniture, kayaks, etc. I then saw the immense possibility for change beyond the few things I had been working on.
Most products people habitually use were in need of redesign. I realized that people needed ergonomic education for their cars, homes,
and office places to assist their bodies so that they can be in more
natural, comfortable and effortless alignment....

About five years ago I went to a patent attorney to see if I could
patent my biomechanical mathematics theory. He looked into it and
called me back with the good news/bad news message. "The good
news," he said, "is that you may have discovered a new law of nature.
The bad news is that, like the Theory of Relativity, a law of nature
cannot be patented. You will have to patent each of your 300 designs."[12]

WHILE WORKING OUT on the beach in the 1920s, Milton Trager,
a teenager from a Chicago slum, independently glimpsed some
of the same elements of habitual movement and techniques of retraining as his somatic forebears had. The young Trager was not only a
dancer and acrobat at the time but also a body-builder and boxer. In
fact, he made his most radical discovery when, reversing roles after a
round in the ring, he decided to massage his manager and sparring
partner instead of being massaged.

Trager discovered that true body-building lay in softening and loosening hard, rigid muscles, rather than in making them tougher and
tighter. He went on to cure his father's sciatica, and then he began to
help polio victims learn to walk again.[13] Later, he enlarged and refined
his techniques into a full somatic system, became a doctor, and combined the practice of medicine with bodywork while working in Hawaii
and, later, Northern California.

He originated a system of Psychophysical Integration, including a
mode of gentle, penetrating manipulation (with a distinctive shaking
of limbs) that has become known as the Trager Approach. "Trager had
discovered that he could release tension from the joints by shaking,
rocking, or gently moving each part of the body in a rhythmic way that
sent ripples through the flesh like a soft sonar wave. Wherever the undu-

lating rhythm stopped or changed, Trager identified some rigidity blocking the natural path of this movement, as if a solid island had stopped a wave in water. He could then shake or manipulate the tension free from the point of the block."[14]

RANDY CHERNER'S WORK combines Swedish movements (his original training) and Lomi therapy with Feldenkrais Method, *aikido,* and craniosacral and visceral palpation to produce a unique modality that some have begun to refer to as Chernerwork. When I studied with Cherner (in a professional seminar between 1992 and 1994), I became disoriented initially by trying to establish for myself the difference between Feldenkrais Method, craniosacral palpation, and Lomi, all of which we learned as discrete systems with repertoires of moves. At one point, I asked for the appropriate circumstances in which to use each of the modalities. He responded by saying that there was no dividing line, only a spectrum in which one was always "following" and stacking tissue layers even when lifting a leg or flexing the whole body so that knees and elbows touched; one was always discriminating movements and habitual rigidities in Feldenkrais' manner; and one was also always encouraging (both physically and verbally) the person's deepening breath. The divisions into systems were solely for training purposes — for learning how to find and palpate somatic axes, lines of reciprocal force, and entrenched patterns of parasitic motion.

Amini Peller, a practitioner in San Carlos, California, trained first in Breema, Zero Balancing, and craniosacral/visceral palpation (with Manocher Movlai, Fritz Smith, John Upledger, and Jean-Pierre Barral, each a pioneer in his field), then learned and integrated Cherner's synthesis, and has since added Polarity, psychic healing, and shamanic vision quest (as taught by Brant Secunda of the Dance of the Deer Foundation in Soquel, California). Never without a hawk feather, mandala, or piece of energized quartz, she attends to the aura, karmic vibrations, and neuromuscular components alternately or simultaneously (sometimes one hand off the body, one hand on). There is no name for

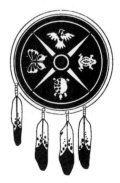

what she does, but everyone who has worked with her knows exactly what it feels like and how it is unique. Far from cluttering one another, the multiple methods are transformed through her personality and therapeutic style into a single healing modality that allows her to bring her full presence to the moment and work at many levels.

The most important feature of *any* somatic modality is to follow an experience where it leads rather than to use each client anew to enact rigid allegiances or always to find the same problems and apply the "house" methods to them. Like meditation and martial arts, somatic work must be continuously reexperienced in terms of what is immediate and functional and reinvented every day spontaneously.

Each new genre emerges naturally from prior ones, much as systems of philosophy emerge from one another. Modalities of "somatic philosophy" differentiate in the way existentialism, phenomenology, Whitehead's "process and reality," neo-Marxism, the Frankfurt School, deconstructionism, etc., did, and continue to, not by proposing new logics or apperceptions but by deriving modes of inquiry directly out of the syntax of prior modes (as well as out of the epistemology of inquiry itself). By comparison to mind-based philosophy, though, somatic philosophy and movement aesthetics are in their infancy. If the Alexanders were its Aristotle and Plato, we can look forward to its Humes, Heideggers, and Derridas.

Moshe Feldenkrais, Ida Rolf, F. Matthias Alexander, John Upledger, Peter Ralston, Kumar Frantzis, Emilie Conrad, and Bonnie Bainbridge Cohen may be regarded as contemporary somatological philosophers inquiring into multiple ontologies of being, body, and meaning. Theirs is a whole new method of philosophy, certain to change our view of human nature and the origin and destiny of consciousness. Pure intellectual analysis of categories, which was transformed initially by the Freudian unconscious and a general biological reconsideration of the physical nature of thought and language, is now subject to recognitions of the consciousness of tissues and organs themselves, living subcreatures that precede both human and cultural identity.

There is one major difference between systems of somatics and the more traditional ones of philosophy. Philosophy is for the most part "noisy," i.e., generative of text; somatics by comparison is silent and text is hard to come by. This is not because philosophy is not also somatic in its origin and somatics is not language-based but because one profession is carried out in words, the other in palpation. Philosophy is concerned with the continuously changing face of existence, the nature of time and space in the context of language, and the articulate obliteration of language. Somatics (like martial arts) is concerned with precisely these same things but insofar as they are expressed mutely in the movement patterns and inner life textures of living organisms.

THE EXTRAORDINARY RANGE of somatic systems can leave one with the sense that almost anything is possible, that any combination of techniques has some critical functional effect. This is not an irrelevant perception. It is likely that untapped realms of somatic philosophy are beginning to open up a vastly wider vocabulary of attention, movement, and touch through which we are becoming capable of being our own shamans and doctors, of experiencing our own innards, and treating one another as peer healers. Nothing could be more timely in the present Western health crisis, characterized by a rapidly aging population and a ridiculously narrow protocol of approved methods for treating disease. In this sense, somatics is not just a branch of alternative medicine but a new paradigm for medicine itself.

The potential multitude of internal somatic experiencing systems suggests an evolving cosmology of health. Not knowing its central principle, we arrive at its almost endless manifestations in the world, each of them represented by a different formalization and core of procedures—in *karate* dojos and dance studios, occupational therapy seminars and zendos—as well as in holistic clinics. These techniques express the different layers of our somatic existence as well as the interpolations of these layers with one another.

Somatic systems literally replicate our own complexity. Thus, there will be no end to new modalities until, imaginarily, we have tapped our full human complexity.

The Body Politic

IN A LETTER to the somatics community dated April 12, 1993, Bonnie Bainbridge Cohen, founder of Body-Mind Centering, challenged the limited public and professional perception of a somatic branch of medicine. She pointed out that, although Bill Moyers, in his just-completed television series "Healing and the Mind," had presented the topic in a "heartful and sensitive" manner, he went all the way to China to demonstrate hands-on bodywork and movement.[15]

"Was/is Bill Moyers unaware," Cohen asked, "of the sophisticated approaches here in the West?"[16]

She then cited modalities listed in the National Institutes of Health Guide, that is, sanctioned categories in which to apply for grant money that Congress made available for alternative medical approaches.

These include: diet, nutrition, lifestyle changes (macrobiotics, megavitamins, diets); mind/body control (art therapy/relaxation, biofeedback, counselling, guided imagery, hypnotherapy, and sound/music therapy); traditional medicine and ethnomedicine (acupuncture, Ayurveda, herbal medicine, homeopathic medicine, Native American medicine, natural products, and traditional Oriental medicine); structural manipulations and energetic therapies (acupressure, chiropractic medicine, massage, reflexology, Rolfing, therapeutic touch, *Chi Gung*); pharmacology and biological treatments (anti-oxidants, cell treatment, chelation therapy, metabolic therapy, and oxidizing agents); and bio-electromagnetic applications (transcranial electrostimulation, neuro-magnetic stimulation, electroacupuncture).[17]

Individual somatic therapies may be included in as many as four of these categories (depending on one's definitions), but the field of somatics is not recognized as a profession. After reviewing this list Bainbridge Cohen asks:

Why in Mind/body control are dance and movement therapies not mentioned (e.g., Dance/movement Therapy, Movement Therapy, Continuum, Authentic Movement, Laban Movement Analysis, Kestenberg Movement Profile)?

Why in Structural manipulations and energetic therapies are the body therapies that include both hands-on manipulations and movement (e.g., Alexander, Feldenkrais, Body-Mind Centering, Aston-Patterning, Trager) not mentioned?[18]

The explanation would seem to be that somatic modalities are still confused with traditionally nonmedical folk and artistic activities and that their direct, systemic challenge to allopathy in its own medical domains is not yet recognized. At the same time, somatic modalities that can be viewed as limited specialties and distinct adjuncts to other forms of medicine are listed, in essence, as mere mechanical or energetic subsystems.

THE ULTIMATE GOAL of somatic psychotherapy,[19] or body-mind works, is to locate the unified whole of a psychosomatic complex—to break into linguistic and life codes and provide transference while, at the same time, releasing, reorienting, and reeducating physiological structures that have developed in concert with these codes. In a modest sense, this is a clinical possibility. In the long run the human race must forge new wholescale institutions to deal with hegemonies rigidified over generations by combinations of emotional compulsion, vacuity, zombiism, economic enslavement, chauvanistic conscription, enforced militarization, and physical armoring. The result of our collective delusions, traumas, pathologies, viruses, exploitations, and sublimations is armies, prisons, institutionalized torture, and religious and political dictatorships. The promise of new modes of body-mind therapy is to release society from the ancestral rites and demons it blindly follows.

Of course, the world arena is not a therapy practice zone; one cannot turn historic process into a clinic. One can, however, build resources for somatic and psychological transformation, and to create an aware-ness of and respect for the body as an aspect of the psyche, the body politic, and the ruling mind.

At very least, body-mind paradigms should enter the dialogue among governments, freedom movements, transnational companies, Amnesty International, *The New York Review of Books,* the World Court, the implementers of the Rio Accord, the World Health Organization, UNESCO, and remediators of child abuse and prostitution, genocide, etc., because without a realization that much damage is done unwill-ingly and in service of gods (and goddesses) long dead, we are bound to repeat the same deeds again and again and produce the same dys-functional societies.

Militant Islam imposed not the heart and ethics of the Koran on the Afghan people but the medieval shackles of macho tribal patri-archy, using military technology and gang precepts. The globalized economy imposes at least as heartless and alienating a set of shackles on the whole developing world. In fact, "developing" has come to mean solely money and goods, not community, education, health, freedom, or spirit.

Right now we tell ourselves that this dynamic is primarily politi-cal—and on one level it will always be—but that is also our addiction, and politics as politics is our favorite excuse. There can also be a post-somatic politics, after the recognition that the body politic *is* the body. There needs to be a post-somatic economy and a post-somatic judicial system too. With the liberation of our bodies from their reptilian her-itage of battlefields and "fight or flight," jailers might someday be released along with the imprisoned. Alienated financiers could be emancipated from the paralysis of their hoarding along with the peasants and factory workers they have robbed and disinherited. Bodies can be freed from their own conscription and ruthlessness only by bodily recognition and radical bodily acts. We must attempt to break the addictive link between the torturers and the tortured because, as things are now, the body and mind of the victim and victimizer jointly return to the site of damage and attempt solely, blindly, to reenact it—even if this process turns victim into victimizer in an endless numb cycle. When there is a gap, a potent onrush of undifferentiated and amorphous desire will forge its own way along the weakest link. A different ritual alone can transform this compulsive cycle into octaves of healing.

Notes

1. Gerda Alexander, *Eutony: The Holistic Discovery of the Total Person* (Great Neck, New York: Felix Morrow, 1985), p. 26.

2. Don Hanlon Johnson, quoted in Bainbridge Cohen letter (see note 15 below), p. 4.

3. Stanley Keleman, "Professional Colloquium, October 29, 1977" in Grossinger (ed.), *Ecology and Consciousness: Traditional Wisdom on the Environment* (Berkeley, California: North Atlantic Books, 1992), p. 25.

4. Don Hanlon Johnson, "The Way of the Flesh: A Brief History of the Somatics Movement," *Noetic Sciences Review*, No. 29 (Spring 1994), p. 27.

5. Ibid., p. 28.

6. Ilse Middendorf, *The Perceptible Breath: A Breathing Science* (Paderborn, Germany: Junferman-Verlag, 1990), pp. 189–90.

7. Stanley Keleman, *Somatic Reality* (Berkeley, California: Center Press, 1979), pp. 90–91.

8. Randy Cherner, remarks during a class, Corte Madera, California, 1990.

9. Joseph Heller and William A. Henkin, *Bodywise: Introduction to Hellerwork* (Oakland, California: Wingbow Press, 1986), pp. 84–85.

10. Judith Aston, "Three Perceptions and One Conception," draft of an essay for Don Hanlon Johnson (editor), *Bone, Breath, and Gesture: Practices of Embodiment* (Berkeley, California: North Atlantic Books, 1995).

11. Ibid.

12. Ibid.

13. Ibid., p. 71.

14. Ibid., p. 72.

15. Bonnie Bainbridge Cohen, letter mailed to members of the somatics community concerning results of a two-day conference entitled "Research in the Field of Somatics," California Institute of Integral Studies, San Francisco, November 1992.

16. Ibid., p. 1.

17. Ibid., pp. 1–2.

18. Ibid., p. 2.

19. This closing section on somatic psychotherapy was rewritten from my essay entitled "Why Somatic Therapies Deserve As Much Attention as Psychoanalysis in *The New York Review of Books,* and Why Bodyworkers Treating Neuroses Should Study Psychoanalysis," in an anthology entitled *The Body in Psychotherapy: Inquiries in Somatic Psychology,* edited by Don Hanlon Johnson and Ian J. Grand (Berkeley: North Atlantic Books, 1998, pp. 85–106). Both the essay and the book address the relationship between somatics and psychotherapy and provide further discussions of the issues in this excerpt.

CHAPTER FOUR

Ground Systems

Eutony

EUTONY WAS DEVELOPED by Gerda Alexander in the context of Eurhythmics and Music Education in Germany during the 1920s and thereafter became a popular and influential system of movement awareness. It is a branch of the original somatic florescence of Western humanities—a forerunner of avant-garde movement practices, human-potential therapy, and behavioral science. Starting with a goal of pure relaxation and the means to accomplish it, Alexander gradually went on to explore bodily sensation, personal expression, artistic improvisation, and the somatic basis of dance, music, and theater. Eutony (literally "good tonus") means learning how consciously to alter involuntary bodily patterns, "to be open and receptive to others without diminishing one's individuality."[1]

Using slow, complex movements, Alexander built a repertoire of reliable exercises to expand "presence" and release tension. These were based not on conscious breathing or formal imitation but recovering inherent biorhythms. They were lyrical, even operatic, in scope. In other sets of lessons, she had clients 1) model human bodies out of clay with their eyes closed, 2) sketch what they felt in their own bodies, and 3) draw human skeletons. Some initially projected harmonious unity; others portrayed cavities, asymmetries, atrophied areas, and gaps. Pupils molded and composed such body images both before and after their Eutony courses.

Over the years most patients came to Alexander for psychosomatic or neurotic ailments (in her words), but she also treated insomnia, circulatory troubles, disc degeneration, lumbago, tics, phantom pains, the after-effects of polio, asthma, and many other conditions. She believed that insofar as Eutony was an open-ended method of dynamic equilibrium finding mind and body in each other, its potential for liberating energy and healing was limitless.

Her somatic principles emphasized "optimal freedom of all joint movements, based on the normal length of muscles at rest . . . , the importance of conscious release of tension . . . , the capacity to use the right amount of energy based on the postural reflex, the bone structure, on tonus adaptation and on optimal circulation and autonomous involuntary breathing, giving maximum strength without strain . . . , and the importance of clear directions and elongations in space for the equalization of the tonus level."[2] The client practices letting go and finding in herself her own parameters of relaxation. If she is not initially successful, the Eutonist uses exercises and images to deepen her sense of her own body and presence. This awareness can carry to the client without direct touch.

Alexander recognized that most people engage the world from superficial to profound sensation, from epiderm to connective tissues and reflexes, so she focused first on the precise contact of the surface of the body with an environment, catalyzing through the vast organ of the skin "the dispersion and harmonization of the tensions of the organism."[3] One method was having clients lie on the floor, feel its resistance, and then roll into different positions bringing heels, calves, thighs, lumbar muscles, etc., into contact with the ground. Tapping the autonomic nervous system by improvisational, latent motions (slight stretches, seated cross-legged bends, and bone vibrations), she guided clients from enhanced surface sensations to methods of shifting and rebalancing striated and smooth muscles that had become rigidified. Then she directed them to their innermost bodily spaces—the outer sheaths of bones and the fluid substance of tissues and organs. From interior sensation and skeletal fulcra they could project outward back into the world. She also developed exercises in which clients contacted the ground indirectly, using bamboo sticks and elastic balls, or even the hands of the therapist. By artifactually enlarging the body's domain, she achieved dramatic releases of tension and coordination of proprioceptive reflexes.

In 1933, as Hitler came into power, Alexander moved her center to Copenhagen. Through her travels and those of her students, Eutony rapidly spread throughout the world. By the time Moshe Feldenkrais developed his own method, Eutony was the most well-known and popular system of movement awareness in Europe, especially among actors, musicians, opera singers, and dancers and also those in academic educational circles. It was training and self-improvement developed *by* performers *for* performers.

Alexander reveals her theatrical bent by quoting Constantin Stanislavski, peerless stage-master, in relation to her system:

> ... [T]he muscular tension impedes the inner life in unfolding naturally. As long as our muscles stay tense, we cannot even imagine the subtle nuances of our sentiments, nor penetrate into the spiritual life of our person.[4]

Eutony is an improvisation of emotions with a priority of dynamic contact in space. It teaches musicians how to harmonize their musculature with their instruments and actors how to "create a real and 'tangible' contact with the audience and other actors."[5] The inner sense of self generates a feeling of "psychosomatic and spiritual unity of the total person."[6] The expanding sensation around one leads to a genuine experience of community, much like a dance company, a mime troupe, a circus, or an orchestra.

Alexander Technique

ALEXANDER TECHNIQUE IS the honorary godfather of twentieth-century independent somatics. It was the first to fashion its own unique set of heuristic exercises out of empirical experimentation. It had no lineal predecessors, and most later systems owe it a debt, either directly or indirectly.

The originator was F. Matthias Alexander (1869–1955), a Tasmanian-born Shakespearian actor, recitalist, and tea-taster who was humiliated by the loss of his voice during plays. He had suffered from asthma and other respiratory diseases during childhood, but his health had generally improved except for a debilitating hoarseness that increased only during performances. Standard medicine offered either "Stop talking and your voice will come back" or gargling with ineffective throat sprays, so, in desperation, Alexander took up his own line of research.[7]

Because his throat was "normal" early in performances and during general conversation, he presumed that something he began to do only *while* speaking caused the malady. Observing himself in the mirror while he recited *The Merchant of Venice*, Alexander noticed (only after many tries) that before he ever uttered a word, his intention to speak initiated an intricate series of events. First, he slightly pulled back his head. The slumping of his head compressed his larynx. Then he began to suck his breath through his mouth in a gasping way. The stress pattern had two ingredients: "(1) a postural one which involved the needless tightening of networks of muscles, and (2) a thought component of repetitive ideas about performing in front of an audience, which identified the network of stress as 'right.'"[8]

Although Alexander could not prevent the compression of his larynx or gasping breath by any direct action, he found that letting his head move not just forward but also upward from his body allowed the larynx to release. When he finally succeeded in inducing his head to move in this manner from his body, his malady was ameliorated.[9] By freeing his neck and releasing his head forward and up, he was able to get his back to lengthen and widen. Subsequently he dubbed the head-neck-back relationship the "Primary Control," because it served as the fulcrum for the entire organization of bodily movement.[10] The head-neck-back relationship is not necessarily more important because of emphasis on the cranial and spinal regions but because released patterns in that nexus invariably transfuse outward (and inward) to the rest of the body.

For the next six years Alexander went on to examine total posture: the dynamic interactions among the head, neck, and torso, and the relationship of these to the way the limbs were deployed, the pelvis held, and the feet kept in contact with the ground. Working with his brother Albert Redden Alexander, he developed a body of lessons and instructions. Together the Alexander brothers spent six years in Sydney and Melbourne teaching their method to others. They were so successful that Matthias decided to transplant his practice to Europe; he left for London in 1904 and set up an office upon his arrival. During World War I he moved to the United States. Subsequently he alternated between continents until establishing a school for children in London in 1925. His practice and training remained in England for the next thirty years.[11]

The Alexander system was communicated in four books published sequentially approximately a decade apart beginning with *Man's Supreme Inheritance* in 1910, followed by *The Use of the Self, Constructive Conscious Control,* and *The Universal Constant in Living.*

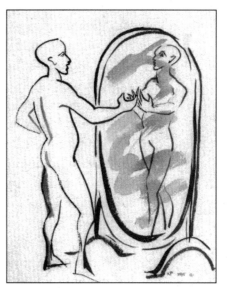

Alexander's method followed the belief that a body moving in balance with minimal effort established natural breathing habits and fluid circulation and relieved pressure on its vertebrae. He claimed not that any particular postures were responsible for people's organizational difficulties, but that *all* repeated postures reinforced rigidifying patterns.

Shaped by years of faulty even abusive teachings about what [Alexander] calls "the use of the self," the adult is not in a situation where he or she can trust judgments and decisions based on unclarified feelings. Everyday sensations of how to sit without back pain, how to keep one's eyes on a golf ball, how to form words without stuttering, even how to make love, are distorted by learned usage within a skewed social world.[12]

Children, for instance, suffer long hours of sitting in chairs in school, which indoctrinate inflexible attitudes. The very attempt to conform to etiquette and remain still leads to muscle tension and a host of emotional compensations. Among adults, lack of exercise, compulsive goal orientation, shallow breathing, apprehension of social embarrassment, and worrying (mentally leaving the present to dwell on past or future) all contribute to putting muscles under stress.

An Alexander Teacher will gently alter the pupil's position in order to release tension

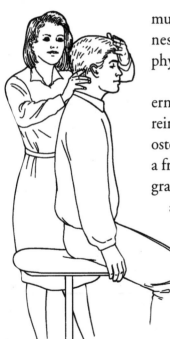

Undetected, these patterns of behavior and response accumulate tensions which gradually result in immobility and sickness. "You translate everything," Alexander said, "whether physical or mental or spiritual, into muscle tension."[13]

The "end sought" (which is an unexamined priority in Western civilization) is not indispensable (or even desirable) if it reinforces a strained and dysfunctional set of habits. Such an ostensible goal must be inhibited—in essence, sacrificed—for a freer, more efficient use of the body/mind. Getting results is gradually replaced by efficient means, relaxed coordination, and unencumbered movements regardless of ends sought.

Then any desired goals—like speaking on stage or riding a bike—become paradoxically more feasible.

Reprinted from *The Alexander Technique Workbook* by Richard Brennan, Element Books, 1992.

THE ALEXANDER TECHNIQUE educates people how to break with patterns of posture and self-organization. Starting with the "Primary Control"— establishing the freedom of the neck and head—one uses this rudder to guide coordination down through the skeleton. Although underlying patterns often seem knotted and permanently immobilized, Alexander believed that one could literally begin coordinating instead of unconsciously discoordinating oneself. He emphasized not merely the learning of techniques but their kinesthetic integration in new patterns of movement—the "means-whereby" leading to the end—rather than trying to skip the means and aim directly for the end ("end-gaining"). He felt that one had to head off habitual movements by constantly halting the preparation for an activity (his "inhibition").

Alexander took it for granted that a client's conception of a movement was invariably misguided, resulting in unnecessary tension and interference with healthy functioning. He developed a variety of ways for people to "inhibit" their preparation for an activity (even as he had learned how to inhibit himself from becoming hoarse). After inhibiting, they were naturally able to make better use of the primary control in their activities.

To be about to do something is not the same as actually doing it. The Alexander Technique rests on this simple discrimination. Through gentle hands-on work and instruction in subtle movements the Alexander practitioner teaches a client how to halt an instinctive action at the moment of preparing to act, prior to actually acting.

Yet the compulsion toward normal proficiency and use is very strong. Alexander himself experienced automatic reversions to old speech habits even after, through great persistence, he had changed his fundamental coordinations and pathways. At critical moments his regimen would betray him, and he would resume dysfunctions tied to accustomed routines (in his words, "misdirections associated with my old wrong habitual use"); he even lost control of his voice again. Given the power of habit, a misapplication of any one of the "dehabituating" exercises can lead to *increased* miscoordination and deepened misuse of self rather than improvement. That is why Alexander came to emphasize continual new habits in place of any mindless repetition of substitute exercises.

The basis of Alexander Technique is learning to trick oneself out of repeating a habitual pattern. First, one inhibits the programming of the primary control (plus any trackable secondary and tertiary controls); then one adopts new intentions in direct response to familiar stimuli. For instance, while intending to speak, a person goes through the process of being about to speak, then remains silent and instead raises a hand. Refusing to pursue a sought-after end provides an opportunity for derailing a poor use of self. Inhibiting a desire to move in a familiar way creates space for a novel way of being, a different experience of one's own identity.

An Alexander session may consist of any of the following: the maintenance of the vertical orientation of the head and body while in a sitting posture, lengthening the arms by extending them parallel to the ground outward from the chest and then raising them above the head and lowering them onto the thighs, the floating upward of the head away from the body while walking, the synchronization of an uncompensated raising of a leg to the point where its thigh is parallel to the ground simultaneous with the floating of the head, the lifting of the toes with the heels on the floor, the raising of the heels with the toes on the floor, the bending of the knees with the hips and ankles held straight and the body perpendicular to the ground, and the efficient transfer of weight to the feet when rising. All of these processes are carried out in series with attention to widening the back and lengthening the limbs, torso, and distal parts of the body, all the while relaxing and releasing tension.[14]

Alexander practitioner Jerry Sontag has objected to the above repertoire on the basis that it "implies a postural focus, or a series of exercises, neither of which are relevant to the Technique."[15] While I would agree that a static list trivializes the system, it does present a working Alexander vocabulary.

More dynamically, the Technique emphasizes breath control, the origination of muscular movement in thought preceding the intention to move, the recognition that actions which habits define as "right"

may in fact be damaging, the understanding that patterns are not always instinctual and reflexive but learned, and the explicit inhibition of habitual movement.

Alexander demonstrated how one could change muscular patterns, as well as mental patterns, by first stopping the old habits, and then "projecting messages from the brain to the body's mechanisms and conducting the energy necessary for the use of these mechanisms." He taught that one could "think" new shapes into the torso by imaging them and directing them through attention. "You come to learn to inhibit and direct your activity. You learn, first, to inhibit the habitual response to certain classes of stimuli, and second, to direct yourself consciously in such a way as to affect certain muscular pulls, which processes bring about a new reaction to these stimuli."[16]

Inhibition of habit is the singular key to the Alexander Technique. Other educational somatic systems (Feldenkrais Method, for instance) are more involved with teaching new and different patterns to replace nonfunctional or self-destructive ones. Alexander decided instead to unpeel the onion. His Technique is about "not doing." If one avoids initiating the discoordinating gesture, then the body will naturally regain its prior harmonic functioning. So if one can learn *not* to tighten the neck, that inhibition alone will free the head and spine and ultimately the organs.

An Alexander practitioner asks his client *not* to do an act. When he says, "I want you not to sit down," he actually means, "I want you to sit down with-

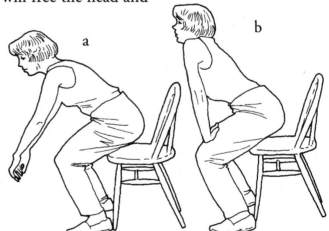

Even when standing up we can put enormous strain upon our entire structure. Beware of swinging up (fig. a) or pushing (fig. b).

Reprinted from *The Alexander Technique Workbook* by Richard Brennan, Element Books, 1992.

out any of the stressful prerequisites you bring to the act of sitting."
But a new version of sitting is not recognized by the nervous system
as sitting, so the therapist has to say instead, "I want you not to sit
down" in order to communicate the revision he is requesting. The first
few times he may guide his client into the chair, holding his head and
neck in such a way that they float free while the spine and pelvis are
sinking. As with kindred systems, the emphasis is on receptivity—the
therapist's touch must not push or bully a person into new patterns. It
must communicate a rational and experiential mode of being which
the patient can gradually make her own.

Next he may take the client slightly off his balance while in the
chair. In fact, he may do this a number of times, pushing him gently
backwards while supporting him. The client must find his balance again
each time. The goal, over several sessions, is to build a new inner sense
of what sitting, standing, and being in balance are, so that habitual versions of these acts don't automatically reimpose themselves. Standing,
sitting, and balancing are chosen not because of any inherent significance but because they are easily demonstrated and performed in a
practitioner's office and because they are customarily repeated with tension many times daily in Western civilization.

Not doing an act leaves space for a new and simpler act. Not doing
an act also allows a person to locate the component of the act which
is dysfunctional, neurotic, or stressful. Sontag describes recommending to a phone stutterer not to answer the phone. That means he is to
let it ring three or four times, trusting that the party will not hang up,
and then, even when he lifts the receiver, he is not to answer the
phone—that is, not to repeat kinesthetically the act his system recognizes as "answering the phone."

IN SUMMARY, the Alexander Technique comprises the following principles and goals:

- "Without awareness, we cannot change."[17]

- "In performing an action, the minute you 'think,' the muscles begin to move."[18]

- Our kinesthetic sense, our ability to tell how we are functioning, is faulty, which causes myriad psychophysical problems.

- The faulty sense occurs because the relationships of the head, neck, and back are not working properly. This limits choice in both movement and thought. "Think about the neck moving in space. Then 'allow' it to move back.... Let the torso lengthen and widen."[19]

- To change our kinesthetic sense to become more reliable, we must consciously stop the old patterns of tension—Alexander's inhibition.

- When these old patterns are stopped, new mental directions can be sent from the brain to encourage movement patterns that are freer and more proprioceptively chosen.

- The benefits of the Technique are an improved kinesthetic sense, enhanced overall functioning, including breathing and movement, a greater ability to maintain one's own health, and an increased consciousness of one's relationship to the immediate environment.

THESE DAYS Alexander Technique might seem of a subset of Feldenkrais exercises. But that is because Feldenkrais is more widely practiced. Alexander was historically prior and actually provided a part of the template from which Feldenkrais built his method (see below). When I mentioned my superficial impression that Alexander was subsidiary to Feldenkrais, a bodyworker familiar with a range of systems objected that they were each entirely self-sufficient, holistic systems with unique orientations. She thought of Feldenkrais as being more earthy, involved with the basic animal, neuromotor processes, bringing people into the thickest core of their bodies, while Alexander was light and puffy, expanding people's movement outward and giving them a celestial kind of airiness. The singlemost Alexander gesture is floating out while expanding across.

Feldenkrais never denied the value of Alexander's lessons, and he was well aware of the importance of inhibition (which played a role in his development of his own method), but he created a much vaster system with a compendium of techniques and applications.

Alexander and Feldenkrais not only met but Feldenkrais received a number of early lessons from Alexander that influenced his own development. When Feldenkrais showed Alexander a draft of the book he was writing, Alexander terminated the tutorial. He felt that *his* own repertoire of inhibitions and recoordinations was sufficient. According to Israeli therapist Mia Segal, "... while living in England and writing *Body and Mature Behavior*, Moshe met Alexander. Moshe used to say that Alexander had the best hands he had ever felt. If I remember correctly, Moshe showed him *Body and Mature Behavior*, and Alexander said, 'Actually you copied it from my book!' This, I suppose, ended the relationship."[20]

ALEXANDER TECHNIQUE HAS been historically popular with artists, musicians, dancers, architects, psychotherapists and intellectuals. The founder taught his method directly to John Dewey, George Bernard Shaw, Sir Charles Sherrington, and Aldous Huxley, the latter of whom extolled the technique in his novels *Eyeless in Gaza* and *Ends and Means*. Dewey lauded Alexander by saying that his Technique "bears the same relationship to education that education itself bears to all other human activities."[21] In "Maximus, to Gloucester" the American poet Charles Olson remembers his experience of being taught Alexander Technique as a young actor in Worcester, Massachusetts:

there we were, three actors,
in a loft above Tarr's Railway
in shorts, in front of her,
doing,
her bidding: "Buttocks
in & under, buttocks"

seeking,
like Euclid,
the ape's line, the stance
fit for crowds, to watch
parades, never
to tire

It was in our minds
what she put there,
to get the posture
to pass from the neck of,
to get it down,
to get the knees bent[22]

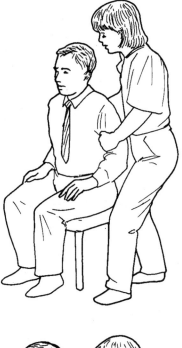

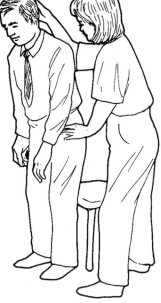

*An Alexander
Teacher helps the
pupil to move in
new ways, putting
less strain on the
body. The teacher
encourages the
pupil to go "up"
when sitting, and
to keep length
when bending.*

Reprinted from *The Alexander Technique Workbook* by Richard Brennan, Element Books, 1992.

Getting into and coming out of the semi-supine position

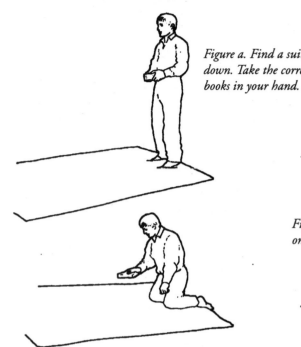

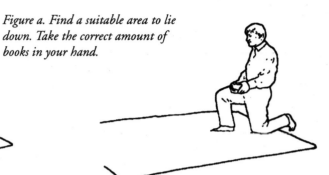

Figure a. Find a suitable area to lie down. Take the correct amount of books in your hand.

Figure b. Maintaining a vertical torso put one leg forward and go down on one knee.

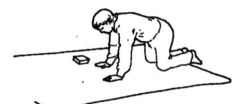

Figure c. Place the books to your right or left, roughly where your head will be when you are lying down.

Figure d. Place your hands on the ground so that you are on all fours.

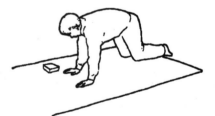

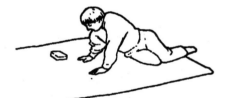

Figure e. Lift yourself up so that you are balanced on your hands and toes.

Figure f. Lower your legs to the ground with your knees pointing to the opposite direction to the books.

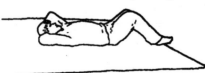

Figure g. Gently roll over onto your back, adjusting the position of the books so that they are comfortably under the back of your head.

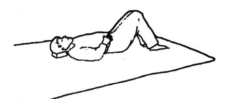

Figure h. Bring your knees upwards positioning your feet so that they are as near as possible to your torso while still remaining comfortable.

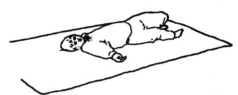

Figure i. After lying down for twenty minutes or so, take a few moments to think about how you can get up while still maintaining the length in your spine.

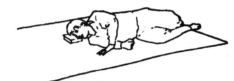

Figure j. Decide which way you wish to get up. Look in that direction and then let your knees roll in that direction. Let your whole body roll off the books.

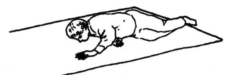

Figure k. Roll over onto your front with the support of a hand and a leg.

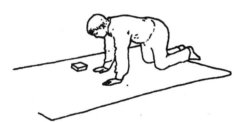

Figure l. Raise yourself until you are on all fours once again.

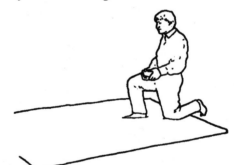

Figure m. Pick up the books and then place one leg in front of the other.

Figure n. Thinking of the head going forward, lean forward and you will naturally come back to the standing position. Note that this is only one of many ways of getting up, but it is useful to start with. It is also valuable to learn to follow a given set of instructions as this will reveal your habits. Experiment with rolling onto different sides while getting up and down.

Reprinted from *The Alexander Technique Workbook* by Richard Brennan, Element Books, 1992.

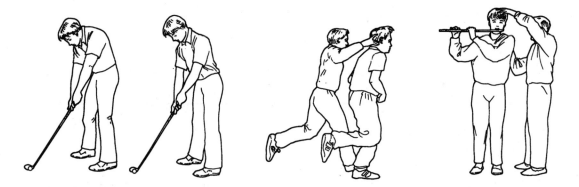

Reprinted from *The Alexander Technique Workbook* by Richard Brennan, Element Books, 1992.

Alexander Technique was also acclaimed by Nikolaas Tinbergen in his acceptance speech in 1973 for the Nobel Prize in Medicine. Tinbergen wrote: "Every session clearly demonstrates that the innumerable muscles of the body are continuously operating as an intricately linked web."[23]

Bates Method

EYEGLASSES HAVE BECOME such a staple of modern civilization that we barely notice the ubiquity of these odd facial props. Goggles to enhance seeing are considered as commonplace as clothes to keep warm. We take it as axiomatic that visual clarity (and lack of clarity) are hereditary and fixed and that artificial lenses are the only recourse for blurs and other nonpathological deficiencies of sight. The entire optometric profession exists to counteract poor eyesight by fitting mechanical aids onto the face. In the late twentieth century this partial prosthesis has been made so unobtrusive and socially acceptable it is no longer a major encumbrance or a stigma. In some circumstances, eyeglasses are even a source of pride and an opportunity to style attitudes and personalities. Many healers and holistic practitioners wear glasses without considering that poor vision might be a synergized aspect of their general

MODALITIES

194

health. They presume that the capacity of the eyes to focus is somehow separate from well-being as a whole. Thus, clarity of vision has become the most conservative bastion of allopathy, the last to yield to somatic holism.

Yet what if visual clarity and blurs are no more hereditary or immutable than the habits of tension and stress explored by Alexander? What if relearning natural patterns of movement underlying sight could dramatically improve just about everyone's ability to see clearly?

This hardly seems likely given the universal acceptance of optometry and the large number of educated and medically trained men and women who themselves wear glasses or contact lenses. Surely they are not all victims of delusion or fraud. After all, how could somatic education alter something as fundamental as the focal length of an inborn lens or the shape of an eyeball?

THE GENERALLY ACCEPTED theory of sight holds that clarity of vision is regulated by the lenses of the eyes and the ciliary muscles around those lenses. In response to the changing distances of landscapes and objects, these muscles recoordinate the shape of the lenses in a manner loosely akin to that of the focusing knob of a camera. A healthy eye, one capable mechanically of being broadly refocused (its muscles adjusting properly), renders sharp images across a range of distances.

By this theory the basic errors of visual accommodation (i.e., responding blurily to objects near and far) are the results of either unfortunate eyeball lengths or a deterioration of the lens from an injury or aging. Distortions include nearsightedness, farsightedness, astigmatism, amblyopia ("lazy eye"), and crosseyedness. Presbyopia, the increasing difficulty people have after approximately the age of forty in focusing objects near at hand, is considered an effect of the gradual hardening of the lens such that it loses its pliability to accommodate for near vision.

Alternate scientific theories base poor vision in part on flaws in the cornea, the retina, and the vitreous chamber, almost all of which are likewise inherited.

BORN IN 1860, William H. Bates matriculated as a prominent New York ophthalmologist and eye surgeon. In the course of examining more than 30,000 patients while adhering to familiar theories of eyesight, Bates began to suspect that the famous "lens model" was not supported by his experience. He noticed that patients' sight fluctuated markedly from day to day and even hour to hour. People with poor accommodation sometimes improved inexplicably for short periods of time. How could this happen if the proposed explanation for poor eyesight were accurate?

Existing orthodoxies made neither physical nor logical sense. Why should presbyopia, as a general hardening of the eyeball, cause only farsightedness? What about people in their eighties who have rigid lenses but still see up close perfectly? How does one explain the plight of those who become farsighted well before the age of forty, likewise those who suffer nearsightedness (but not farsightedness) after the age of forty? Why, when there is no physical connection between the two eyes, do most people suffer the same distortion in both eyes at the same time? Why, if one constructs a pinhole with a fist and stares through it at a previously blurry object, does the object come into sharp focus? Why should a movie on the screen be blurry and sharp at different cinematic distances when these actually are all at the same distance from the viewer? These events, considered collectively, indicate that deficiencies of eyesight may originate not in the eyes themselves but in subtle and profound links among the eyes, the rest of the body, and the mind.

Challenging what he called "theories, often stated as facts,"[24] Bates set out to discover the actual causes of clear vision. From the turn of the century he embarked on an elaborate course of experimentation, eventually summarizing his findings in 1920 in the landmark book *Perfect Sight Without Glasses.* The opthalmological profession was outraged, and he was dismissed from his position at the New York Postgraduate Medical School. Predicting that an "incalculable amount of human misery"[25] would result from the rejection of his theories and the continuation of ophthalmological delusion, he spent the rest of his life continuing to study eyesight and teaching his method.

Today, eyeglasses set at one focal length (or bi- and multi-focal lenses) remain virtual requirements for correcting poor eyesight and are universally recommended, while Bates' techniques are considered fallacies or quackery. Yet through these "fallacies" many people, even ones who were legally blind, have improved their vision to a level where they are no longer required to wear corrective lenses to drive a motor vehicle. Bates teacher Tom Quackenbush's myopia and astigmatism, which resulted in a 20/100 diagnosis at age ten and deteriorated to 20/500 by the time he was thirty, improved by 90 percent after he began practicing the Bates Method.

I N PLACE OF traditional explanations for the errors of visual accommodation, Bates established to his satisfaction that blurs and similar distortions were caused almost solely by strain and tension in the extrinsic muscles of the eye (as opposed, for instance, to inherited eyeball shape or the pliancy of the lens or intrinsic ciliary muscles). In proper visioning, the six muscles around each eyeball automatically change its shape to effect clarity (Bates' mechanism of focus can be approximated by squeezing and stretching a rubber model of an eye between one's fingers). The muscle cords literally squeeze the delicate, watery organs to appropriate focal lengths. Their compression is not particularly deep, but a deformation of millimeters has a dramatic effect on the clarity of images passing through a tiny, soft eye.

In the case of near vision, the two oblique muscles above and below the eye wrap around it from left to right and cause it to lengthen (they squeeze the eye long so that the cornea has a higher curvature and the image falls further back in its chamber and is larger). For far vision, the four recti muscles originating way in back of the eyeball near the brain extend forward and wrap, respectively, around the top, bottom, left, and right of the eyeball. In these positions they can pull the front of the eyeball back against the fatty tissue filling the hollow bony orbit cushioning the eye, causing it to foreshorten. The curvature of the cornea is reduced, and a smaller image lands closer to the front of the eye. For middle vision all six extrinsic muscles combine to round the eye into a sphere. The image lands midway and is of medium size.

If the two oblique muscles remain chronically contracted, the recti muscles cannot squeeze the eye short to focus far objects more clearly. The result is nearsightedness (myopia). Lucid near sight is permanently fixed. Likewise, if the recti muscles are chronically contracted, the two oblique muscles cannot stretch the eye to see near objects more clearly. This leads to farsightedness (hyperopia). The eye becomes a rigid telescope. Laser surgery can accomplish this too.

As Bates observed the actual changing shape of the eyeball in response to proximate movements of nerves and muscles in the spinal column, he determined that the muscles altering the shape of the eyeball were the sole direct cause of successful or unsuccessful accommodation. Blurs of nearsightedness, farsightedness, and astigmatism, and other symptoms of poor vision were caused by these muscles gripping too tightly in one way or another. Crosseyedness was caused by their being twisted out of position. Thus, natal eyeball shape and lens pliancy are secondary to the movements of extrinsic muscles in determining clarity of vision.

S INCE EYE HABITS are not fixed at birth, they are quite mutable. If the muscles can become chronically tense, they can also be relaxed. Once relaxed, they adjust the eye properly; naturally clear vision should result.

Bates' proposition was both simple and radical. He argued uniquely that improving vision had nothing to do with ophthalmological or optometric attention to the eyes themselves. On the contrary, it had everything to do with the muscles around the eyeball and the contingent neuromusculature of the neck. Since all of the dynamics connecting these tissues were at least partially disorganized by stress and other psychosomaticized habits, Bates looked solely to non-ophthalmological techniques for improvement of vision. He did not want to do anything to the eye itself, either by surgery or optometry. He sought only to get the extrinsic muscles working again autonomically.

To restore natural movement to the neck and muscles is much more efficient than to stabilize poor vision at selected focal lengths of corrective lenses. Additionally, tension in the extrinsic muscles is often made worse by the wearer's unconscious attempts to see through eyeglasses at distances different from those for which they were prescribed. Thus, eyeglasses and contact lenses can become a self-fulfilling prophecy, making vision worse by freezing dysfunctional patterns (and thus requiring ever new, stronger prescriptions). Chronically tense muscles also squeeze the retina and ultimately damage the eyeballs.

People are encouraged to think that their worsening vision is the effect of age, hence that they need glasses. As both vanity and worry over aging influence their attitudes, they strain harder to see, to convince themselves they are not losing clarity. Straining to see immediately makes their vision deteriorate. After glasses are prescribed and they begin to see more clearly, they are convinced they have a good doctor and are on the right path.

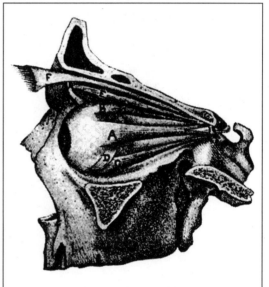

Extrinsic Muscles of the Eye

A. External rectus muscle   B. Superior rectus muscle
C. Inferior rectus muscle   D. Inferior oblique muscle
E. Superior oblique muscle   F. Levator of upper lid

However, the glasses and laser surgery themselves lock in poor vision, the latter permanently. This scenario has now become a boondoggle of major proportions.

Bates improved accommodation by teaching new neuromuscular habits through educational paradigms not unlike those of Matthias Alexander and Moshe Feldenkrais. All of his techniques in one or another way introduce movement into the eye-neck relationship and challenge

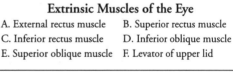

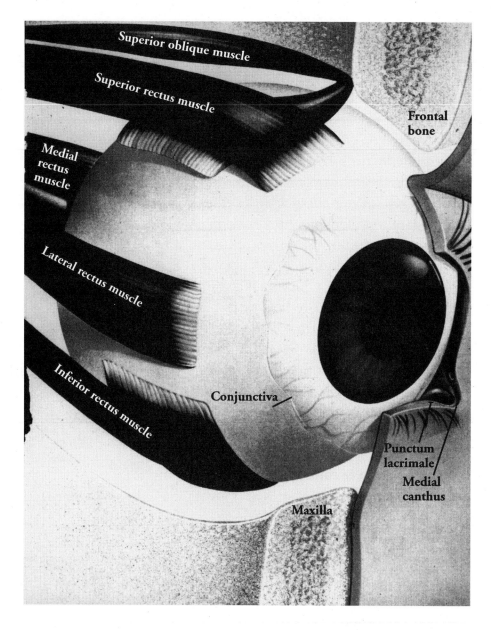

kinesthetic stagnation. His central practice is called "shifting," which is
little more than the collective motions of natural relaxed vision. Shifting means keeping the eyes moving and centralizing, focusing one point
at a time. The eyes graze freely about a landscape. They "see" as they

focus single objects sequentially. They do not stare, and they do not diffuse. They do not glaze over into seeing "nothing," and they do not try to see too much at once. In fact, Bates argued, too many people try to see more than one point at a time with the result that everything is out of focus. The retina comprises photosensitive, achromatic night receptors (the rods) and a highly sensitive plate with focal color capacity (the cones). Only the cones, located in an extremely small pit (the fovea centralis) at the back center of the retina, focus sharply. The more abundant rods, distributed in membranous layers throughout the retinal periphery, enhance night vision and detect movement, but they do not register sharpness of detail. Chickens, with only cones, pick grains from dust in the daytime but are sightless after dusk. Owls and bats, with only photosensitive rods, rouse at dusk but otherwise shun bright light and cannot see unblurred detail. Trying to see too much means attempting to focus with rods, which are incapable of accommodation, hence a blur.

Its indented morphology exposing its cones to photons of light, the fovea centralis occupies less than one percent of the total area of the eyeball. The exposed cones are not only limited (for all practical purposes) to this tiny pit, but they are even more concentrated in its minute center. Thus, sharp vision comes solely from moving the fovea centralis to each object of interest. Super-sharp vision comes from shifting the center of the fovea centralis. Objects may be as remote from one another as a ship on the horizon and a watch on one's own hand, or as tiny as indentations on a grain of rice in which a Tibetan monk is carving a Buddha. The human eye is capable of remarkable feats of clarity and microscopy, but only if the cones move, centralize, and track.

Centralizing means bringing the cones of the eye to the object ones wishes to see. People with excellent vision merely centralize and shift rapidly, seeing things in sequence. They do not have a larger visual field than others even though it might seem as if they do.

Inhibition of both staring and diffusing is central to the Bates Method. Inhibition means putting an end to attempts to focus with the periphery. Shifting and centralizing are simply *not* staring and diffusing. They are natural acts of "seeing."

Bates insisted that staring not only always strains the muscles and reduces vision, but it is the result of a series of dysfunctional attitudes. People stare and diffuse because they want to escape. They want not to be present in uncomfortable situations. Diffusing, the consequence of attempting to hold too large a visual field in focus, "spaces" a person out. Blurry vision is automatic when one tries to see lots of different things at once or strains to focus one's peripheral vision.

The principles of the Bates Method can be learned in less than an hour, but it takes many classes and much practice and reinforcement for most people to unroot their subtle habits of staring. A person tries to ease tension by first tracking—doing an internal inventory of her body—and then relaxing any "held" muscles one by one. She is letting go her neuromuscular "stares" and unparking her eyes. Stares come in many forms, both blatant and subtle. Staring, diffusing, and centralizing are also universal states. Vision is merely their most apparent metaphor. For a person truly to achieve clarity means to eliminate (or reenergize) all stares—first, obvious fixed stares, then minute "micro-stares" camouflaged in habit, attitude, and shallow breathing, and finally stares of the mind itself which can occur with virtually no ocular effect.

The most imposing hurdle is the fixation of mind. Often a well-trained person is able gradually to relax every palpable point of tension, both gross and subtle, and yet still experiences a knot of underlying tension. She releases all her micro-stares and sketches freely, yet still experiences a fixation of mind patrolling through superficially darting eyes. This stress center has a profound hold on the body and seems to pour out of the center of "mind" like a dead, diffusing light. It marks the seam where mind and body meet.

Eyes are pure brain tissue honed into landscape-replication by the effects of sunlight. It should be no surprise that they express basic char-

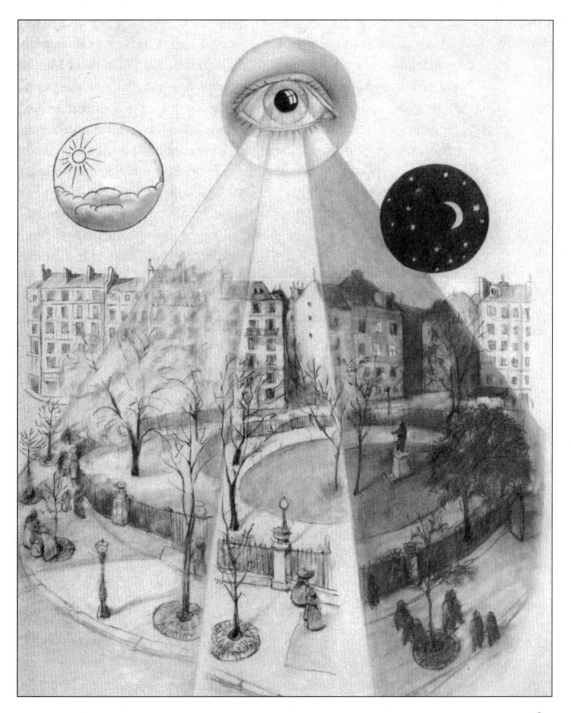

acter, attitude, and interest. Symptoms of stress, anxiety, and depression often manifest directly through the neuromusculature of vision.

Acts of staring are mini-phobias. To stare is to attempt to hold reality in place, to be unmoved and invulnerable, to be locked in anxiety or fright. To stare is to be drawn magnetically and obsessively toward single things and away from one's own center and mobility. The stares that lead to poor vision habits and blurs are symptoms of modern life. They represent alienation, fear, boredom, and dependence on electronic representations of images. They are the opposite of relaxed vision in open sunlight (practiced by all tribal societies). Glasses are their artifact and validation.

When a person loses interest in the environment, she begins to stare rather than sketch. Natural quick movements of alert, clear vision are replaced by degrees of resistance to events, people, and tension. The environment is not exciting or safe enough to encourage active vision.

Transitions from centralizing to diffusing are so gradual and subliminal that one is not even aware of the process. It seems as though the eyes themselves are losing acuity.

B ATES PRACTITIONERS USE any method they can to get an individual to relax and make vision unstrained again. Some are tricks, some are visualizations, some are puzzles or games, and some are mnemonic devices for forming new habits.

Contemporary vision teachers prefer a form of shifting called "sketching" or "brushing" in which a student imagines, for instance, that she has a short pencil or feather attached to the end of her nose—not a soft pink plume but a sleek pointed feather. She then sketches or brushes objects with it, touching them imaginarily as she selects them for seeing: her own fingers, a friend's face, a stranger's hat, a fence in the distance, a tree at the horizon, clouds, the Moon. Brushing *is* seeing. Instead of needlessly straining the eyes to focus better, brushing consciously uses the nose as a compass and the muscles of the neck as a clarifying rod.

Brushing places the fovea centralis right on the object being viewed. The precision of this act can be illustrated by a reverse phenomenon. On a dark, preferably moonless night, try brushing single stars. Effective brushing should make each star disappear at the moment the nose-feather touches it. As acutely as the cones register detail in daylight, they are blind at night. Thus, if one can accurately impose the viewing field of the cones on a night form without the assistance of the rods, that object should disappear. The fact that each brushed star vanishes demonstrates that the effective area of visual clarity is as fine as the arc of a single star.

For this reason, brushing cannot be a mere exercise. It must become a subliminal habit, like any serious self-improvement practice or Dzogchen meditation. It would be far too distracting to brush every object one wished to see. As Tom Quackenbush enjoys commenting, "You only have to practice what I teach twenty-four hours a day."[26]

If one is brushing, they can't be staring. Thus brushing is effective first in tricking the mind into not trying so hard to use the eyes to see and second in allowing the mind to exert another, more relaxing fulcrum to achieve clarity. The object attached at the end of the nose feather indirectly loosens the contraction in the ocular region. It also centralizes.

"Swinging" is initiated by setting the feet approximately a foot apart and then turning the body to the right while lifting the left heel. The head and eyes remain stationary, and the apparent movement of motionless objects is ignored. As the left heel returns to the floor, the body turns to the left, and the right heel is raised. This sequence of alternately raising right and left heels and turning is carried out for about five minutes in order to recoordinate movement and vision.

Effect of superior oblique muscles on eye movement

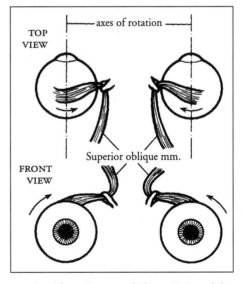

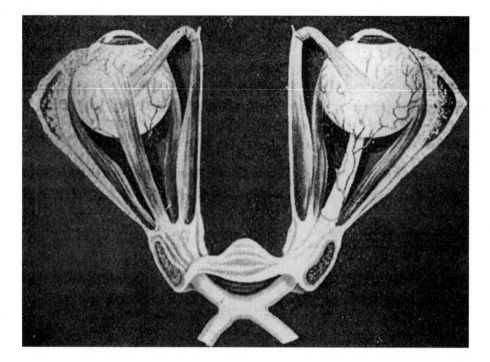

*The relative
positions of
the eyeballs,
muscles, and
nerves*

THE BATES METHOD is an attempt to educate people to regain natural habits of good vision most of them had at birth (and in the
sightless realm of the womb). The fact that the dispelling of stares and
"micro-stares" enhances metabolism, immunity, and emotional states
makes the Method more than just vision improvement. It is a form of
holistic healing grounded in the mechanism of the eyes and ocular
habits. It is based on locating and healing the mental patterns that give
rise symptomatically to misuse of the visual apparatus and to a cycle
in which poor vision habits lead to rigid, phobic thinking, and vice
versa.

The Bates Method differs from other somatic learning techniques
insofar as it is the invention of an ophthalmologist, is based exclusively on the role of vision in systemic health and organization, and
thus deals specifically with improving eyesight. Its goal is not so much
to teach the body new overall patterns of organization as it is to restore

the single act of seeing to a subliminal level. Other organs then respond to the neuromuscular fluidity of the eyes. The vestibular system becomes more cohesive and coordinated; digestion improves; stress is taken off the intestines and heart.

Bates techniques can never be mere isolated mechanical remedies. Since the eyes regulate so many interpersonal functions and aspects of personal identity, the regaining of natural movement in their extrinsic muscles generally means an improvement in overall mental and physical health. Likewise, neurotic patterns must precede poor eyesight. The eyesight becomes weaker when a person doesn't want to relate, perhaps because his job or environment imposes stress, perhaps because there is nothing joyful to see. Relearning to see is relearning insight, intimacy, and sensuality.

Insofar as Bates practitioners acknowledge the holistic aspects of eyesight and its kinesthesis, they respect Alexander and Feldenkrais work. However, they deny that these can have any lasting effect on vision because they do not address the muscle patterns in the eyes pragmatically and thus can deal with vision only secondarily as an aspect of somatic organization. These systems miss the single point of relaxing the six extrinsic ocular muscles, so they improve eyesight only by chance or because they train a general harmony and the eyesight follows.

Today the Bates Method is used in collaboration with many other somatic therapies, often to treat serious injuries affecting eyesight. An osteopath may correct an underlying spinal lesion while a Bates practitioner teaches ocular relaxation. This combination has worked well in instances of near blindness after car accidents and muggings.

M ANY OF BATES' other techniques are obvious to the point of syllogistic, and all of them involve relaxation. The simple process of "palming" was something Bates came upon quite accidentally when, one day, he removed his own glasses and cradled his head in his hands, cupping his eyes. The resulting darkness was so restorative and calming that he kept his eyes covered for about fifteen minutes. Upon removing his hands he noticed a new vibrancy of color throughout the office. Later he formalized "palming" as a soothing placement of one's own cupped palms over the eyes with fingers crossed on the forehead to avoid touching the eyes themselves. In Bates' time the hands were usually rubbed together first to generate heat. Nowadays forming a *"chi"* field between separated rounded palms is more popular. The palmer can also summon up internal landscapes and play his eyes over these, focusing alternately on imaginary objects near and far—closed-eye "sketching."

Another elegant therapeutic method Bates called "sunning." This involves closing the eyes and rotating the head slowly from side to side so that the sun lightly massages the outer surface of the eyelids. Sunning rebuilds light tolerance and color intensity and restores some diurnal/nocturnal vision resilience. Natural light passing through the eyes is a nutrient for the whole body (see "Healing by Color" in Chapter Eight).

Bates also recommended self-massage, fuller breathing, and conscious blinking. In fact, he urged blinking softly (like a butterfly's wings) every two or three seconds until it becomes a habit. This naturally lubricates the eyeball and antidotes the scourge of visual accommodation: staring and "dry eye syndrome."

Such exercises should not confuse the basic issue. Conscious sketching, breathing, and blinking will never in themselves restore clarity. They are approximations of an extremely subtle mechanism that must be activated unconsciously. Thus, a person in the process of learning the Bates Method may find himself at the theater unable to see the characters on stage clearly. Having already improved his vision over seven weeks of classes, he may struggle to sketch, breathe, and blink, and be disappointed when the figures remain blurred. At such a point it would be better for him to accept his blur and stop straining because the thing that ultimately restores clarity is not sketching, breathing, and blinking as he knows it. It is a deeper and subtler rendition of these acts. The blur, at least initially, is correct. When the so-called exercises of clear vision are carried out as goal-oriented strategies they cannot work. Remember, it is precisely such straining that undermined good vision in the first place.

Seeing happens at the speed of light and thought; thus any actions meant to enhance seeing must sink to such an autonomous level. Only when these acts become natural again does clarity slowly return. The key to the Bates Method is not in learning techniques of focus. It is in retracking the system to the point where natural, primordial coordination takes over. At the end of his life Bates summarized his training in precisely these terms:

> The importance of practicing certain parts of the routine activities at all times, such as blinking, centralizing, and imagining stationary objects to be moving opposite to the movement of the head, is emphasized. The normal vision does these things unconsciously, and the imperfect vision must first practice them consciously until they become unconscious habits.[27]

Feldenkrais Method

MOSHE FELDENKRAIS IS one of the founders of twentieth-century somatics. Born in Poland in 1904, he immigrated to Palestine as a teenager and lived there for ten years before moving to Paris to study physics at the Sorbonne. He fled to Britain just ahead of the German invasion of World War II. There he worked for the Admiralty on the science of submarine detection and anti-sub warfare.

> He was required to be on a ship every day. Ships at sea pitch to and fro and the constant jostling was wreaking havoc with his knee injured years earlier in a soccer accident. His wife, a pediatrician, introduced him to one of the best surgeons in England. The surgeon concluded that an operation would probably prove successful. Feldenkrais asked what he meant by "probably successful." The surgeon gave Feldenkrais 50–50 odds that he would walk normally and 50–50 odds that he would have to spend the rest of his life walking with the help of a

cane. Feldenkrais replied that 50–50 odds were no better than mere chance and that in designing experiments he would look for something like a 98–2 probability; otherwise it was a waste of time.[28]

He told the astonished surgeon he would repair his own knees. The surgeon assured him that he would be back within six months begging for an operation. From such a gauntlet the system of Functional Integration emerged. Individuals with strong wills make quantum leaps when challenged and motivated. History is replete with such accomplishments. Feldenkrais' discovery of the somatic principles of behavior and function came from a similar process to Johannes Kepler's calculation of planetary orbits.

First, he began his own study of existing kinesiological literature and texts of developmental anatomy. Nothing suited his standards. From what he gleaned he began to try subtle manipulations of his knee. Keeping careful records of his attempts, he would note the effect during the manipulation, then thirty seconds, a minute, five minutes, an hour, and a day after. He gradually found the right combination of mechanical adjustments to restore his knee to functioning. Or so he thought.

> Walking on a sidewalk in London, Feldenkrais hailed a cab. Stepping off the curb into what he assumed would be the street, he in fact stepped into a storm drain. The added distance jarred his knee and reinjured it. Feldenkrais realized, in his words, "I was like every other idiot who fixed a part and didn't look at the whole system. . . ." He began an inquiry into the activities of daily life. This inquiry led to his greatest realization: that whether one walks "poorly" or "gracefully," unless one knows the "how," both are equally mechanical. . . . As Feldenkrais began again the project of restoring functioning to his knee he now knew that he had to proceed very differently.[29]

Gradually, by slow trial and error, he rehabilitated himself again and at the same time tracked his stages and developed a teachable "method." Returning to Israel to test, practice, and teach the new principles, he established a training center (the Feldenkrais Institute) in Tel Aviv. After his work became known internationally, he traveled widely to lecture and give demonstrations, including a legendary stint at Esalen Institute in 1972. Feldenkrais died in 1984.

LIKE MANY OTHER somatic innovators, Feldenkrais did not invent every element of his system; he grafted many of them from existing techniques and practices. Yet his method stands totally on its own, transforming its components so that they take on new identities and applications in terms of the logic in which he rearranged them. Among the somatic areas he studied were auto-suggestion, hypnosis, neuroanatomy, yoga, Alexander Technique, the martial arts, and the teachings of G. I. Gurdjieff. He was familiar with prevailing European movement traditions, including Eutony and the work of Elsa Gindler (which led directly to the practices of Marion Rosen and Charlotte Selver in the United States). Gindler taught a system of sensory awakening which, in defiance of Hitler's demands, she refused to name. Her radical experiments in sensing included hours of sitting, standing, or jumping, all trying to develop pure attention to function and recover an immediacy of experience. Selver later called her work "Sensory Awareness." This same mode of inquiry guides Feldenkrais' development of what he called Awareness Through Movement.

While also clearly influenced by Gerda Alexander, Feldenkrais contended that Eutony relied on random nonspecific explorations as opposed to a logical scientific inquiry. This is true only by comparison to Feldenkrais and later methods. Alexander's practices were quite complex empirically, given their development at such an early stage in the history of movement awareness. In fact, for some people today, they function precisely in place of Feldenkrais exercises for some of the same learning experiences.

FELDENKRAIS METHOD FUNCTIONS as a science of living thermodynamics for mammals. Disciple Jack Heggie has fantasized that the founder, using common kinesiological principles, combined the structural essence of Shaolin martial arts with Taoist energy practices.[30] Advanced Taoist practitioner Kumar Frantzis noted, "In the West, it has been the author's observation that the Feldenkrais Method is the only method which has principles in common with *Chi Gung* therapy in terms of re-educating the body's physical tissue and central nervous systems." However, Frantzis adds, "The Feldenkrais system does not have a *chi* component in its diagnostic or treatment methods. . . . The *Chi Gung* therapy methods are not derived from only the genius of one man but from thousands of years of refining consistent research and development."[31] Still, that such a dedicated promoter of *Chi Gung* would even consider Feldenkrais in the same league as the entire lineage of Taoist masters is high praise indeed!

Feldenkrais work does not notably resemble *Chi Gung* except in cultivating awareness of minute components of movements. Yes, it is an empirical, kinesthetic tracking system written in the language of awareness exercises, but it concerns habit and psychosomatic restriction not intrinsic energy. We will discuss this issue further in the section on *Chi Gung* in Chapter Six.

The Method does not resemble American Indian shamanism either; yet after Brooke Medicine Eagle trained in Feldenkrais work and returned to the Northern Cheyenne reservation, she observed the activities of the medicine men through new eyes. "Now," she declared, "I saw what they were doing."[32] Even though the Feldenkrais technique does not specifically deconstruct cross-cultural rituals, Medicine Eagle had learned the effectual subtle components of *movement itself* and thus could relate to shamanic gestures on this basis. As Feldenkrais himself said at the outset of his North American training in 1975: "I am going to be your last teacher. Not because I'll be the greatest teacher you ever encounter, but because from me you will learn how to learn."[33]

In principle he taught people how to learn

Chi Gung as well as how to stop overeating and form words after a stroke. By contrast, a *Chi Gung* teacher transmits or demonstrates "something"; whether his student can use his example and instruction to locate her own *chi* or can't, he has no way of relating success or failure to particular sensory-motor habits. He can define *chi* only by its putative existence and its existence by his own spontaneous discovery and utilization of it. Thus, it may be argued that, while a hypothetical student might never find *chi* by mere Feldenkrais lessons, the lessons could teach her states of being that would make her receptive to *Chi Gung* training. Without the prior Feldenkrais work, she might in fact organize away from experience of *chi*.

FELDENKRAIS WAS THE SON of a family of rabbis, a direct descendant of Pincas of Koretz, elder of the innermost circle of Hassidic Judaism. In fact, Feldenkrais' gravestone in Israel identifies him solely by this genealogy, ignoring his international renown as a master of somatics. In a certain sense Feldenkrais performed first as a Hebrew mystic, second as physical educator. His entire Method is one more subset of a vast qabbalistic puzzle; legend has it that his exercises tap an ancestral heritage of secret Hassidic dances paralleling extant Taoist techniques. At the very least, his work embraces and dissects "Russian, German, French, English, Yiddish and Hebrew ways of being embodied."[34]

One should not underestimate the role of Feldenkrais' expertise in physics. Like osteopathic grandfather Andrew Still, he operated on the basis of a thorough comprehension of engineering principles. Having worked in the Paris laboratory of Nobel laureate Frederic Joliot-Curie, he "had a very contemporary systems and field theoretical approach to the physical world"[35] that flouted a mechanistic and Newtonian view of nature and the body. His somatic "laws" were based on relativistic and psychological understandings of structure and movement.

Whether he uncovered the age-old fighting principles of the Shaolin Temple or not, Feldenkrais became an adept enough judo practitioner to write books on the subject. In fact, he earned one of the first European black belts:

> In judo one's posture must permit without prior readjustments movement in any of six cardinal directions—up/down, forward/backward, left/right. Most attackers or defenders move in one plane, e.g., forward or back, left or right, up or down. They become predictable targets.... Counting time, the martial artist moves in four dimensions or rather becomes four-dimensional. The personal self, which is time/space bound in a cultural matrix of lower dimensionality, disappears. Intentional multidimensionality, closely linked with what Feldenkrais called awareness, is one by-product of changing our way of moving.... By educating, differentiating and integrating the movements of the lower torso and upper legs—the so-called "center"—one apportions strength to the strongest muscles, freeing the limbs for expression and sensitive contact. With action organized from the center the skeleton becomes a means for transferring force from the lower torso outward to the extremities. Additionally, one learns how to utilize and turn the strength of another against him, how to transform the fear of falling into rolling, how to "re-educate" the opponent rather than destroy him or her.[36]

Elizabeth Beringer, a contemporary practitioner and teacher, told me that she conceives of the Feldenkrais Method primarily as the dynamism of judo fused with the rigor of physics.[37]

FELDENKRAIS' NETWORK OF neural reeducation is comprehensive, with myriad elements operating at different intellectual and somatic levels. Its repertoire includes a highly structured but flexible sequence of lessons taught to individuals as Functional Integration and to groups under the name Awareness Through Movement. Their emphasis is on sensory-motor experience: reintegrating functions and becoming aware of previously unperceived areas of the self while connecting them one to another. The techniques range from methods of gentle manipulation—often to relieve pressure from a particular zone and allow a client to move in a more efficient way—to games of practical anatomy so direct and playful they could be taught in primary schools.

What stands out about the Method is the degree to which it is involved in proprioception as well as manipulation—that is, conscious learning and not just adjustments from the hands of a practitioner. Feldenkrais devised his lessons to show people on simultaneously kinesthetic and cognitive levels why they moved in the ways they did, where the restrictions they felt were located, and, starting from the ground up, how to evolve new patterns of movement and activities.

He had no ambitions to train "improved" behavior in a rigorous sense. Conscious awareness and freedom rather than performance were at stake—how people build modes of "being" out of the rudiments of their own sensations. As there are no sets to learn, no prototypes, no formally sequential protocols, the Feldenkrais system is a limitless alphabet. Using the basic model, therapists conceive new methods of treatment and ingenious variations on familiar exercises almost daily.

After years of doing this work, Dennis Leri finally concluded:

> Throughout the many hundreds of ATM (Awareness Through Movement) lessons, with all their varied themes, there are two general injunctions: 1) Move only in one's comfort zone. Work smarter rather than harder ... 2) Carry out the instructions only as long as one is able to attend to what one is doing. If the mind begins to wander, if the movement becomes mechanical, stop.[38]

FELDENKRAIS TURNED AROUND the traditional paradigm of physical therapy. Instead of asking, "What can I touch to change this person?" (as most therapists do), he wondered, "How can I initiate the transformative effect of awareness itself?" Once again, the Feldenkrais Method is first and foremost a learning model. The therapist is trying to create a situation in which a client can learn a new way of doing things.

For instance, like Matthias Alexander, Feldenkrais found that interrupting preexisting patterns was extremely useful both in diagnosing impediments and in developing new possibilities of movement. It didn't matter whether these patterns were kinesiologically "successful" or not. Novel behavior always emerged from their dissolution.

Feldenkrais applied this principle variously to bodily rigidity, relanguaging, bed-wetting, and obesity. He instructed one very overweight woman at a seminar always to leave one bite on her plate, one spoonful in her bowl. Since no previous diet had worked, he was instructing her to change her habits of eating instead.

He taught nonhabitual movements to trick people into giving up their habitual patterns. Simply interlacing one's fingers with the right thumb on the outside (if the left thumb is habitual in that position) is enough to challenge basic kinesthesia throughout the body. Interlacing one's toes is even more radically nonhabitual. If the eyes are closed and the muscles moving them are held consciously to one side (the extreme left or right or directly up or down), then the head may be moved independently of the eyes. After one direction is completed to satisfaction (a few circuits are usually sufficient), the other side may be attempted. After all four directions are completed, they may be smoothed and liquefied into several full orbits of a circle. For the more advanced student, the eyes and the head may be tracked in opposite circuits—one clockwise, the other counterclockwise, or vice versa. That is, each attempt rotates these neuromuscular components simultaneously and smoothly in opposite directions. A parallel set of exercises may be carried out holding the head in place and shifting the eyes. In subsequent rounds the shoulders may be integrated into a series in which any two of the three (eyes, head, or shoulders) progress in one direction while the third is tracked in the other direction. This constellation of techniques is startlingly effective in extending range and orbit of movement, relieving head, eye, and neck pain, and reducing the frequency of headaches. What is more astonishing (less so if one accepts deep reciprocality throughout the body) is that the exercises may also increase the range of motion of the arms or

pelvis, not specifically moved during the session. Conversely, restriction in the head area can be relieved by pelvic and leg exercises. *Somatics*

Feldenkrais generally believed in indirect treatments to unlock the core:

> I never deal with the affected member or articulation before an improvement in the head-neck relationship and the breathing has been brought about. This, in turn, cannot be achieved without a betterment of the spine and thorax configuration. Again the pelvis and abdomen must be corrected. In practice the procedure is a successive series of approximations, each one allowing a further improvement in the segment just dealt with. . . .
>
> The head movements must have no predilection for particular directions. The "normal" head should have easy access to all directions of the anatomically possible range. The limiting factor should be the skeletal structure and not the muscular impediments. . . .

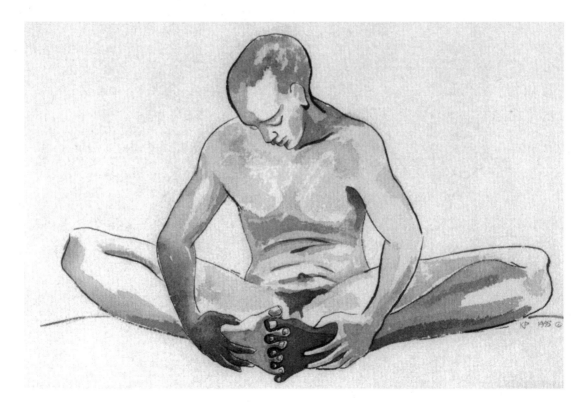

The healthy coordinated movements of the body as a whole obey the mechanical principle of least action, while the muscles work in step and perform their task with the least expenditure of metabolic energy.[39]

Getting people to differentiate between languaging mannerisms and actions was one of Feldenkrais' gateways to affecting deep habitual behavior. You could not reeducate function unless you persuaded people to sever their unexamined bond between clichés of thought and clichés of action:

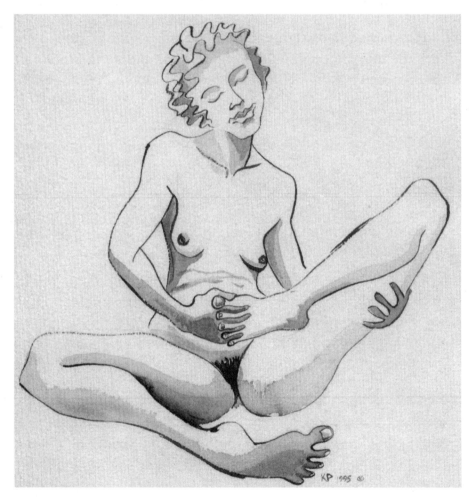

Linguistic articulations, verbal and non-verbal codings, make mute the protean somatic articulation from which they emerge. Our body broken by language is reassembled with conjunctions. We say the hand *and* the wrist *and* the arm *and* so on, creating a body of thought apart from our organismic body. To make language a part of our biology we need to be able to read, access, and utilize the organismic body's "alphabet," "grammar," and "vocabulary".... Any learned behavior [including speech, reading, and writing] obscures the learning processes used to construct it. Feldenkrais lessons access and recombine the patterns of somatic learning used to construct any meaningful behavior.[40]

Feldenkrais favored the creation of double binds and paradoxes in order to force students to abandon their familiar patterns and improvise new ones. He liked to pose purposely ambiguous instructions in order to see how class members would interpret them and put their bodies to different uses. In this manner, he was able to expose the often rigid relationship between languaging patterns and somatic activities. During one exercise reminiscent of Matthias Alexander, he instructed:

Don't breathe.... Don't hold your breath either.... Just don't breathe. Don't breathe in any way that you know to be breathing.... Don't hold your breath.... Don't make efforts.... Don't breathe with your chest.... Don't breathe with your abdomen.... Don't do any of the things that you know.... Just don't breathe, that's all.[41]

For Feldenkrais, differentiation was crucial—differentiation of each part of the body from its contiguous parts and differentiation of one axis of movement from all others. For instance, rolling one's head and pelvis on the floor in opposite directions breaks an integrated motif; this movement can then be used to invent more complex, less rigid patterns. Without differentiation, there is no alphabet of behavior.

Differentiation is the embryogenic and historical way in which the primitively forming tissues locate themselves in space and in relation to other tissues and thus know how to shape fascia, bones, and viscera.

How the embryo forms in layers of tissues becomes how the infant learns primary motor skills, always discriminating similar motions and aptitudes until they are fully distinct from one another. Morphogenesis continues to arrange and educate tissues and give cells new identities.

FELDENKRAIS' INITIAL CHALLENGE to new clients is to lie on the floor. People in a group feeling the contact of the ground with their bodies will each perceive points of solid connection—floor against self—and points where the connection is broken, intermittent. Simply becoming aware of each of these sensations and what they represent teaches a person which muscles are overworking to hold irrelevant parts of the body up from the floor. If these are released, even partially, one's overall use of the skeleton is improved. This is how Feldenkrais made Eutony more empirical, less random. He brought the same analytic precision to "reinventing" Alexander's technique.

Sitting in chairs is a great deadener of the proprioception of the hip joints. Feldenkrais explains:

The awareness of the location and function in these joints is non-existent compared with that of people who sit on the ground and not on chairs. The chair sitter is almost without exception completely out of place when locating the hip joints. Moreover, he uses his legs

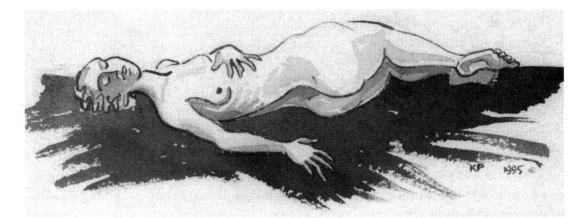

as if they were articulated at the points where he has them articulated in his body image and not where they are.[42]

Styles of presence in modern life are based on the tensions between our idealized images of self and what would be anatomically elegant. In order to be more present, we must become more aware of the ways in which we embody these strained characters, at the expense of our natural, motile selves.

As we compel our living bodies to carry out the imaginary functions of nonexistent abstract bodies, these become our character states, ridiculously stylized masks or caricatures of systemic ambivalences, parading as normal stances and acts. Where imaginary functions depart from actual anatomy, we become ineffective and must compensate both physiologically and emotionally.

FELDENKRAIS' GUIDING TENET was that people are born with a capaciousness of movement, much of which they inhibit. Like Freud and Reich, he presumed a cognitive, emotional cause underlying this crisis, but unlike them, he did not accept the inevitability of trauma in the formation of deep neurosis or character armor. He believed that many blocks were the incidental result of habituated mislearning, and that others were deep-seated not from the force and static content of a traumatic moment but because of an ultimately trivial and unnecessary repetition of a dysfunctional or restricted pattern of movement, or of an essential kinesthetic ambivalence that continually furnished opposed sets of behavior. They were ruts—pure and simple—historically tangled without deep-seated charge.

That is, whereas Freud presumed that people had complicated emotional reasons for their neuroses, Feldenkrais believed that while resistances were legitimately retreats into positions of imagined ego security, the neural energy binding them was no more cathected and trenchant than, for instance, the unwillingness to speak a new language (like French) before one knows enough of it to express oneself.[43]

I cannot emphasize enough how important this point is. Whereas Freud said, "We need a trauma to become neurotic or dysfunctional," Feldenkrais said, "A bad habit is enough to do it." If we "practice" a dysfunctional movement again and again, even without a trauma (perhaps simply from a neurological confusion or dyslexia-like displacement), the mere repetition of that movement will gradually cut deeper and deeper into the organization of our whole body/mind, sometimes leading to physical and mental disease from the blocking or distorting of natural visceral and neuromuscular functions. Yet there may be nothing more behind it than an innocent, happenstance mistake.

In fact, even in deep trauma-based patterns of fright, stress, or paralysis, the functional debilitating element is not the original trauma but the way in which the body/mind reacted to it, internalized it, and continues to reenact its habitual protection pattern in an attempt not to have the experience again. This is the basis of many new psychoneurological systems of treating trauma, including the seminal "Waking the Tiger" work of Peter A. Levine.

MOST PEOPLE, when asked to carry out a simple motion like raising their eyebrows, will move many other unrelated parts of their body at the same time: the jaw may open in the other direction, the forearms tighten slightly, the rib cage contract, the toes may even curl—all seemingly to aid the raising of the eyebrows. These other movements are "parasitic" and contribute nothing; in fact, they detract from the intended movement. Arrays of parasitic movements throughout our bodies at all times accumulate in multiple levels of pain, uncoordination, numbness, lack of differentiation, and, ultimately, counterproductive behavior. Feldenkrais writes in *The Potent Self:*

> Many people fail to recognize the true cause of their inability or failure. The cause is very often not lack of ability, but improper use of self—there must not be too little an urge to do, a desire to act, nor too much. Now, we may not be able to influence our inheritance [i.e., our genetic anatomy], but we have a large measure of control

over our urges and over the means of freeing them from inhibiting agents of which we are rarely aware. We can learn to adjust our body tensions and the state of the nervous system, so that self-assertive and recuperative functions alternately dominate our frame. In this state of unstable balance, we find ourselves able to enact what we want more expediently.[44]

That is, by learning to carry out sets of initially destabilizing and confusing movements, we can rewire our neural and psychological patterns. The goal is—note—not some imaginary perfection, but an "unstable balance" free always to change into something else. Feldenkrais continues:

> We may be in a state of inability to enact any projected idea, from writing a letter to loving. Impotent rage and impotent love have a great deal in common. In both, the *desire* to do is excessive, and prevented from expression by extraneous and contradictory motives of equal intensity. . . . [Yet] that which is formed through personal

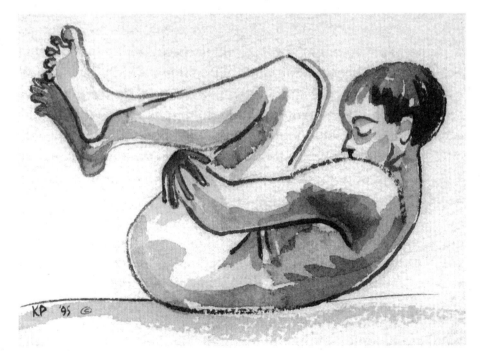

experience is essentially alterable and, *a priori*, capable of being influenced by a new personal experience.[45]

Elsewhere in the same book he writes:

The apparent ability of all of us is far below our latent ability, as contradictory motivation diminishes and tempers most of our actions. . . .

My considered opinion is that in general we only use a fraction of our latent capacity in most walks of life. The rest is buried in habitual contradictory motivation, to which we have become so accustomed as to be unable to feel what is happening.[46]

ALTHOUGH THE DESIRE to change is important, contradictory motivation doesn't just melt under the force of instruction and will. If double binds were that mutable, they would not become rigidified simultaneously in the brain, the neuromusculature, and the personality. "Each and every person, via the agency of their nervous system, makes the best choices possible given their perception of choices. . . . Granting intelligence to someone's personal history validates it. The practitioner's task is to create conditions for more choices. It is not to correct errors, right wrongs or straighten people out."[47]

The genius of the system is that, without invalidating or indicting present behavior, it provides schematic body-movement instructions for differentiating one's motivations and activities and unlocking the behavioral grid in which they are trapped.

When asked sarcastically by a frustrated student how to become "a genius like you," Feldenkrais answered with the wise restraint of a koan-master:

Most people spend their whole lives using their strengths to cover up and hide their weaknesses. They expend tremendous energy in keeping themselves a house divided. But if you surrender to your weakness therein lies your pathway to genius. A person who knows and utilizes his true weakness and uses his strength to include it is a whole person. He may seem rough around the edges, but there are so few people like that that they lead their generation.[48]

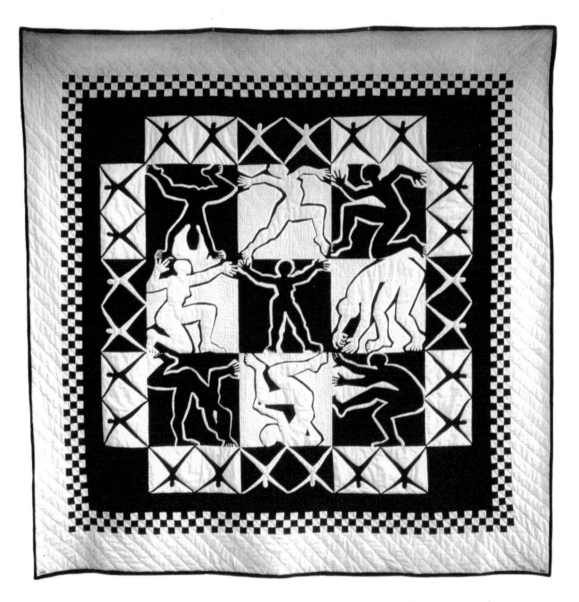

WITH A NOD to osteopathy, Feldenkrais developed an explicit palpative method of going with distortions until they released on
their own. Working with a person with scoliosis, he might instruct
him to lie down and then take the shorter leg on the thicker side and
stretch it toward the head. While this makes the leg all the shorter, it

also prevents the psoas muscle (that has been pulling the leg) from continuing to strain. Because the student is making the leg shorter than the muscle can pull, the muscle relaxes. Then the counter muscle can be stretched even longer. Both muscles now have new information, are in balance and communication with each other, and at the same time stimulated by fresh blood.[49]

> In another situation, Feldenkrais worked with a small boy with cerebral palsy whose knees pressed spastically together as he walked. He worked on the boy with his hands until his knees were "slightly separated, no longer locked in place." Then:
>
> Feldenkrais makes a fist, places it in the new space between the knees. "Now Ephraim," he says. "Please, can you press your knees against my fist." Then: "Come on, you can do better than that! Close your knees on my fist as hard as you can." He keeps it up, and Ephraim, no longer relaxed, is now straining mightily with the weak muscles on the inside of his thighs, an unaccustomed workout. Soon, "listening" carefully with his fist, Feldenkrais is satisfied that the time is right.
>
> "All right, Ephraim," he says, "you don't have to close your knees anymore. You can open them now." With clear relief, Ephraim relaxes, and opens his knees—all the way.
>
> "See how much easier it is to have your knees open? To close them requires work. To keep them open, you don't have to do anything at all." The boy moves his legs in and out, in apparent disbelief, then bursts into a peal of delighted laughter....
>
> In this session, Feldenkrais did not "contradict the nervous system" by trying to stretch the knees apart but utilized instead the boy's spastic pattern of holding his knees together. By exaggerating his "symptom," Ephraim was able to learn to make an involuntary movement voluntary.[50]

This feature of "not contradicting the nervous system" sets Feldenkrais work apart from many other forms of adjustment and manipulation in which practitioners try to antidote dysfunctional patterns by imposing new ones. It was not that Feldenkrais lacked concrete goals; it was that, in order to improve the likelihood of their successful outcome, he chose to impart them to each organism in a series of proprioceptive puzzles.

F UNCTION (AND HEALTH) are marked by unrestricted and facile movement within the limitations of the skeleton. "Correct coordinated action," to paraphrase Feldenkrais, is elegant action. To the outside observer and from the inside, such movement seems effortless, though there may be a great deal of actual work involved in sustaining it. Motion becomes more graceful the more it is felt. What is not felt, axiomatically cannot be changed.

Even victims of severe diseases, such as Parkinson's and multiple sclerosis, or paralyzing strokes and accidents can learn alternate neuromuscular pathways to seemingly lost behavior (walking, speaking, cognizing colors and faces). But the pathways must be fashioned step by step. Forced uncoordinated thrusts at the impossible only habituate overefforting and a sense of defeat. New coordination is invented by the body learning all over again how to move and enact functional behavior and record it in nervous tissue, much as it did in partnership with the mind in the first place.

The medical "meaning" of Feldenkrais' work is validated by his success in re-laying neural templates. For a stroke victim to be able to talk and write again is not dismissable as mere "pop psychology." Of one patient he treated successfully, Feldenkrais wrote:

> Nora, like every one of us, was not aware that the functions she had lost [by her stroke] were originally learned and not inherited as was her digestion or temperature regulation. Were these latter lost, then life would come to an end, but she had lost learned organization and like everybody else saw no difference between the *Homo sapiens* part of her and the animal part. She could not help herself and neither could anybody who was not aware of the difference. Many of the evils from which we suffer are rooted in our conception of human education as the training of a complete being to do this or that, as though we were making a computer perform a desired activity.[51]

What Feldenkrais discovered in the treatment of those who had severely damaged nervous systems was tantamount to a realization that all of us operate as if we were victims of neurological disorders. He sought a compassionate and scientific way for us to extricate ourselves from the dilemma of our own trap, basing his entire hope for the future of *Homo sapiens* on the belief that human beings had *just begun* to learn the range of things they were free to do.

ON THE ONE HAND, Feldenkrais Method is the work of a single man and thus a pale shadow of a millennial system like *Chi Gung*. On the other hand, it is also a millennial system, for it encompasses the entire history of Western civilization, from the first anatomical experiments of Hippocrates and Apollonius of Cyprus and the philosophical ontology of Aristotle to the early scientific research in neurology and phenomenological psychology.

Feldenkrais discovered processes of reeducating movement and breaking habitual patterns that no prior scientists had considered, let alone enacted, at least in part because they themselves were in such trances they were not even aware of the habitual patterns in which they proclaimed their freedoms and the primacy and objectivity of their science. As Dewey declared in praise of Matthias Alexander, education at this level bears the same relationship to education that education itself bears to all other human activities.

The Feldenkrais Method is thus much more than just the system of Moshe Feldenkrais. It is the primary method of Western (and possibly human) sensory-motor education. As such, it sits at the beginning of its historical development, and its potential and ramifications are limitless. Its final success, generations from now, would be a planetwide reorientation to the fact that we all need to learn new habits in order to make a more functional society. Then, long after people knew the name "Feldenkrais," each generation could set about inventing its own appropriate life lessons.

Rolfing

Like Moshe Feldenkrais, Ida Rolf developed her method of body work relatively late in life only after engagement in a number of other professions. In Rolf's case a Ph.D. in organic chemistry from Columbia University was followed by extensive instruction in yoga, osteopathy (including William Sutherland's cranial work), and homeopathy. While in London learning the Alexander Technique, she participated in a Gurdjieffian group at which she met Greta Garbo and Georgia O'Keefe, both of whom were, years later, to become part of her. She also studied Alfred Korzybski's General Semantics. However, the osteopathic influence was by far the most extensive and fundamental. According to historian of somatics Don Hanlon Johnson:

> Ida spent nearly fifty years of her professional life within the community of osteopaths and chiropractors. Her first encounter with that work occurred when she was a young adult on a camping trip to the Rockies in 1916 after graduating from Barnard College. While she was tying up her gear one afternoon, her horse kicked her. The next day she developed pneumonia. Within a very short time her breathing became so impaired and her fever so severe that she had to be taken to a small Montana town for help. To her surprise, the doctor prescribed a treatment from the local osteopath. After a . . . manipulation of her spine, her fever was immediately reduced and her breathing became normal. . . .
>
> The Montana osteopath's simple act of adjusting her spine was to have a lifelong impact on her conceptions of healing. It dramatically convinced her of the truth of the basic osteopathic principle enunciated by Andrew Still that structure determines function.[52]

The system devised by Rolf is an explicit hands-on method of improving health and changing dysfunctional behavior by altering structure. Rolfing could have been a branch of osteopathy, but it was not for a variety of reasons. First of all, Rolf devised her protocol of manipulation out of physical therapy and yoga, and she did so more

Ground Systems

229

as a biologist than as an osteopath. Secondly, she practiced at a time of far more rigid boundaries between fields and disciplines than prevail today; thus, she kept her own method distinct from osteopathy, Feldenkrais Method, and other techniques she respected and studied because she did not want to infringe on their turf and she wanted her own trademarked territory. Thirdly, she was never actually permitted by the osteopathic establishment to study their system as an outsider (so curious was she about the training and techniques that she volunteered as a secretary and went under cover to meetings in order to learn what was being taught).[53] Thus, while it is impossible for there not to be a major complement of osteopathy in Rolfing, Rolfing is a separate invention—and the entrepreneurial undertaking of an ambitious and independent-minded physical therapist.

Feldenkrais emphasized gradual reeducation; by contrast, Rolf developed an actual practitioner-imposed regimen for reorienting the parts of the body in relationship to one another so that they would function efficiently in the field of gravity in which we all exist. This meant first establishing a central vertical axis—the collective centers of gravity of all the centers of gravity in the body. The "Line" of gravity would be straight if all its centers were properly organized in relationship to one

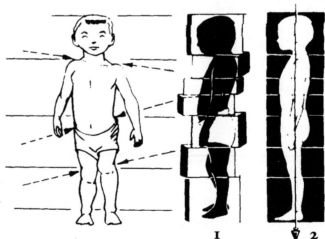

All bodies may be analyzed by seeing them as aggregates of blocks. The blocks have direct attention to the levels of rotation and therefore greatest strain on the body. To transform Johnny 1 into Johnny 2, whole blocks, not merely individual vertebral segments, must be realigned.

Reprinted from *Rolfing: The Integration of Human Structures* by Ida P. Rolf, Ph.D., Harper & Row, 1977.

another. To Rolf, the healthy body described by medical kinesiologists and even most osteopaths was actually poorly organized and functionally compromised. Eyeballing how the Line might look if a patient were integrated—and then carrying out the manipulative procedures necessary to approximate if not achieve this—was her method in a nutshell. It was heavy-duty remolding and structurally reimprinting the cellular masonry of connective tissue.

> If man weren't a standing, two-footed animal, he would have fewer problems. But he is standing, he is walking as best he can. He's been doing this since he was a kid—climbing up the side of his playpen and somehow getting his legs under him. Possibly he got his legs under him very badly, but he wasn't paying attention to that. He had one goal: he wanted to be like big brother, and big brother was able to walk.....[H]e didn't care how he did it, he only cared that he did it ... any old way.... Any old way disorganized his pelvis, disorganized his ribs, disorganized his head, disorganized the whole overlying structure.[54]

Massage, light adjustments, and exercises alone were inadequate to this task. Conventional osteopathy needed to be supplemented by a direct and explicit structural technique to address disorganization of the skeleton under the relentless vertical assault of gravity.

Rolfer Jeffrey Maitland says:

> The struggle with gravity and form is the human struggle. Our fondest theories about freedom and the transformation of consciousness are empty fantasies unless we realize that freedom at every level is always a matter of liberating our bodies. And liberating our bodies is a matter of creatively appropriating gravity. We cannot change gravity, but Dr. Rolf discovered and created a system of manipulation and movement education that can transform the way our bodies move and balance by transforming our relation to gravity....
>
> Beginning with the insight that the human body is a unified structural and functional whole that stands in a unique relation to the uncompromising presence of gravity, [she] asked this fundamental

question: "What conditions must be fulfilled in order for the human body-structure to be organized and integrated in gravity so that it can function in the most economical way?"[55]

The present rationale behind deep tissue work is that if the organism knew how to break its dysfunctional patterns of behavior, it would. It doesn't, so a somatic therapist must support—and even carry out—the feat. Rolf believed that verbal instruction and light, energetic touch (as was common in cranial osteopathy and Feldenkrais work) could not penetrate the full depths of the somaticization of character armor.

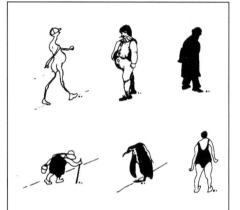

Many of our fellow citizens might be cartoons rather than patterned human energy fields. Their body language betrays their misuse of gravitational energy.

Reprinted from *Rolfing: The Integration of Human Structures* by Ida P. Rolf, Ph.D., Harper & Row, 1977.

The trained Rolfer quoins mainly mesodermal tissue to whatever degree of depth is tolerable to and integratable by the patient (and a little beyond, some might say). The goal over a number of such sessions is to accomplish a thorough and dynamic reintegration—a change in structure sustained at skeletal and cellular levels.

Rolfing uses the elastic qualities of the fascial connective tissues found everywhere in the body—these are the substructure of muscle fibers themselves bundled in fascia and surrounded by fascia, and the tendons, cartilage, and bone that grow from muscles as the body shapes itself in three dimensions. Made up of collagen fibers, fascia responds to injury, emotional trauma, and other pathology by shortening and becoming static. It loses its basic fluidity. Fascia invariably holds the strain patterns in the body as it struggles to find its most comfortable alignment in the gravitational and social field. But fascia can change form as well as maintain it, so it becomes collectively the vehicle for redesigning and reestablishing the architectural integrity of the body. Correctly applied tactile pressure can restore an initial state of fascial mobility and literally resculpt the body in it.

Writes Maitland:

> An organized body will ... exhibit an orthogonal order observable as horizontal and vertical lines/planes throughout the body's tissue. Fascial strain patterns are observable as twisting and/or oblique patterns or lines in the tissue. As these lines of fascial strain are eased through Rolfing manipulation, you will actually begin to see horizontals and verticals [lines and planes] in the tissue.[56]

Despite its reputation, Rolfing is not simply an engine of force; it is a mode of somatic education. Feldenkrais stated this unambiguously when he wrote to Rolf on the occasion of her eightieth birthday:

> Structural Integration and Functional Integration have much more in common than the word that connects them. Indeed, in the case of humans, structure and function are meaningless, one without the other.... [W]hen you integrate structure ..., you improve functioning.[57]

FULL INTEGRATION WITHIN the gravitational field marks the development of Rolfing as a mature system. However, in the early days, in 1942, after years of osteopathic study, Rolf began her new method of working with a far more modest first principle: "moving the soft tissue toward the place where it really belongs."[58] Slowly, day by day shifting the tissue of a forty-five-year-old friend who had been crippled from age eight as the result of an accident, Rolf got

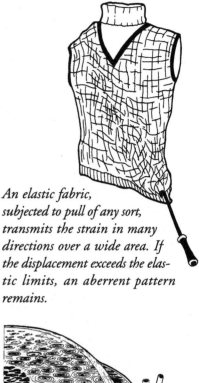

An elastic fabric, subjected to pull of any sort, transmits the strain in many directions over a wide area. If the displacement exceeds the elastic limits, an aberrent pattern remains.

Bone structure seems unitary although it is a patterned aggregate whose elements are unified only by their collective derivation from connective tissue. This is impregnated with deposits of calcareous salts that qualitatively and quantitatively vary according to age, mobility, exercise, etc.

Reprinted from *Rolfing: The Integration of Human Structures* by Ida P. Rolf, Ph.D., Harper & Row, 1977.

The Pelvis Has
Many Facets

Components
of the pelvis.
*While the function of
the bony pelvis can be
summarized as that of
a bony basin, it should
be remembered that the
development is from
several smaller bones.
Lateral views show the
fashion in which these
bones coalesce to form
the pelvis and how the
relative size of the individual segments alter
and shift to form the
pelvis from child to
adult.*

The pelvis is a bony basin.

LUMBAR
VERTEBRAE

SACRUM

COCCYX

ILIUM

PUBES

ISCHIUM

*Child
Lateral view*

*Adult
Lateral view*

Reprinted from *Rolfing: The Integration of Human Structures* by Ida P. Rolf, Ph.D., Harper & Row, 1977.

her on her feet and walking. To accomplish that she used whatever part
of her own body presented the most effective tool—fingers, fists, and
elbows—massaging not to relax and soothe but to change structure
even if the pressure was painful. "The manipulation is slow and often
extremely deep, the fingers going all the way through the abdomen,
for example, to touch the psoas muscle which lies directly in front of
the spinal column. Or behind the hard into the soft palate of the mouth,
even up into the nasal passages."[59]

MODALITIES

234

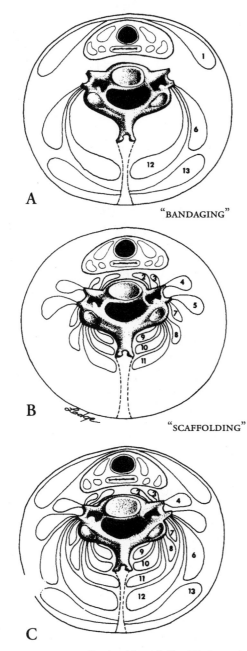

A

"BANDAGING"

B

"SCAFFOLDING"

C

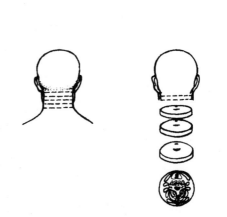

All three of these schemata are cross sections through the same upper cervical vertebra. A pictures muscles of the superficial level (in our terms, the extrinsic level), which act as bandaging and protection. B is the deeper level (in our terms, intrinsic), which as scaffolding maintains the position and spacing of vital cervical structures—autonomic nervous plexi, glandular units (thyroid, parathyroid), etc. And C is a combining of A and B. These muscles, attached horizontally to the bony vertebral structure at one end only, are directionally oriented by planes of fascia. Like all fascial planes, they are plastic and by slight elongation or shortening can change the tone of the related muscle. In so doing, they lessen or exaggerate pressure on vital structures. This changing pressure is the clue to migraine headaches—in fact to all headaches. Key: 1. Sternocleidomastoid. 2. Cervicis longus. 3. Longus capitus. 4. Scalenus anterior. 5. Scalenus medius. 6. Levator scapulae. 7. Costocervicalis. 8. Cervicis longissumus. 9. Multifidus. 10. Semispinalis cervicis. 12. Semispinalis capitus. 12. Splenius. 13. Trapezius.

Reprinted from *Rolfing: The Integration of Human Structures* by Ida P. Rolf, Ph.D., Harper & Row, 1977.

Years later, Rolf developed the skill of intuiting in a snapshot-like glance the alignment of a body and likewise its misalignment through fascial strain. As she recognized what was needed, she developed her famous *modus operandi* for reintegration. The process of resilient granulation might begin with the practitioner molding thoracic and clavicle musculature, freeing the patient's rib cage to enhance general breathing. Deep-tissue massage around the hips, hip joints, and thighs discriminates the legs from the pelvis. Later the fascia of the back is loosened, leading to release around the neck and also the crest of the ilium. In subsequent sessions the legs, ankles, feet, shoulders, and the rest of the back are stretched and sculpted into relationship with one another. The therapist might hammer out the legs by starting from the buttocks and working thumbprint by thumbprint down their dorsal musculature, at times instructing the client to resist her movements (which refines the sculpting and also provides dynamic recoils). The goal here is to open and give length to the entire body much like elongating out a coiled worm. In a still later session she might work the

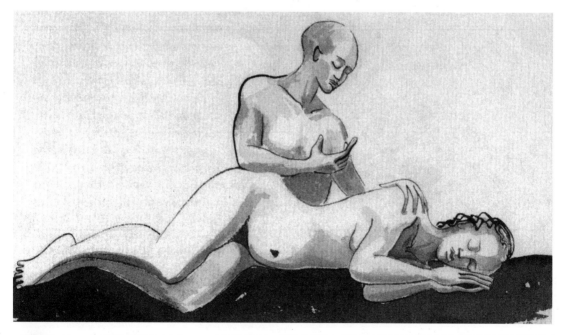

fingers and palms in along the forearms (right side, then left side), uncurling and freeing tissue around an imaginary bowl into the chest and ribs. Each week a different region is molded or a prior sequence is repeated depending upon how much of the imprinted architecture endures. The direction is always expansion, like octopus arms underwater, relieving pressure while spreading radially from the core.

Sometimes poisons are dislodged and flush out through bodily fluids, leaving a bitter taste and stench. On that level Rolfing is also a cleansing of the stream of blood and viscera, the one such connective-tissue-oriented mode. As in strikes from the Zen master's staff while one is sitting zazen, the pain serves as a reference point, a way for tissues to learn how to inhabit new postures. Pain also provides a margin of safety between the therapist and the client. The process must not go so fast that nothing is learned. The most skillful Rolfer works at the edge.

The sensation of being Rolfed is its most fabled aspect. Rolfing *does* hurt but as the fallout of pulling open blocks, restoring feeling, and

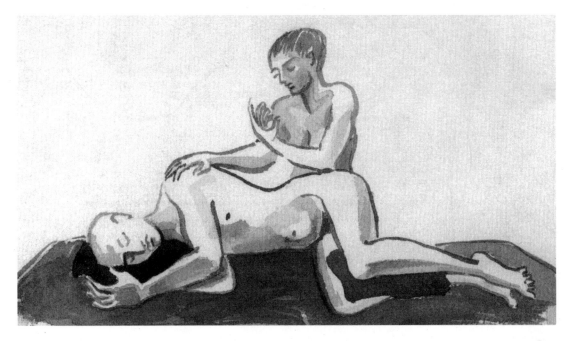

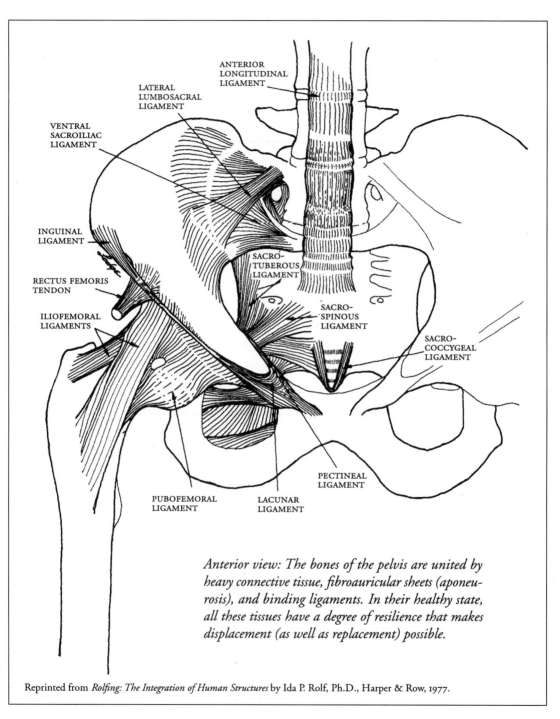

ANTERIOR
LONGITUDINAL
LIGAMENT

LATERAL
LUMBOSACRAL
LIGAMENT

VENTRAL
SACROILIAC
LIGAMENT

INGUINAL
LIGAMENT

RECTUS FEMORIS
TENDON

ILIOFEMORAL
LIGAMENTS

SACRO-
TUBEROUS
LIGAMENT

SACRO-
SPINOUS
LIGAMENT

SACRO-
COCCYGEAL
LIGAMENT

PECTINEAL
LIGAMENT

PUBOFEMORAL
LIGAMENT

LACUNAR
LIGAMENT

Anterior view: The bones of the pelvis are united by heavy connective tissue, fibroauricular sheets (aponeurosis), and binding ligaments. In their healthy state, all these tissues have a degree of resilience that makes displacement (as well as replacement) possible.

Reprinted from *Rolfing: The Integration of Human Structures* by Ida P. Rolf, Ph.D., Harper & Row, 1977.

238

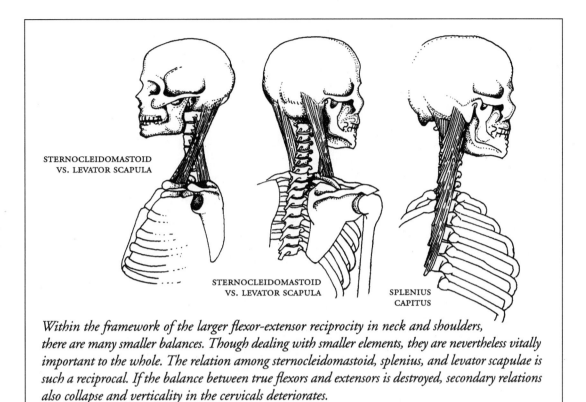

STERNOCLEIDOMASTOID
VS. LEVATOR SCAPULA

STERNOCLEIDOMASTOID
VS. LEVATOR SCAPULA

SPLENIUS
CAPITUS

Within the framework of the larger flexor-extensor reciprocity in neck and shoulders, there are many smaller balances. Though dealing with smaller elements, they are nevertheless vitally important to the whole. The relation among sternocleidomastoid, splenius, and levator scapulae is such a reciprocal. If the balance between true flexors and extensors is destroyed, secondary relations also collapse and verticality in the cervicals deteriorates.

Reprinted from *Rolfing: The Integration of Human Structures* by Ida P. Rolf, Ph.D., Harper & Row, 1977.

working back through old pathology according to the Hippocratic law of cure. It makes the body feel like crumbling clay coming to life. An electric rubbery sensation refreshes one's whole neural grid and leaves one full of breath, empty of thoughts, and embodied. At spots (for instance, around the pelvis and at the sacrum) the Rolfer's deep penetration may be like electric shocks which (ideally) dissolve into sensual tingles. It is a pleasurable pain, though that doesn't necessarily make it comfortable at the time. Many Rolfees tell "war stories," but it is usually with the pride of someone who has been through a shamanic battle zone.

I N THE DECADES that followed her development of a template, Rolf continued to expand her system, developing a training program and

Ground Systems

educating a lineage of practitioners. Ultimately she proposed a four-part protocol:

> 1. Consider the body as an aggregate of larger segments of weight (head, thorax, abdomen, pelvis, legs, feet) moving in the field of gravity.
>
> 2. The relationships among the segments (a person's unique body structure) are a function of balance and tension in the connective tissues that bind the segments into a unity.
>
> 3. Those tissues—fascia, tendons, ligaments and muscle groups—are plastic, capable of radical change.
>
> 4. The direction of this change can be either in the direction of entropy due to aging and trauma, or, through sensitive manipulation and educated self-awareness, in the direction of balance and harmony with the vertical field of gravity.[60]

IN THE EARLY YEARS the inner circle of practitioners of Structural Integration was small. Prior to the introduction of her techniques into the counterculture, Rolf spent some forty years teaching them solely to osteopaths, physiotherapists, adventurous orthopedic physicians, and others in seminars and developing her reputation from work with autistic children and within the general rehabilitative and physical-therapy community. Gradually she lost some of her standing within this guild because of her existential notions of personal freedom and her rejection of all medical models as too confining. But she became legendary in her own right. What she developed wrote its own insignia. Her very name defines a unique process and became a full-fledged verb expressing a deep visceral agency while ironically commenting on countercultural excess. This shows how both "wondrous strange" and utterly ridiculous the act of manually imprinting new memory in tissue appeared to popular culture. It wasn't massage; it was a mythic feat of body-molding (and a parody of well-intentioned torture) carried out by a charismatic woman—Rolfing.

Through the Human Potential Movement of the mid-1960s Rolf's work flowered and became widely known to the general public. The success of one of her early pupils in treating the serious heart condition of Fritz Perls, the founder of Gestalt, led to Perls bringing Rolf to Esalen Institute. There she found an eager group of trainees, many of them already advanced in radical psychiatry, diverse genres of bioenergetic manipulation, meditation, and holistic modes of healing. Among these students Rolf became an elder statesperson—at once seer, medicine woman, grandmother, and uncompromising mentor. Although she ascended to the level of a "Human Potential" guru, she was never comfortable with the blending of her work into Gestalt therapy, Reichian analysis, and avant-garde bodywork. She considered herself an elite Structural Integrationalist, and she did not favor the egalitarian philosophy of the counterculture. Toward the end of her life, she viewed Rolfing as a means of sculpting a new humanity according to a perfect Line—hardly a way to pass muster in today's "politically correct" holistic environment.

The rigidity and provinciality of Rolfing are reflected in its culture-bound notions of movement, body shape, and wholeness, and her failure to accommodate the wide variety of body types and movement styles practiced by non-Western peoples across the planet. The depth and humanity of Rolf's teaching, however, resonate in her emphasis on "harmonious spiritual consciousness" and tireless attempts to keep her students from trying merely to replicate functional cures. Contemporary Rolfers have unabashedly crossed the boundaries of this provinciality. Some, as noted, combine deep-tissue release with Taoist or Polarity energy work; others blend Rolfing's direct, linear techniques with the more indirect, nonlinear vectors of osteopathy and various craniosacral modalities. Jeffrey Maitland has merged Rolf's body-mind inquiry with the zazen of Buddhist meditation. The renowned Rolfer R. Louis Schultz has taken Rolfing into the forbidden territory of male genital work. The *corpus spongiosum* in the front of the penis and the *corpora cavernosa* at its back, extensions of mesodermal fascia, almost uniquely carry the imprint of men's sexual projections into their own tissue. The attempt to derive pleasure, sometimes forbidden, sometimes displaced, sometimes desperate, puts an enormous weight on the organ through which the erotic projections flow. Gentle Rolfing can unravel some of these kinks and distortions and balance the genital with the rest of the body.[61]

Interestingly, Rolfing of the penis makes its flesh feel just like any other bodily tissue, an unfamiliar and therapeutic state to men who tend to genitalize emotions. There are also Rolfers who work with female genitalia, but they do not publicize their work to the degree that Schultz docs. Not only is genital work with either gender an extension that would have appalled Ida Rolf, but it is also opposed by most Rolfers and illegal for all bodyworkers.

IDA ROLF WAS trapped at many levels of paradox and contradiction. She suffered the dilemma of teaching a doggedly physical system in the context of pluralistic and transcendental conceptions of mind, body, and spirit; she also held old-fashioned ideas about authority, discipline, and hierachy of transmission. At times, though, she stepped aside from reputation and orthodoxy and flouted her own pure mystery:

> One morning . . . Ida Rolf clumped into her living room at Big Sur where about twenty of us were assembled. "Word's going around Esalen that Ida Rolf thinks the body is all there is. Well, I want it known that I think there's more than the body, but the body is all you can get your hands on."[62]

Notes

The section on the Bates Method has been developed through discussions with Thomas R. Quackenbush, founder and director of the Natural Vision Center of Ashland, Oregon. See also *Better Eyesight: The Complete Magazines of William H. Bates,* edited by Thomas R. Quackenbush (Berkeley, California: North Atlantic Books, 2001), and *Relearning to See* by Thomas R. Quackenbush (Berkeley, California: North Atlantic Books, 1997).

1. Gerda Alexander, *Eutony,* p. 8.

2. Ibid., p. 168.

3. Ibid., p. 54.

4. Ibid., p. 148.

5. Quoted in Gerda Alexander, *Eutony,* p. 149.

6. Gerda Alexander, *Eutony,* p. 168.

7. Nevill Drury, *The Healing Power: A Handbook of Alternative Medicines and Natural Health* (London: Frederick Muller Ltd., 1981), p. 16.

8. Don Hanlon Johnson, *Body, Spirit, and Democracy* (Berkeley, California: North Atlantic Books, 1993), p. 65.

9. Richard Brennan, *The Alexander Technique Workbook* (Rockport, Massachusetts: Element Books, Ltd., 1992), pp. 2–3, 9–11.

10. In these descriptions I received help from Alexander practitioner Jerry Sontag, whom I gratefully acknowledge.

11. Brennan, *The Alexander Technique Workbook,* pp. 3–4.

12. Johnson, *Body, Spirit, and Democracy,* pp. 65–66.

13. F. Matthias Alexander, quoted in Brennan, *The Alexander Technique Workbook,* p. 12.

14. Drury, *The Healing Power,* pp. 16–17.

15. Jerry Sontag, notes on *Planet Medicine,* 1994.

16. F. Matthias Alexander, quoted in Brennan, *The Alexander Technique Workbook,* p. 67.

17. Ilana Rubenfeld, "Alexander: The Use of the Self," in Leslie J. Kaslof (editor), *Wholistic Dimensions in Healing: A Resource Guide* (New York: Doubleday & Company, Inc., 1978), p. 223.

18. Ibid.

19. Ibid.

20. Mia Segal, interview in *Somatics* (Autumn/Winter 1985–86), p. 10.

21. Quote supplied by Jerry Sontag.

22. Quoted in Rubenfeld, "Alexander: The Use of the Self," p. 224.

23. Charles Olson, *The Maximus Poems* (originally 1950) (Berkeley: University of California Press, 1979), pp. 64–65.

24. William H. Bates, quoted by Thomas R. Quackenbush, personal communication, Berkeley, California, 1995.

25. Ibid.

26. Quackenbush, personal communication, Berkeley, California, 1995.

27. William Bates, quoted by Quackenbush.

28. Dennis Leri, "Learning How to Learn," unpublished draft used as the basis for a variety of published articles.

29. Ibid.

30. Jack Heggie, personal communication, 1994.

31. Bruce Kumar Frantzis, *The Tao in Action: The Personal Practice of the I Ching and Taoism in Daily Life,* unpublished manuscript.

32. Robert Spencer, personal communication, 1994.

33. Quoted in Leri, "Learning How to Learn."

34. Leri, "Learning How to Learn."

35. Ibid.

36. Ibid.

37. Elizabeth Beringer assisted me by writing notes on this section and a critique of my earlier version which I have drawn upon for the current version.

38. Leri, "Learning How to Learn."

39. Moshe Feldenkrais, quoted in William S. Leigh, *Bodytherapy* (Coquitlam, British Columbia: Water Margin Press, 1989), pp. 54–55.

40. Leri, "Learning How to Learn."

41. Moshe Feldenkrais, quoted in Mark Reese, "Moshe Feldenkrais' Verbal Approach to Somatic Education: Parallels to Milton Erickson's Use of Language," in *Somatics* (Autumn/Winter 1985–86), p. 27.

42. Moshe Feldenkrais, quoted in Leigh, *Bodytherapy,* p. 56.

43. Moshe Feldenkrais, *The Potent Self: A Guide to Spontaneity* (Berkeley, California: Frog, Ltd., 2002), p. 130.

44. Ibid., pp. 3–4.

45. Ibid., p. 4.

46. Ibid., p. 28.

47. Leri, "Learning How to Learn."

48. Quoted in Leri, "Learning How to Learn."

49. Leigh, *Bodytherapy,* p. 56.

50. Moshe Feldenkrais, quoted in Reese, "Moshe Feldenkrais' Verbal Approach to Somatic Education," p. 28.

51. Moshe Feldenkrais, *The Case of Nora: Body Awareness as Healing Therapy* (originally 1977) (Berkeley, California: Frog, Ltd., 1993), p. 64.

52. Johnson, *Body, Spirit, and Democracy,* pp. 81–82.

53. Michael Salveson, personal communication, Berkeley, California, 1974.

54. Ida Rolf, *Ida Rolf Talks About Rolfing and Physical Reality* (New York: Harper & Row, 1978), p. 70.

55. Jeffrey Maitland, *Spacious Body: Explorations in Somatic Ontology* (Berkeley, California: North Atlantic Books, 1995), pp. 142–143.

56. Ibid., p. 167.

57. Moshe Feldenkrais, quoted in Leigh, *Bodytherapy*, p. 23.

58. Ida Rolf, quoted in Johnson, *Body, Spirit, and Democracy*, p. 84.

59. Johnson, *Body, Spirit, and Democracy*, p. 85.

60. Johnson, *Body, Spirit, and Democracy*, p. 87.

61. R. Louis Schultz, *Out in the Open: The Complete Male Pelvis* (Berkeley, California: North Atlantic Books, 1999).

62. Don Hanlon Johnson, *The Protean Body* (New York: Harper and Row, 1977), p. 140.

CHAPTER FIVE

Osteopathy and Chiropractic

Bone

THE SKELETAL FRAME of the body is made of the same material as its blood, retina, and heart. Cells within bone share an immediate, direct ancestry with cells of muscles and organs. Of course, all cells in a body originate from the single sperm and egg, and those that become skeletal must pass through visceral phases before crystallizing. Mesenchymal cells do this by sliding frictionally, dessicating, and packing more closely together, not by altering their animate nature.

Bone is living, changing tissue—fluid, neuromuscular, sensual. It is biochemically active and participates in metabolism and immunity. To engage bone therapeutically is to work not just at a skeletal level but in depth and at core. Anthroposophically, bone is the hardened state of the first wave of spirit to encounter the realm of matter. Raw soul, entering the force field created by the embryo, is whorled deeper and deeper in a physical dimension until it resembles stone—a fascial cave of accreting lime. In the singular deed of grounding spirit, tissue becomes osseous and electromagnetic, a quartz doll along the axis of the body's manifestation. This creature state develops unique characteristics, even as hydrogen and nitrogen manifest new qualities when liquified or frozen. In the case of bone it is a psychosomatic liquifying and freezing, and the effect is alchemical. Bone is body/mind's transsubstantiating medicine bundle. It is an active field of morphogenetic shear planes and visceral, energetic potentials. Bones are not only structural girders but wands and generators. Multilingual, they distribute biodynamic codes.

Systems of therapeutics based on the handling and palpation of bones are core therapies. They can be more intrinsic and effective than the most powerful drugs and radiation. The impression that they are superficial and mechanical is an offshoot of the unexamined belief that bone is fixed and inert—a stony lattice for the "real" biological functions of brain, blood, and kidneys. Though not all osteopathic professions acknowledge skeletal vitality, all are based (at least in part) on the fluidity of bone and its essential faculty of transmitting protean medicine into the entirety of body/mind. The medicine itself may be an actual biological substance (an enzyme or trace mineral), an electrical signal or subcellular rune, or an energetic adjustment that spreads globally.*

An adjustment of bone is an adjustment of character and the unconscious self. The failure of psychoanalysis to recognize this has forestalled a possible healing discipline of unprecedented effectiveness combining cranial osteopathy and Freudian transference.

However categorized, osteopathy is still a foundation psychosomatic medicine, a complete route-map through body/mind, and a holistic vehicle for the embryogenic transmission of *prana*.

Bones serve as discrete pathways to the neuromusculature, immune system, and psyche in a number of ways (that are probably different versions of one another). They build up, store, and transmit the tension of displacement from morphogenesis and environmental and internal bumps and torques. They impinge upon and support and restrict

---

*I am using the term "osteopathy" in two simultaneous contexts here: the specific therapeutic discipline developed by Andrew Taylor Still in the nineteenth century and a diverse range of manual medicines and musculoskeletal, myofascial, neurovisceral palpation techniques practiced traditionally on bones, muscles, and nervous systems before Still's declaration of a science.

viscera and nerves. They manufacture stem marrow. They transfuse a sense of either organic wholeness or fragmentation.

In skeletal therapies, bone is used to simplify confused systemic tendencies, sort crossed motivations, establish deeper unity, and transmute sensation into meanings. Bone energy is discharged through dreams, dances, diseases, desires, and personae. By another interpretation each individual bone (atlas, sphenoid, sacrum, pelvis, etc.) is a puzzle piece within the wholeness of the organism. This means each bone in terms of its gross shape but also in terms of the subtle variations of angle, density, and design that separate one person from another and one species from another. Bones are signatures and amulets of identity and dialect.

A comparison of mammalian bones (see illustrations on the following pages) reveals a network of declivity leading to the evolutionary functions of individual creatures—i.e., the way in which each uses its shape to engage the world and express its particularity. Each human atlas, sacrum, and pelvis likewise contains an imprint of lineage and life experiences. Precisely the subtle and discrete equivalents of anatomical differences that occur at the level of species discrimination are what an osteopathic therapist attempts to locate and reenergize at a systemic level within individuals.

What is fixed and artifactual in a nonphilosophical beast can become symbolic and characterological inside a human aura. A species of animal loose on the prairie or in the sky can become a dream or a "disease" inside a person, and a cure as well. A skeleton is an autochthon, a totem (as American Indian doctors implicitly understood). The map of mammalian bone variations is a map of character and (metaphorically) a chart of both successful and unsuccessful styles of self-healing (survival) in us. Each totem contains within it a charge powerful enough to make the difference between a bobcat and a squirrel and the domains they master in nature. Clearly then it has the power to restore locally pathologized tissue grids to a vital state.

PELVIS

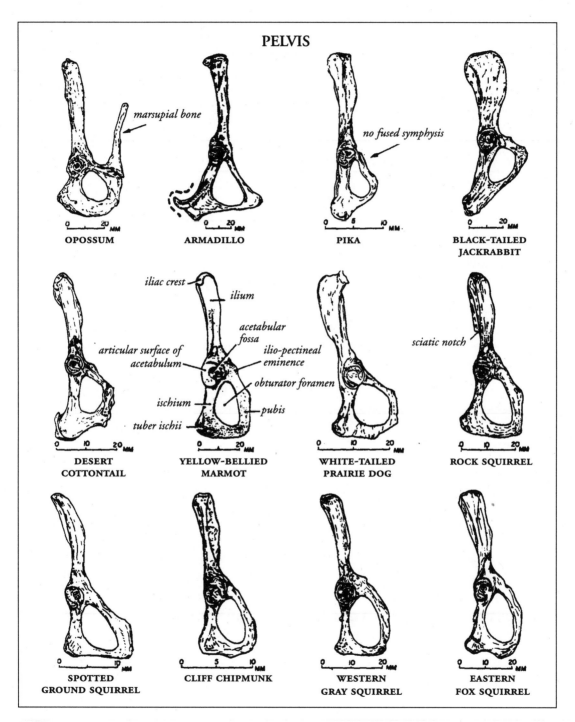

marsupial bone

no fused symphysis

iliac crest

ilium

acetabular fossa

articular surface of acetabulum

ilio-pectineal eminence

obturator foramen

ischium

pubis

tuber ischii

sciatic notch

OPOSSUM

ARMADILLO

PIKA

BLACK-TAILED JACKRABBIT

DESERT COTTONTAIL

YELLOW-BELLIED MARMOT

WHITE-TAILED PRAIRIE DOG

ROCK SQUIRREL

SPOTTED GROUND SQUIRREL

CLIFF CHIPMUNK

WESTERN GRAY SQUIRREL

EASTERN FOX SQUIRREL

SACRUM

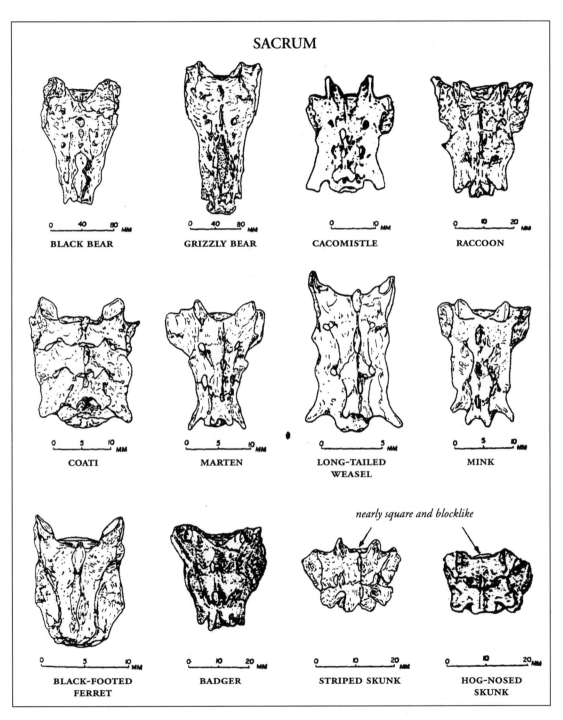

BLACK BEAR

GRIZZLY BEAR

CACOMISTLE

RACCOON

COATI

MARTEN

LONG-TAILED
WEASEL

MINK

nearly square and blocklike

BLACK-FOOTED
FERRET

BADGER

STRIPED SKUNK

HOG-NOSED
SKUNK

ATLAS

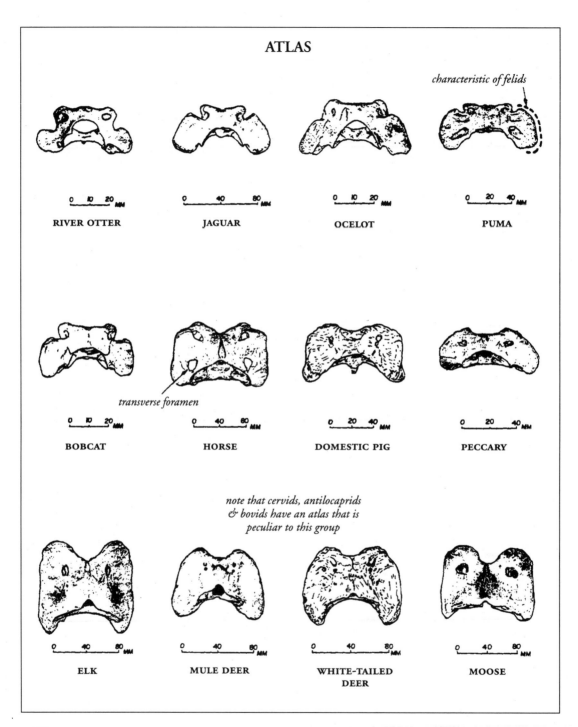

characteristic of felids

RIVER OTTER   JAGUAR   OCELOT   PUMA

transverse foramen

BOBCAT   HORSE   DOMESTIC PIG   PECCARY

*note that cervids, antilocaprids
& bovids have an atlas that is
peculiar to this group*

ELK   MULE DEER   WHITE-TAILED DEER   MOOSE

Osteopathy

Historically a nineteenth-century scientific manual medicine, osteopathy has become a relativistic system for energy transduction. Osteopathy is also a rebirth of an original mechanical medicine practiced with a million variants by groups from tribes of Africa and the rain-forest bands of South America to island peoples of the Pacific and folk doctors of Europe. It provides an intact model for the role of ancient manual therapies in the development of new alternative modalities.

Osteopathy-like folk traditions of "trampling in the fields," "weighing salt," and "the shepherd's hug" arose worldwide and hearken back to Neolithic and probably Palaeolithic times (see "Mechanical Ethnomedicine" in Volume One, Chapter Five). Sailors at most Third and Fourth World ports still find remarkable native manipulators and bonesetters practicing these crafts, passed from generation to generation, on the streets. These heal organic diseases as well as skeletal ones; they have no written tradition, no formal school, no medical theory, and no contact with one another from Tahiti to Mexico to India to Madagascar. Andrew Still's later invention of osteopathy as a system and Daniel Palmer's chiropractic variation were revivals of traditional bone-setting and healing touch. They systematized manipulative lore according to a version of intellectual anatomy and physics and provided a mainstream arena for the fusion of all tribal and ethnic modalities of therapeutic adjustment and palpation under one tent.

Weighing salt, one of the oldest somatic techniques on Earth

By now, both osteopathy and chiropractic have been enlarged and transformed to incorporate an even greater variety of native and Oriental bone and visceral-energy techniques.

The osteopathic paradigm has helped birth many major somatic disciplines, including Polarity Therapy, Rolfing, craniosacral therapy, and Zero Balancing. In its holistic mode, osteopathy has contributed subtle-energy and palpation techniques directly to a spectrum of hands-on methods, including visceral adjustment, lymphatic drainage, hydraulic application of stillpoints, strain-counterstrain, fascial triggerpoints, and the general psychosomatic transfer of kinetics out of body blocks and traumas into functional flow.

Osteopathy embraces a profound original contradiction. It would appear that A. T. Still, while proposing rather mechanical and material medical precepts, inadvertently discovered *another* system and, without realizing it, tapped into the vital organizing life current. Samuel Hahnemann stumbled upon homeopathy's energetic microdoses because he did not realize that high molecular dilutions were chemically inert; thus, he applied them medicinally as if they were extremely elevated potencies of matter and ascribed dynamic effects to them. Still entered a realm of mysterious visceral energy by not understanding that his mechanical model was merely the entry point into the meta-mechanical complexity of organized cells. While stacking weights and densities of tissues and balancing fascia, he invented a system for conducting energetics within living fields of bones and tissues. Osteopathy, which began as physics-like equations of mass and surgery-like manipulations, spawned techniques as vitalistic as those of Reiki or homeopathy.

An offshoot of the bone-setter's unique method of feeling and interrogating anatomy and disease, osteopathy was reinvented, named, modernized, and formalized by Still; subsequently it developed its own new lineage. On the surface, the osteopathic perspective is Solidist and Rationalist (see Volume One, pp. 265–281), viewing the body as a dense geometric grid supported by a skeleton, activated by nerves, and permeated with channels flushed by systolic and diastolic motion. Trained academically as an engineer, Still could not help but initially view the organism as another dynamic system, one that occasionally developed congestions and blocks. He improvised corrections based on his intuition of mechanical relationships among its parts (i.e., bones, fascia, circulations of fluids). The son of a doctor, he had once attempted allopathy and given up on it:

> I was born and raised to respect and confide in the remedial power of drugs, but after many years of practice in close conformity to the dictation of the very best medical authors and in consultation with representatives of the various schools, I failed to get from drugs the results hoped for and I was face to face with the evidence that medicine was not only untrustworthy but dangerous.
>
> The mechanical principles on which osteopathy is based are as old as the universe. I discovered them while I was in Kansas. You can call this discovery accidental or purely philosophical. I was in the practice of medicine and had been for several years. I treated my patients as other doctors did. A part of them got well and a part of them died. Others both old and young got sick and got well without the assistance of the medical doctor.
>
> As I was an educated engineer of five years' schooling I began to look at the human framework as a machine and examine all its parts to see if I could find any variation from the truly normal among its journals, belts, pulleys, and escape pipes. I began to experiment with man's body as a master mechanic would when he had in his charge any machinery which needed to be kept perfectly adjusted and in line in order to get perfect work. There are many ways by which a machine may be adjusted. An osteopathic operator is not expected to depend on any one method or manipulation for the adjustment of a bone.[1]

Still did not. During the 1870s he cultivated modes of treatment based on ever more subtle analyses of anatomical relationships. "We, as engineers, have but one question to ask," he asserted: "What has the body failed to do?"[2]

Osteopathy works by asking concrete questions of pulsating, dynamic bodies, by engaging in manual, subtle-energy dialogues with tissues. It begins with basic structure and flow.

The philosophy of manipulations is based upon an absolute knowledge of the form and function of all bones belonging to the bony framework of the human body.... Simply to know that our heads are situated upon the atlas and the atlas on the axis, that we have seven bones in the neck, twelve in the dorsal region and five in the lumbar is of little use. We must have a perfect image of the normal articulations of the bone or bones that we wish to adjust. We must be critically certain that we know all articulations of the bones in the whole system. We must know how blood is supplied and when that arterial blood has done its work we must know how it returns and what would be an obstruction to prevent its return.... Nature is a living critic and the answer must be yes or no....[3]

A T THE TURN of the twentieth century, most other manual therapies were sectarian and segregated by modality. They did not influence mainstream therapeutics and were isolated from one another. Some were breathing-oriented or exercise regimes associated with spas. Some were orphans of both hermetic and quasi-scientific vitalistic schools employing theories of magnetism and life-force stimulation. Others involved linear applications of manipulation or calisthenics to skeletal and muscular defects, or they undertook corrections of culturally defined weaknesses of the body by adjustment and exercise. Amateur surgeries in the context of phrenology and other metaphysical systems of diagnostic anatomy also informed early osteopathy and chiropractic.

Underlying all of these was the empirical legacy of an ancient guild of doctors who treated the body directly, maintaining a rigorous protocol of techniques and using all available somatic tools and insights. Members of the original clan of healers, these medicine men and women shared an identity and work-ethic through the evolution of society with carpenters, boat-builders, cooks, nurses, and hunters. Blue-collar at heart, they did not join the early elitist guilds of philosophers and scientists that became professional medicine. They may have participated at some level in the Hippocratic synthesis in Greece, but they were back on their own by the time of Galen's formalized anatomical theory that laid the foundation for allopathy.

The empirical hands-on tradition did not ignore mainstream medical technology and the advent of surgery. Anything that contributed to manual cures they either considered or adopted; thus, their system so closely paralleled professional medicine as to be almost indistinguishable from it even to the point where today osteopathy remains a twin to allopathy. Many osteopaths are essentially allopaths with a manual specialty. Meanwhile, some older allopaths continue to apply manual principles by habit, though such ecumenical practitioners are now sadly dying out. Earlier allopaths in general were not as far removed from manual medicine and "feeling" the living, energetic aspects of tissue as later medical-school graduates because they did not have anything like the present-day array of technology and synthetic drugs to incorporate. They *had to* palpate structure and intuit what was right or wrong. They were decidedly outcome-oriented rather than theoretical.

Insofar as the critical kinetic junctions among bones, muscles, and nerves are more or less obvious, there is no reason to question the potential effectiveness of osteopathy in the treatment of injuries, strains, sciatica, or even constipation. In this context osteopathy is no more or less than an expanded version of therapeutic massage and maternal care-giving. But Still gradually enlarged his system to address pneumonia, diabetes, mumps, hysteria, alcoholism, mental disease, and the like. Even though he also employed pharmacy, diet, hygiene, surgery, and verbal therapy (he meant his osteopathy to be a complete system of medicine rivalling allopathy), his emphasis was primarily on understanding and reorganizing anatomy, not only in the gross sense but at ever more subtle levels of hormonal and fascial microanatomy until he had mastered the entire anatomicophysiological mechanism.

Although there was no consistent formula to Still's techniques, he did generally seek by pressure and movement to restore blood supply and nerve responsiveness in afflicted areas; he worked from the perspective that natural flow would lead to the organs' reestablishing their original dynamic relationships and harmonics. He did not have to try to antidote every germ and flush out every toxin because a kinetic system regaining its own efficiency would accomplish all that without further toxic interference.

Still gradually came to endow the kinetic life system with almost magical properties. He perceived that the circulation of fluids, energy, and substances through the body was so subtle and highly complex that it occurred on many levels simultaneously, including not only arterial, venous, nervous, lymphatic, and cerebrospinal components but also others foreshadowing axoplasmic flow. What he could not explicitly assign to a level of circulation, he assigned to the collective circulatory mechanism. Beginning as an ardent materialist, he ended up describing the lungs as "organs, beings or personalities of life . . . the functions of the heart . . . imparting life and knowledge to the blood."[4] He likely strayed upon some of the same ostensibly vital reactions that *Chi Gung* therapists and Hippocratic doctors attributed to causes specified by their own paradigms. While his treatments activated ever more discrete and discriminative layers within the body, he stuck patriotically to his mechanical epistemology:

> To the osteopath who understands the human body as the engineer does his engine, all the mysteries disappear. . . . He squares, plumbs and levels all foundations, journals and boxings. He examines all pulleys to know that they are in place and position. He examines the belt to see if one side is longer than the other. He corrects and goes on. . . . With the square and plumb he adjusts the drive wheels, pulleys and journals, then he inspects all pipes conducting water to his boiler and all pipes conducting steam to the chest.[5]

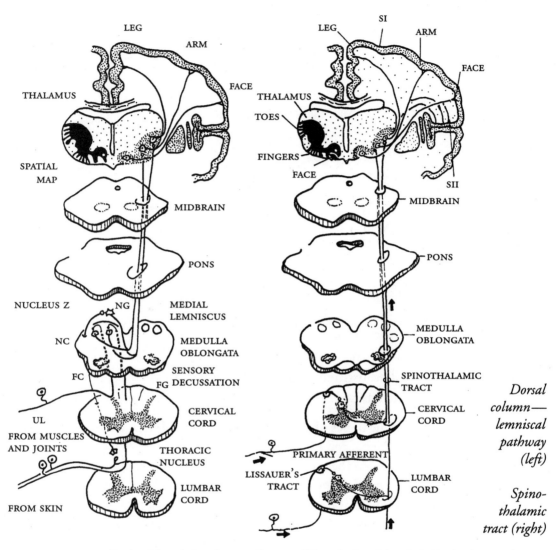

Reprinted from *An Introduction to Craniosacral Therapy* by Don Cohen, D.C., North Atlantic Books, 1995.

Still's trademark was his emphasis on diseased conditions originating in the head, neck, thorax, abdomen, and pelvis, with particular concern for encumbrances in the pelvic zone, all of which ultimately engaged organs like the kidneys, spleen, lungs, and heart. His mechanical treatments are models of ingenuity, and they were responsible for much of osteopathy's early success. For instance, he explained pneu-

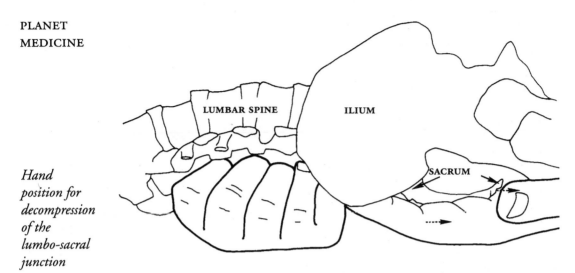

*Hand
position for
decompression
of the
lumbo-sacral
junction*

monia as a constriction of the thoracic/pulmonary system leading to
stagnation of the venous system and impure blood, curable through
sequential adjustments of different bones. In the case of a cataract of
the eye, he advises:

> Adjust the bones of the upper spine, ribs and neck and re-establish
> normal nerve and blood supply. Then make a gentle tapping of the
> eye to loosen the crystalline lens a little. With one finger give a few
> flips or gentle taps on the back of another finger the soft part of
> which is held against the side of the eye. This tapping should be just
> strong enough to make the eye ache a little. Without any surgical
> interference whatever I have been rewarded in a majority of cases by
> the disappearance of that white substance in the eye called a cataract.[6]

For constipation:

> ... [W]hen the pelvis is crowded and impacted with bowel, uterus,
> bladder, fecal matter or any foreign growths he [the osteopath] must
> get a free return of the venous blood with a normal action of the
> lymphatics, in order that they may throw off the water fluids to sup-
> ply the intestines. He can expect normal action of the bowel to appear

very soon after the drawing up of the viscera from out of its impacted condition in the pelvic cavity.[7]

For drunkenness:

> I found the ribs in the region of his left shoulder pushed upward. I threw his arm up putting the ribs on a strain and placed them back into position, and then said to him, "Now go into the saloon and come back, and if you do not want to turn sick at the smell of liquor I will pay for the whiskey."[8]

Osteopathy rests more upon a working set of intuitions and empirical discoveries than upon an explicit logic of disease causation and cure. Still himself was forced to revise even his own primary axiom. According to critical medical historians:

> ... [W]hen it was made clear to him that any spinal dislocation large enough to block the artery would give rise to a complete paraplegia, if not instant death from rupture of aorta, he changed this "Rule of the Artery" to pressure on a nerve, disease now resulting from the cessation of vital force transmitted to an organ along the nerve-trunk. This idea has scarcely been modified since....[9]

That is not true. The "meaning" of osteopathic adjustment was never unidimensional. It has been modified from decade to decade and is now in the service of a psychodynamic and holistic paradigm, casting its lot with other so-called "quantum medicines." The nerves have become merely a metaphor for the transfer and transmutation of a substance more resembling *chi* than synapses. The reference to "nerves" among osteopaths is now a subtext for a "feeling" or homeostasis that in some fashion lies at the basis of most health and pathology.

Osteopathy is post-Newtonian Hippocratic medicine carried out with trust in touch, dexterity, and intuitions of anatomical pathways rather than by disease classes and pathological cause and effect. It features the physician more as juggler, *bricoleur,* and martial artist than as laboratory technician and surgeon. The initial prejudice is to think that osteopathy cannot be the same as medicine or as therapeutic because it lacks sophisticated tools and intellectual categories and utilizes mere mechanical and skeletal adjustment or visceral massage—as though to stroke the intestinal region could cure a cancer as effectively as to cut into the very tissue.

But if we view the osteopathic principles from a different perspective, we can see that osteopathy is also a complex and complete medicine. It proposes treatments based as much on mechanical cause and effect as allopathy, though it translates the burden of mechanical correction to the already-functioning organism, which is viewed as perfect. Osteopathy doesn't need heavy equipment because, like other "homeopathic" treatments, it relies on the viscera to respond self-curatively to a quantum of energy directed appropriately in the right spot.

Allopathy, with its more entropic view of the universe, takes account of the grand array of parasites, germs, viruses, bacteria, toxins, and "bad" genes and assumes constant remedial work is needed for each of us even to survive. In a sense, modern medicine boggles itself with the complexity of the universe to such a degree that diagnosing and correcting defects become substitutes for ordinary living. Daily life has become commoditized and medicalized, and health has become an oracle and superstition, even a fetish, rather than simply the fact of our being.

Osteopathy, by contrast, assumes that most pathology can be reversed by simple mechanical stimulation or manipulation, that the body is already working well enough to solve most of its problems but will respond favorably to a sensitively directed adjustment. Like a dancer catching the beat of music, the organism picks up the curative vector.

If the latter example approaches gross medical oversimplification, the former risks the fallacies of hygienic obsession and thermodynamic reductionism. We do not actually understand the true underlying principle that links cells together and induces them to conduct chemical cycles and metabolism functionally.

Many of the theories common to allopathy are also employed in osteopathy (isolation and neutralization of pathologizing tissue complexes and pathogens)—yet from a tissue-sensitive and stimulative perspective, less surgical and antibiotic, almost always simpler, less microbial and viral—because osteopathy premises that we exist primarily and self-organizedly at the level of interrelationships of bones, fluids, and viscera. It considers most of the synthetic chemical, radiational, genetic, and surgical modalities dangerously invasive, for they undermine an ontologically prior level of function and self-healing and seek to penetrate, according to a purely conceptual and idealized paradigm, the molecular realm where disease products supposedly originate and spread.

By the allopathic line of reasoning, atomic and subatomic medicines must one day take over tracking the origin of all diseases and curing those that can be cured. But what if none of this is possible, efficient, or even necessary? What if the molecular and atomic realms are not the functional dimension of life? What if these contain mere subsidiary effects of events originating elsewhere, their core inalterable (or inalterable on a level of matter separate of mind)? What if creatures have all the requirements for health fully and holistically integrated at a tissue level? What if the cohesive synergy of cells is the sole active psychosomatic level of life?

By this line of reasoning, osteopathy is not only directly medical but in some ways more medical than surgery. Far from being superficial, its touch is exquisite, as the physician works his way into the patient's system by assessing complex reciprocal forces, stacking lines of tension and immobility, meeting and incrementalizing tissue resistance, and following sensations and distortions to their exact sources. What could be more empirical? Why valorize surgery such that it is declared automatically more scientific and profound than guided manipulation? Who established a rule that you have proximally to contact and incise actual disease products in order to heal tissues? If actual illnesses are the consequence of deeper imbalances rather than the source of the diseases they give names to, then orthodox medicine would be regularly attacking the effects of pathology rather than its causes. It would be invading nonlinear homeostatic systems with one-dimensional vectors.

Along these parameters, surgery is not a technological advance but a retreat from pure science of some hypothetical twenty-fifth century—a refuge only for the entrenched allopath who does not want to consider the whole holographic system and its interrelationships as much as he wants to find shortcuts to produce temporary but dramatic results. His access to a machinery of overkill and his allegiance to the lineage of that machinery leads to his removing structures that may have future use. Still writes:

> I am proud of osteopathic surgery which never uses a knife for the removal of tumors of the breast, abdomen or any other part of the body, until the arterial supply and venous drainage have failed to restore vitality and reduce the system and its organs to their normal functioning. Through the arterial supply and the venous drainage a large percent of tumors of the abdomen and breast will vanish in the hands of a trustworthy and philosophical osteopathic doctor.[10]

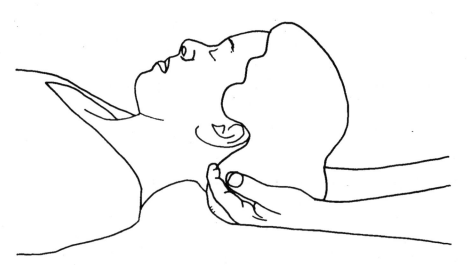

*Occipital
decompression*

Reprinted from *An Introduction to Craniosacral Therapy* by Don Cohen, D.C., North Atlantic Books, 1995.

THE MEDICINE OF sensitivity and vitality Still initiated is not fully realized even today. There is a prevailing illusion that osteopathy was accepted and accreted into mainstream medicine decades ago and no longer exists in its traditional form. Yes, a large number of former osteopaths abandoned the aspect of their trade that made them holistic doctors and became allopaths. In that form, osteopathy as an empty name made it into the mainstream. As energetic medicine, it all but disappeared. Allopathically oriented osteopaths now have their own medical schools and practice in allopathic hospitals. This outcome speaks neither to the success nor failure of Still's and Sutherland's science but to the effectiveness of the AMA in bullying its unorthodox practitioners into submission. Osteopaths who maintained their own specialty went into hiding and practiced only secretly. Old-school doctors had to know a person really well before they would treat him with their real repertoire. Otherwise, they practiced a superficial massage-like "parody" of osteopathy, ever in fear of medical police. Many refused to sell their books and destroyed their unpublished writings at death. Some privately published texts and distributed them one by one. It took lawsuits citing the First Amendment simply to make the writings available to the general public in the 1960s.[11]

Osteopathy has ironically become a profession in which those bearing its name (osteopaths by shingle) don't practice it, and those who practice it (craniosacral therapists, visceral manipulators, drainers of lymph, etc.) are not "osteopaths" and are ignored or actively boycotted by the osteopathic profession.

Early twentieth-century osteopaths did not foresee this defeat; they naively sought official recognition and sanction for their treatments. They tried to get into regular medicine. After all, they had successful cures, happy patients, and a solid mechanical, thermodynamic paradigm. Yet, like homeopathy, osteopathy violates key allopathic taboos. It cures the sick but cannot define precisely why or how. As a team of orthopedic historians smugly recounts, initial British attempts at legitimization were a disaster:

Curiously enough, the osteopaths ... tried to establish themselves
legally, as practicing an alternative system of medicine, by an application to the House of Lords in 1935, but their answers to the medical questions put to them at the hearing brought them into a number
of impossible situations. In the end, their position became unten-
able. Small wonder; for they denied standard tenets built up during
centuries of research by doctors all over the world, without putting
forward a shred of disproof, and affirmed an alternative creed without offering any evidence in its favour. They claimed to practise a
complete and revolutionary alternative system of medicine, but when
the Lords asked on what grounds these remarkable assertions rested,
none was put forward. This ventilation was an advantage; for the
osteopaths were shown in their true light, not only to doctors and
the public, but also to themselves. As a result, few even of the most
bigoted now claim to cure *all* diseases by manipulating the spine....[12]

In truth the claim that all diseases can be cured by manipulating
the spine is merely the historical launching point for osteopathy (if
even that)—at best, a ritual to which only the most poorly trained
osteopathic hacks still cling. True artisans continue to treat a wide array
of diseases by manipulating not only the spine but the viscera, fascial
tissue, and other bones. And "manipulate" is an understatement; they
assay, interpret, and follow tissues to their sites of compromise.

Yet one can certainly understand the mainstream outrage at pub-
licized osteopathic claims insofar as the more pedantic osteopaths and
their cousin chiropractors do little more than adjust bones from a world-
view that simple subluxations restrict healthy flow and cause all pathologies. It is one step from these pedants to practitioners who produce
exploitative X-rays and feign improvements of these by fake adjustments (which, if authentic, would also accomplish little or nothing).
They are neither grass-roots bone-setters in a folk tradition nor skilled
vitalistic physicians in a contemporary energetic paradigm. They are
trapped between these poles in a middle ground made up of the worst of
primitive medicine (crude linear manipulation) and the worst of

technological medicine (X-ray simplification of disease etiology). They want to be doctors without taking the necessary courses, or they are amateur doctors who want to be creative osteopaths but lack artistry for diagnostic and therapeutic touch. When I propose a future holistic osteopathic medicine, I mean the palpative skills and intuitions of the pure osteopath combined with the medical training of the contemporary scientific physician. I mean the best of both.

Although the above-cited orthopedic critics would have little sympathy for such a profession, most understand the separate realms of manipulative physiotherapist and M.D. and acknowledge the need for at least manual auxiliaries to standard physicians:

> The family doctor would no longer be forced either to manipulate himself, perhaps hurriedly with unskilled assistance, or covertly to advise recourse to some layman. He would send the patient for manipulative physiotherapy; this would be faithfully carried out as a matter of course by an auxiliary fully trained in these methods and accustomed to working side by side with the medical profession. The arrangement has already been established in Norway, where a special register of those skilled in manipulation is available to doctors.[13]

This trend has continued to develop into the twenty-first century with separate, highly esteemed fields of physical therapy and integrated manual medicine.

From my viewpoint, reducing osteopathy to physical therapy is a halfway measure that, while recognizing the importance of manipulation, attempts to limit it to a subset of exactly the linear and Solidist viewpoints that doomed original osteopathy never to become a full medical system. It is an attempt to claim the most superficial aspects of manipulation for the medical hierarchy (those aspects that cannot threaten it) and discard the innovative systems that arose from them.

Insofar as manual practitioners treat serious visceral diseases and psychopathologies, they do not regard their techniques as merely musculoskeletal (engineering-based); they view palpation as a means of accessing the core mechanism of life. Later osteopaths such as Jean-Pierre Barral and John Upledger continue to arrive at innovative modes of working with the interrelationships of bones, nerves, viscera, blood flow, cranial pulse, and psyche. A continuity of invention and institutionalization of its own techniques finally sets true osteopathy apart from all other manipulative medicines, prehistoric and modern, and makes it, on the one hand, a quasi-academic medicine with specialized branches of research and application much like allopathy, and on the other, a totally new paradigm in body-mind relations and complexity-based life dynamics.

Cranial Osteopathy

PALPATION AS ENERGY MEDICINE owes a good part of its development to William G. Sutherland. A student at Still's College of Osteopathy in Kirksville, Missouri, Sutherland was familiar with the school's famous mounted disarticulated skull— a specimen in which the individual cranial bones were pulled apart and wired into positions true to their original structure yet revealing the complexity of their sutures. In 1899, "glancing at the Beauchene skull, he became transfixed by the squamosal suture of the temporal bones, the rolling-overlap joint between temporals and parietals. The words 'Bevelled like the gills of a fish, and indicating articular mobility for a respiratory mechanism' flashed into his mind."[14] At the time, even among osteopaths, the cranium was presumed to be a fixed, interlocked dome (to this day there is no clear recognition of the pliability of the bones of the skull in most American medical texts).

It was not until his fifth year of practice in Minnesota that Sutherland got to explore his intuition. He purchased a football helmet, small pieces of India rubber, leather, straps, shoemaker's buckles, and sewing materials and turned the helmet into a device for restricting the individual bones of skull and thus testing their ranges of motion. That is, he immobilized his own supposedly immobile bones and, to the dis-

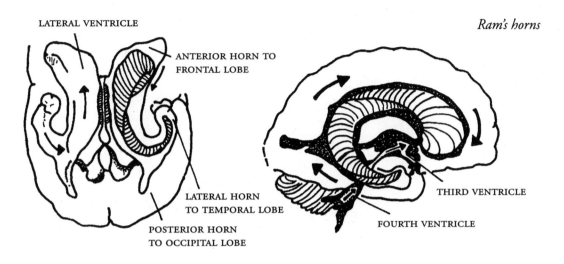

LATERAL VENTRICLE

ANTERIOR HORN TO
FRONTAL LOBE

Ram's horns

LATERAL HORN
TO TEMPORAL LOBE

POSTERIOR HORN
TO OCCIPITAL LOBE

THIRD VENTRICLE

FOURTH VENTRICLE

Reprinted from *An Introduction to Craniosacral Therapy* by Don Cohen, D.C., North Atlantic Books, 1995.

The design of the temporal bones provided the original inspiration for William G. Sutherland's concept of cranial bone motion. He noticed that the temporal sutures are "bevelled like the gills of a fish" and the bones swivel around a rotatory horizontal axis in a spiraling fashion that in flexion flares the anterior aspects laterally, like gills, and approximates the mastoids. The motion of the temporals reflects the "ram's horn" configuration of the lateral ventricles.

tress of his wife, induced an astonishing array of mental and internal ailments. Their naturally occurring counterparts would later lend themselves to cure through cranial manipulation.

Taking his cues from the sensations of immobilization, Sutherland explored the sinuous and minute cycles of motility among the many tiny articulated bones; he painstakingly remapped the cranial skeleton as dynamic tissue. Then he developed a variety of means of manipulating and balancing the skull's individual zones, always with great precision because of the subtle properties of such miniscule fields of articulation. He soon built a practice based on treating a variety of emotional and physical disorders, including migraines and various emotional maladies, all through cranial osteopathy.

*Osteopathy
and
Chiropractic*

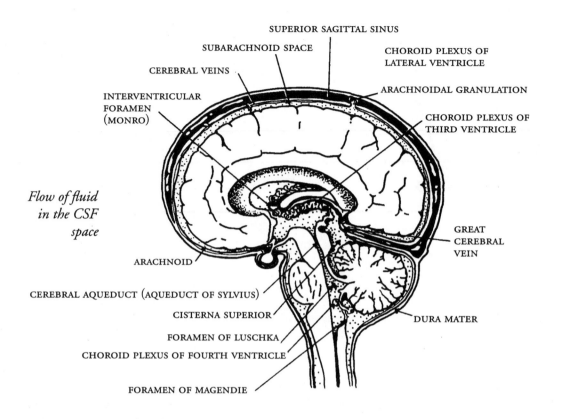

Flow of fluid in the CSF space

SUPERIOR SAGITTAL SINUS

SUBARACHNOID SPACE

CEREBRAL VEINS

INTERVENTRICULAR FORAMEN (MONRO)

CHOROID PLEXUS OF LATERAL VENTRICLE

ARACHNOIDAL GRANULATION

CHOROID PLEXUS OF THIRD VENTRICLE

GREAT CEREBRAL VEIN

ARACHNOID

CEREBRAL AQUEDUCT (AQUEDUCT OF SYLVIUS)

CISTERNA SUPERIOR

FORAMEN OF LUSCHKA

CHOROID PLEXUS OF FOURTH VENTRICLE

DURA MATER

FORAMEN OF MAGENDIE

Reprinted from *An Introduction to Craniosacral Therapy* by Don Cohen, D.C., North Atlantic Books, 1995.

Sutherland was curious to find out what happened when he tied down all the straps at once. In this profoundly uncomfortable headlock (which, all the same, should have been entirely static from the standpoint of most medical theories) he was astonished to feel his sacrum begin to oscillate rhythmically while becoming warmer. He had penetrated what was to become the "core link" of cranial osteopathy, the energetic and mechanical conjugation between the occiput and the sacrum through the supple spinal dura. "Indicating articular mobility for a respiratory mechanism" indeed!

[Sutherland] told of lying down, his head in the V-shape head rest; of imposing compression by gradual tension of buckle and strap. He described the sensations he had experienced as he approached near-unconsciousness. And that although weakened, he had succeeded in releasing the leverage strap. "A sensation of warmth followed," he explained. "And also a remarkable movement of fluid up and down the spinal column, throughout the ventricles.... Fantastic!"[15]

He later described the experience of listening to the cerebrospinal fluid—Still's "great river of life"—irrigating the central nervous system "like water going under ice." He ascribed the onset of many diseases—either causally or symptomatically—to the "inactivity of the cerebrospinal fluid, lymph, and blood."[16] He eventually developed a phenomenological anatomy based on system hydraulics.

> In [my] experiments of controlling or directing cranial respiratory movement, it was found that the diaphragmatic respiratory mechanism changed its rhythm to that of the cranial. Hence the conclusion that the diaphragmatic respiratory system is secondary to the cranial....
>
> This hypothesis views the lateral ventricles as dilating during the period of inhalation; the convolution of the hemispheres in the meantime expanding. During this same period the third ventricle dilates in a V-form manner, the fourth ventricle in a lozenge form, while the spinal cord is drawn upward; and the CSF fluctuates within the sub-arachnoid spaces and the ventricles. During the period of exhalation, the convolutions relax, the ventricles contract, the spinal cord drops downwards, and the CSF again fluctuates within the sub-arachnoid spaces and ventricles.[17]

Ultimately Sutherland came to rediscover the body as a relativistic, fluid form, combining respiratory, circulatory, skeletal, emotional, and other properties in a series of interrelated ripples and vibrations.

According to contemporary Sutherland disciple Franklyn Sills, the cranial rhythm flows as a deep, long tide with subtides and wavelets inside it, conducting it and also radiating from it. The long tide forms the central vortex of the body, maintaining its biodynamic equilibrium.

This grounds the power of hydraulic palpation. The separate subwave and wavelet forms continue to assimilate unresolved experiences and autonomic functions within the central nervous system. These too may be treated by various osteopathic techniques.

The crises and unruly energies of tissues and the unconscious impressions of living creatures imprint themselves from the cells and nervous system in the cerebrospinal fluid to be cleansed and transmuted. Palpation enhances this process, thus evokes the deepest autonomic, embryogenic elements of biological existence. Riding the cerebrospinal pulse, Sills says, is like placing hands gently on a bird taking flight, as the practitioner attempts to awaken or enhance the spark of transmission of the Breath of Life to all the tissues and organs.

By now, osteopathy has become a tool for entering the Breath of Life, the tides of cosmic *prana* and oceanic flow internalized by evolving animal entities on this planet. The combination of Still's and Sutherland's anatomicophysiologies has led to a complete post-modern medical system. As contemporary osteopath Rollin E. Becker wrote to Sutherland in 1949:

> The more I study Osteopathy, the more it seems to boil down to a Highly Intelligent fluid surrounded and held in shape by fascial membranes.
>
> Allow the fascial strains to correct what might be present, allow the fluid to resume its normal TIDAL mechanism, and all associated pathologies in the muscle, skin, blood vessels or nerves *will correct themselves*. Bend to the oar through the fascia, and ride the TIDE to the shore by way of the fluid.[18] [italics mine]

THE MODERN DEVELOPMENT of osteopathy since Sutherland emphasizes riding the tide: light over heavy adjustments, tissue dialogue over mechanical movement, and psychospiritual integration over structural repair. Osteopathy is still a manual medicine based in thermodynamics—informed touch is the starting point for all procedures—but

it has also become a vitalistic, psychotherapeutic modality.

Since the late 1980s one of the major events among alternative therapies in general has been the development and spread of systems of *nonverbal* dialogue (at the relative expense of more familiar neo-Freudian models based on verbal or semantic components). Techniques prioritizing cognitive insight, mere neuromuscular mobility, and the cause-effect realm of the central nervous system (ranging from classical psychotherapy with its gestalt and bioenergetic branches to a New Age diversity of visualization techniques) have been merged with those emphasizing the subtleties of the autonomic nervous system, visceral motility, and the hydrodynamics of bodily fluids (Applied Kinesiology, Body Electronics, craniosacral therapy, Continuum, etc.). In fact, therapists of many persuasions are now gradually incorporating dialogues between internal somatic rhythms on the one hand and skeletal, muscular, emotional, and spiritual aspects of tissue on the other. I do not mean to imply here that such therapies were invented during the 1980s, only that their range has increased, the practice of them has become more sophisticated (in terms of their relationship of both scientific anatomical and psychological components), and they are providing quite unexpected paradigms of disease and cure. The methods themselves—remember—are either very old or have their origin in systems that are very old.

Probably the most significant single factor in the advance of autonomic therapies has been the shift of focus within schools of osteopathy, following Sutherland, from musculoskeletal modalities to visceral and craniosacral ones.

Late in the twentieth century, energetic osteopathy not only reestablished itself outside AMA-approved manual medicine but expanded as myriad modalities. The basic principles of mechanical palpation sensitive to the body's various densities, layers, cavities, fluidities, stress lines, organizational principles, and unexplored electromagnetic and other fields have spawned a variety of osteopathic subdisciplines, most of them cranial (i.e., Sutherlandian) by orientation if not literally cranial physiologically. Visceral manipulation, lymphatic drainage, mechanical link, myofaction, and Zero Balancing are but a few. Sutherlandian osteopathy has joined with the *chakras* of Polarity therapy, the tissue molding of Rolfing, the channeled intention of Reiki, the potentized succussions of homeopathy, the biochemical saturation fields of Body Electronics, and the symbolic conversions of shamanic psychoanalysis to produce a new body-mind medicine, in fact a new life science.

As noted many times, the prime—in fact, the only—capacity medicine has is to hitch itself to the embryogenic process. If a single cell contains the whole plan of an organism and a mechanism for enacting it, how can a physician rival or replicate this? He can assist it, catalyze its sluggishnesses, and attempt to remove more blatant impediments in its way, but he cannot sculpt or congeal anything resembling a lump of protoplasm let alone a breathing, conscious, philosophizing organ. Thus, medicine aboriginally is meant to awaken the goddesses and totems that lie at the heart of development, to encourage their miracles to go on happening in this strange and compelling world. In this dance, Antelope Shamans and osteopaths can be as effective as—or even more effective than—surgeons and internists.

F ROM ITS IMPLICIT (experiential) comprehension of self-organizing life fields, quantum density, decoherence spin networks, and tensegrity of cytoskeletons, osteopathic palpation is no longer limited (at best) to possibilities of manipulating proximate and contingent tissue; it is now considered plausible to attempt to change cell shape, structure, relationship, and even heredity by activating a range of morphogenetically inductive factors. Cranial and energetic disciplines have thus been legitimated to explore the entire universe of soma, psyche, health, and disease as a relativistic, post-cybernetic modality, beyond the Ages of Solidism, Materialism, Physicalism, Quantity, and Commodity. The fusion of touch, intention, and energy-channeling portends a possible medical science of indeterminate scope and breadth. Today's quantum palpation was not something that Still could specify from a nineteenth-century theocratic perspective that understood physical energy only nonmolecularly and nonholographically.

In a future age, some version of Sutherlandian osteopathy may lead to the much-sought transmutative, alchemical, telekinetic science, bridging the imaginary gap between mind and body, energy and matter. That such a discovery will hearken back to the oldest Stone-Age modes of touch, manipulation, voodoo, and totemic conversion will be entirely appropriate. Post-materialistic magic may regain the vitality of prescientific magic, with the additional cogency of having passed through the heart of matter, the atomic nucleus—the very birth and death of the universe— and come out the other side.

IT IS NOT UNUSUAL for intellectual and technical systems to gravitate toward their opposite pole. Psychoanalysis began as language and linguistic therapy, then gravitated toward the "body as shadow" with Reich, and now propounds mainly drug therapies. Homeopathy, vitalistic characterology at its beginning, is now a kind of statistical biodynamics and nanopharmacology. Allopathy began as intuitive systems of coction and evolved through vivisection, microanalysis, and genetic technology. A system does not necessarily continue to address the world at the level it initially proposes. Its subtexts take on their own lives.

Still was an engineer. He construed the organism as a divine machine of flesh and bones. His strategies for repairing that machine originated in familiar technological metaphors. He was confident that the Architect of the machine was of Christian and progressive persuasion and would welcome the improvements of science as a celebration of His own design. He did not anticipate the transformation of body architectures into resonant and scalar waves or new thermodynamics going past quantum uncertainty limits into autonomous phase states. Yet once Still (and his followers) began grabbing bones and fascia by their protrusions, following their tissue resistance, and draining energy like a sponge, they entered into the unfathomed realm of the body's reciprocities, dimensionalities, grammatologies, hologrammatic transition fields, and the subtle impregnation of mind in organs. They were dealing with a machine perhaps, but it was a trans-cybernetic, nonergodic machine of an order that had not yet been imagined. The biosphere, after all, is fundamentally different from the geosphere or gravity organizing stars.

Osteopathy opened a whole realm of hands-on energetic medicine embracing the reciprocal mechanics and equilibria of manipulation but also moving beyond them into realms of innovative chirokinetic healing. The first osteopaths devised an engineer's robotic model for palpation as a mechanical technique; then they set a biological priority of hypersensitive diagnostic touch. The original physical projections of Still keep providing osteopathy with an empirical anatomical basis (even as external research in a laboratory makes allopathy scientific). This is therapeutically critical, for intuitively palpated energy forms occupy the same spaces as tissue structures, and informed diagnosis and treatment must acknowledge the actual densities and shapes of organs.

Even if it is possible that all of the functions of the body are reducible to fulcra, levers, pulleys, and pumps, the living anatomico-chemical mechanism functions as extremely complex gradations of kinetic energy between gross and subtle levels, with motion and potential constantly flowing downwards from the skeleton to the cytoskeleton and upwards from the molecular nucleus to the neuroviscera. Cells and molecules, after all, also have tiny fulcra, pulleys, pumps, etc. The overall machinery of the body is multidimensional, nano-mechanical, kinesthetic, and phenomenological, and within the domain of mind, fluctuates as surely as photons between waves and particles.

Still set a living machine in motion, and the resonance he kindled continues (through the present osteopathic disciplines) to be distributed down to the subtlest levels of flesh and intention and to return from there. Yet, no matter how the operator/practitioner behaves, the machine can never be run as an assembly-line robot. Soft and sentient in every aspect, it takes vectors imposed onto it and transposes them into other vectors which generate yet others.

Matter also generates energy, especially in living tissue. It resonates with its own emergent waves of sentience. However, the fully realized art of palpating by following energy did not take hold until John Upledger "reinvented" osteopathy as CranioSacral Therapy. Until then, osteopaths were chiropractors and manipulators by history and training. Even late in his career, Still carried around a special stick to whack vertebrae into structural compliance. This was the heritage of the system, and it was hard to buck until Upledger came along.

What Still did not fully perceive was that the force he directed into the body from the premise of a machinery was received by that machinery as nonlinear impulses and hologrammatic currents. The same was true for Sutherland; his (albeit delicate) clockwork of cranial osteopathy was also a transfusion of imagery and energy of an indeterminate nature. Thus, osteopathic palpation reinvented itself as highly precise articulate mobilities. Matter was Still's landmark, but energy was his medium and guide. The original machine has not been discarded; it continues to occupy space with its exquisite architectures, to translate simple into complex energy. It is the kind of machine that, once it perceives the mind of a therapeutic conductor, leads him transpersonally into its own plan.

Today osteopathy is both a manipulative medicine (in fact, *the* pure manipulative medicine) seeking legitimacy under the blanket of professional health care and supporting manual medical trainings that mirror conventional internal ones, and an innovative paraphysical science tracking quantum currents in alive fabrics and fields. It has become, for many, a mode of placing hands through skin on bones and viscera and touching the soul.

Chiropractic

D ANIEL DAVID PALMER was a trained osteopath, faith healer, and grocer in Iowa who learned ancient bone-setting from European immigrants. Finding himself successful in his treatments, he broke away from Still's orthodoxy, asserted himself as the true heir to Hippocratic medicine, and initiated his own manipulative training program in the late 1890s—it was more linear, concrete, musculoskeletal, and purely mobility-oriented ("move dem bones") than osteopathy.

In developing chiropractic, Palmer proposed that three factors influenced the chronic skeletal-dislocation patterns (subluxation) in patients. They were deep-seated traumas, poisons (including autotoxicities), and autosuggestions (or self-hypnosis). All of these generate self-replicating cycles through which the organism loses its inherent "cure" capacity; they literally deplete the natural potential to transmit healing oscillations and sub-signals.

The resulting facilitated segment, as defined by the chiropractor, is a level of spinal cord that has become hyperactive or hair-triggered from postural and emotional stress and, while perpetuating itself, numbs potentially therapeutic impulses en route to surrounding muscles and skin, which consequently become restricted and amorphous. That is, a vertebra becomes subluxated; in this condition it impinges upon nerves, blood vessels, and lymphatics traveling through the intervertebral foramen; the conduction of autonomic neural pulses is impaired; and parts of the organism subject to that vertebra's nervous tonus become predisposed to disease. The facilitated segment comes to represent essentially a dynamic, dysfunctional interaction between the somatic system, the viscera, and the autonomic nervous system on the one hand and the mind on the other.

The chiropractic formula for adjusting such subluxations is: the minimum force, in the correct direction, at the maximum speed. Each movement is enacted with an elegant jolt that transcends its gross mechanics. The cranial osteopath likewise uses the least pressure necessary to induce a reaction, but then, instead of compelling the bones and viscera into a presumed normal path, he follows their intrinsic movement. Both systems emphasize intention over pressure, though traditional chiropractic tends to prefer (often to the exclusion of directly palpating the viscera) direct torques with immediate energetic outcome.

For the modern chiropractor, disease is not simply a matter of bones out of alignment, but the exact vectors of such tilts and restrictions and what they indicate about the life and responsiveness of the patient. Any good physician must interpret the signaling errors from a holistic point of view, not jumping to conclusions that the body's lethargy or asymmetry *per se* are functional statements of illnesses. He may adjust skeletal tissue to restore health, but, remember, the original tilt was carried out by a disease or injury which set the biomechanical charge for such realignment. Chiropractic is to that extent "homeopathic," since its remedies reenact aspects of diseases. They go toward the direction of the block and then release back. They do not try to budge anatomy into the right position. Even allopathic surgery is unintentionally "chiropractic" insofar as it attempts to "outdo" a disease on its own plane, imposing its precise disfigurement and adding its didactic "wound" to the pathology.

That so many chiropractically defined lesions and osteopathic restrictions and energy cysts are imperceptible to orthopedic surgeons may scream unabashed fraud to the medical establishment, but this might also indicate layers of subtlety and nonlocalized organizational principles in the body itself. Chiropractors and osteopaths might see "diseases" that slip through even the most rigorous allopathic exams because conventionally trained M.D.s look for familiar anatomical landmarks and intellectual rubrics.

Sometimes when a surgeon fails to recognize anything pathological on an MRI and finds no clinical basis for dysfunction, and when anti-inflammatories and other mechanical treatments (such as orthotics) have no remedial effect, yet the patient is in such pain he cannot walk or type, the reason may be that the condition exists only on multiple psychosomatic levels, expressing its discohesiveness and restriction on no one level completely enough to be diagnosed there. The pathology is dynamic, holistic, and single.

*Osteopathy
and
Chiropractic*

279

The conventional doctor cannot locate it because its visceral or skeletal symptoms by themselves are not sufficiently impacted to leave telltale scars, and the psychiatrist cannot track a deep-seated emotional cathexis in fascia and neuromusculature. Thus, no one is able to give a name to the condition—or to help.

This is why osteopathy and chiropractic have found their niche in medicine between surgery and psychiatry. People are often in pain for "no reason" allopathically. What the chiropractor feels with his hands (allowing him to venture a treatment), as concrete or energetic as it seems and as acceptable the results of his subsequent adjustment to the patient, cannot be located or named either before or after in allopathic terms. Even if there is an allopathic disease, it is by definition a different energetic complex. The prescribed regimen likewise may vary so much as to require, for instance, immobilization allopathically and induction of movement chiropractically. It is like the difference between traction vertically and traction horizontally or between compressing in and diffusing out.

The same contradiction exists on the axis between psychoanalysis and chiropractic. A headache with weeping would seem psychiatrically to have its origin in a personal event, whereas a chiropractor might find its agitation at the fifth vertebra, making the psychological origin incidental to his quick and efficient adjustment cure. Ten years of psychoanalysis would accomplish nothing, at least vis-à-vis that ailment, though it might generate other therapeutic results. Sometimes psychosomatic penetration of character shares more with the chiropractor or acupuncturist than with the psychiatrist.

Bone adjustment can be like standing on a very high mountain, looking at everything far away. That's how bones are. They create a sense of the vast, in fact cosmic, space the body encloses. If a bone is damaged or shifted out of place, even infinitesimally, the disorientation is vast; identity becomes shapeless. At the moment the adjustment takes place—the famous bone cracking—there is not so much pain as immense surprise. The spacing within shifts and the muscles momentarily hang on nothing. Energy releases electrically through the system and toxins flush. Viscera respond instantaneously. The stomach expands and fills its own hollowness and sensations of sadness. Lungs and chest surge with air as if it were magnetically drawn into them. They expand and contract easily and fully; the breath rushes into them as into deliciously deep, sucking cavities.

In acupuncture, by contrast, needles go directly into the body's mind. They feel like bee-stings, but their actual locations are redistributed by the field they create. It is not so much the pain of the needles that is uncomfortable as the overall sense of being out of alignment, of being torn among multiple selves. Even thought hurts, for the same thoughts can no longer travel in the old way. From a chiropractic standpoint acupuncture is a kind of subcellular adjustment.

Fundamental reorientation of bones may activate anxiety too, but a very faraway fear, as a shape seen from a mountain. At the moment when the bones crack and right afterward, the sensation is as though the person is standing above a river, a river which rushes between his legs, limitless in both directions. Suddenly he is lifted above the river and dropped on both sides of it at once. He struggles to his feet, but he is on both sides, he is on opposite sides, he is on the wrong side from himself and must somehow cross over in order to get back together, but as each half tries to cross, so does the other half. There is a momentary amnesia that he has ended up on the wrong side and he cannot get back. Then the effects settle, and the new side becomes

Osteopathy
and
Chiropractic

281

the right side. In fact, it is familiar as the right side from long ago, before the loss of function.

One makes a flesh grid for the river of his or her own being. After the treatment the river will gradually shift toward its familiar bed, but it will have been slightly redirected. Over time, through recurrent needle treatments, herbs, *t'ai chi*, Feldenkrais work, or other remedies, the

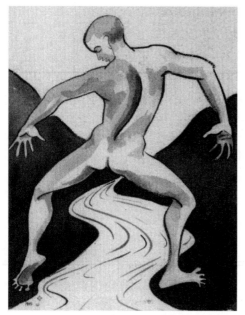

river may forge a fresh channel. Whatever this river is made of—nerves, meridians, blood, *chi*, mind, or synergistic fluidity—it carries the organs with it. At every juncture of therapeutic experience an alteration of current is felt because the entire field of the meridians is being realigned.

In the end, it does not matter what side of the river one is on or what happens when the tingling stops. Life continues from there, as whatever life is.

Various contemporary modalities of chiropractic are usually subtler and more yogic and isometric than Palmer's spinal jolts. They are like exercise regimens and stretches with a little extra tug or recoil of bony tissue at the opportune occasion. Osteopaths also use recoils, though they are more often visceral (in soft tissue) than musculoskeletal and bone-oriented.

With chiropractic now more osteopathic and osteopaths employing chiropractic adjustments (and with both systems sharing roots in Still's osteopathy), the distinction between the two techniques may seem arcane to the novice. And not just to the novice. I have been convinced more than once that I grasped the essence of their difference only to slide subsequently into even greater confusion. In revising the chiropractic section for this edition, I enlisted the aid of numerous mainly chiropractic practitioners, but their own standards of discrimination varied in ways I found irreconcilable. To further complicate the matter, a wide spectrum of physical therapists trained in allopathic medicine have not only adopted chiropractic techniques but contributed new generalized forms of manipulation, some of them hybridized with conventional chiropractic techniques.

My presumption that chiropractic has matured well beyond the sectarian physiognomy and bone movements of Palmer, while enthusiastically endorsed by some chiropractors, was challenged by others. The concept that osteopathy is gentler, more energetic, and less skeletal and structural than chiropractic was likewise popular with some chiropractors (and many osteopaths) but unpopular with most contemporary practitioners of Palmer's art. "Palmer did 'laying on of hands' and magnetic healing too," one wrote me with some pique.

When I tried to advance the idea that modern chiropractic is really a new field combining some of Palmer's diagnostic and therapeutic techniques with other, more scientific methods developed by physiatrists, orthopedic doctors, and manual therapists, some chiropractors again agreed and others disagreed.

"It is a mistake to describe these treatments as chiropractic," explained one objecter. "They are physical therapy using manipulation. They are not specific to one vertebra at a time, as chiropractic is. Generalized manipulation in a region of the body is a totally different approach."

Yet another offered, "There is no chiropractic or osteopathy any more in the old sense of either of them. They were systems of their time and are both antiquated. Everything now is subtler, more indirect, less dogmatic. Even Rolfing has changed. Rolfers don't just do the deepest tissue work clients can stand. They are more in dialogue with the body, more indirect now. Everyone borrows techniques from everyone else. We are close to a generalized manual medicine, and that manual medicine has even begun to find its way into the mainstream of physical therapists and M.D.s."

I DISCOVERED CHIROPRACTIC long before I had any experience with osteopathy. As a graduate student in anthropology in 1969, I began a study of alternative medicine, mostly in Eastern Maine, using chiropractors. I quickly encountered a bizarre array of self-identified Palmerites who x-rayed every patient, seemed to find serious problems in all of them, simplified most diseases to subluxations of vertebrae, and specialized in heroic lurches and yanks. One proudly referred to his trade as bone-snapping; another was a Pentecostal minister. None of these were holistic in any sense of the word. A friend also pointed out the strange coincidence of many of their names: Bendbow, Crick, Collison, Riggle.

Although I abandoned the study after a month, I later wrote a critique of chiropractic in the form of a book review in the Portland daily paper. My feeling then was that patients needed to be warned about such abuses. Chiropractic to me was a disingenuous scam.

However, while working on the first edition of this book in 1976, I met other, very different chiropractors who *were* holistic. A series of positive treatments, along with my interviews and reading, caused me to revise and even reverse my opinion of the system. My description of chiropractic from that time survives more or less intact into this edition. Many chiropractors who read it, however, found that I retained a subtle prejudice against chiropractic: "Referring to adjustments as 'bone-snapping' or jolts is inflammatory and condemning. You will alienate the chiropractic community with that description. It sounds barbaric and frightening."

I was surprised at this reaction because I presumed that everyone knew about the sorts of "bad" chiropractors I ran into in 1969—the ones who called themselves "bone-snappers." I didn't think that holistic chiropractors would resent my flagging them and making a distinction between the two discrepant poles of Palmer's kingdom. I was wrong.

Most chiropractors consider Bendbow, Crick, *et al.,* a myth. "There are incompetent and dishonest practitioners in all systems," was a typical comment.

Yet, at some level I felt a responsibility to protect readers from "doctors" who call themselves chiropractors, have credentials from Palmer-oriented schools, but do only x-rays and heavy, nondiscriminating adjustments.

"Chiropractic is the most utilized alternative health-care system in the U.S.," a chiropractor asserted when I tried to justify my reporting of the word "bone-snapping" as good oral history, even if not a fair description of his profession. "Funding for basic research and clinical studies is rapidly expanding, and the efficacy of manipulation is being demonstrated again and again. Your unfortunate experience thirty years ago shouldn't color people's perceptions of what I do."

But it was real at the time. I assume that simplistic, mechanical chiropractors still practice in many parts of the world, especially in rural North America, though I have no current experience of them and no desire to investigate further. Instead I have tried to put both my old prejudice and modern chiropractic in fresh perspective.

I WILL OFFER, with some misgivings, that chiropractors utilize a short-amplitude, high-speed manipulation directly into a restriction barrier to release it, while osteopaths rely on indirect techniques to palpate away from a barrier. Some (but not all) chiropractors rely on a rote formula—a precise vertebra to be adjusted at one site on one of its sides in a prescribed direction to release any diagnosed restriction.

"Not so," challenged an osteopathic reader. "Many osteopaths are very direct and do adjustments that cannot be distinguished from chiropractic. And I know chiropractors who are more indirect than most osteopaths."

Once again, the umbrella of unified manual medicine catches both systems overlapping.

Another generalization that does not apply to either all chiropractors or all osteopaths is that the former tend to deal directly with the hardened gelatinous basis of the body and to release energies through skeletoneuromuscular shear planes, while the latter tend to engage the watery basis of the body and to activate ripples and eddies from light palpation. Thus, chiropractic is more akin to elemental fire—igniting dormant potentials and charging inert spaces. Conversely, osteopaths presume that the fluidity of the body will carry even the tiniest motions along currents inward to the core.

Two aspects of chiropractic treatment, however, seem to define the core modality satisfactorily for most practitioners: the spine and joints as the sole (or major) originating cause of restrictions leading to illnesses, and direct manual techniques to relieve spinal blocks and release joints. Certainly some chiropractically trained practitioners who use the spine for diagnosis and a direct trajectory of adjustment also incorporate osteopathic procedures, *Chi Gung,* or other indirect movements. In the alternate version, a chiropractic map is traversed using non-chiropractic or quasi-chiropractic techniques. When the spine as a compass and a direct method of adjustment is abandoned, the modality is chiropractic in name only.

So-called Network Chiropractic, which is based on stimulating reflex points to expedite energy movement in tissues and bones, is not considered chiropractic by most Palmer-educated chiropractors. In fact, Wisconsin has refused to certify such "nonforce" practitioners, and I have been told that the name of this system may be changed to Network Spinal Analysis.

Many other techniques of muscle energy, fascial adjustment, and skeletally-based tissue release sometimes end up under the shingle of chiropractic, perhaps because the practitioner got his or her degree at a chiropractic institution. These would better be called "naturopathic manual medicine" or even physical therapy. Otherwise, the name chiropractic means simply somatic adjustments in a historically chiropractic context.

Lauren Berry, a Northern California physical therapist and mechanical engineer, trained many chiropractors and future chiropractors in his own system of soft-tissue manipulation (called Swedish movements) during the last quarter of the twentieth century. An aggressive manipulator who liked to do high-speed adjustments, Berry theorized that since all soft tissues in the body hold mechanical positions in relation to joints and their distortions, their lesions should be treated too. In the case of rounded shoulders and slumped posture, the anterior deltoid muscles roll forward, so Berry taught the practitioner to massage and manipulate them posteriorly.

When I researched the first edition of *Planet Medicine,* one of the "chiropractors" I interviewed and from whom I received treatments was actually a disciple of Berry's and had no chiropractic training. Yet, as a neophyte, I frankly could not distinguish his work from that of a trained chiropractor. They both asked me to relax and hold my breath; they both balanced my torso in their arms and shifted it slightly back and forth, feeling for their pivot; they each then made a sudden, startling torque.

Tom Hendrickson, a student of Berry's who later completed the full chiropractic curriculum, has developed his own system of orthopedic massage for identifying and resolving imbalances and restrictions in soft tissue, including hyper- and hypo-tonicities and inhibitions caused by muscle tensions and weaknesses. Hendrickson interweaves techniques from a variety of therapeutic traditions: chiropractic, Berry's positional work, fascial release, James Cyriax's transverse friction massage, muscle energy (see Applied Kinesiology below), and many other sources, including Proprioceptive Neuromuscular Facilitation—a modality that was developed out of neurology and used originally to treat polio and stroke victims. As pressure is put on tissues in specific planes, the patient is asked to resist it. Sequences of resistive techniques are then blended with other direct executions and chiropractic manipulations. The goal is to dissolve adhesions, normalize the position of soft tissues and release their torsion, lengthen connective tissues, hydrate joints to a natural lubricative phase, and release entrapment of peripheral nerves.[19]

Many physiatrists, neurologists, orthopedic surgeons, and other manually disposed M.D.s have developed their own direct "chiropractic-like" techniques to deal with skeletal lesions and disc deterioration. Gerald Hirschberg, a Berkeley M.D., employs a variety of corsets and body jackets in combination with exercises to treat intradiscal pressure and nerve compression in the lower lumbar region. He also uses a painful skinrolling massage for fibromyalgia and has had diagnostic and clinical success with injections of lidocaine at the iliac crest for lower-back pain of uncertain etiology. In general, "uncertain etiology" encourages complementary or allopathic experimentation with direct manual techniques, leading to a new version of meta-chiropractic medicine.

After reading this paragraph, a chiropractor faxed me: "Hirschberg is *very non*-chiropractic in his approach. He places a high value on exercise and posture, which distinguishes him from a surgical approach but does not make him a 'meta-chiropractor.'"

It is both true and false to conclude that chiropractic, having blended with physical and manual therapy and neurology, is beginning to evolve into a new complementary discipline, rooted in Palmer's lineage but expanding exponentially beyond the guild. Perhaps I would like to hasten a reinvention of chiropractic in the context of physical therapy as well as a transformation of physical therapy in the context of chiropractic, and then both of them in the contexts of cranial osteopathy, *Chi Gung,* and other energy-based, holistic systems. I like synthesis, reconciliation, and evolution. I would prefer that everyone shake hands and agree to share secrets and work together. That is why this book is called "Planet Medicine." But I have been warned to keep my traditions plain and clear.

Applied Kinesiology[20]

AT THE HEART of Applied Kinesiology is kinesiology (biomechanics), the study of how nerves signal muscles to contract, resulting in postures and movements. Discoveries in biomechanics have taught scientists and therapists how to use the body most effectively, with applications in the fields of sports (optimal performance), industry (increase in productivity and reduction of worker injuries), and medicine (the design of prosthetic limbs and techniques of rehabilitation).

Manual muscle testing is a main diagnostic tool of kinesiology. To perform the standard muscle test, the doctor has the patient place his or her body in a position in which the muscle to be tested is partially contracted. The examiner places his hand upon the patient's limb (or other body part) in such a relationship as to provide static resistance against further contraction. Then the examiner asks her to contract that muscle as fully as possible. His counter-pressure, however, impedes any movement. Once the examiner ascertains that the patient has maximally contracted his muscle under compromising circumstances, he pushes or pulls on the patient's limb in an attempt to extend the muscle. If the patient can muster the additional strength to resist this pressure, the muscle has tested strong. If the muscle cannot contract sufficiently and the limb extends, the muscle has tested weak. Weakness is defined as collapse and flaccidity.

Muscle testing is not just an alternative technique; it is a standard medical diagnostic tool. For example, after an injury to the spine, a doctor will test the muscles that are enervated by nerves that emerge from the damaged area of the spine. If the muscles do not provide adequate resistance in the test, this is evidence that the nerves supplying the muscles have been damaged.

In 1964, Dr. George Goodheart, a chiropractor living in Michigan, made an interesting discovery. While working on a patient with a peculiar problem—one of his shoulder blades did not lie flat but rather jutted out from his back—Goodheart remembered reading (in Kendall, Kendall, and McCreary's classic on kinesiology*) about conditions of the serratus anticus muscle which holds the shoulder blade down upon the back. Using protocols from this book, he tested the muscle. On

---

Muscles—Testing and Function, Baltimore: Williams & Wilkins, revised third edition 1983.

the unaffected side the patient could tighten his serratus anticus strongly and hold his arm up undeterred during a muscle test—but on the affected side, the patient could not adequately tighten his muscle; as a result, his arm fell when Goodheart pulled upon it.

Goodheart palpated the muscle. It was equally large and well developed on both sides of his patient's body. Though Goodheart could find no reason for it to test weak on the affected side, further palpation revealed small beebee-sized lumps at the origin and insertion, the two extreme ends of the muscle, on the weak-testing side only. When Goodheart firmly massaged one of these, it vanished. So he massaged all of them. They gradually softened and disappeared—and, much to his surprise, the scapula pulled down firmly against the back. The muscle tested strong on both sides of the body. This serendipitous discovery of a method of re-fortifying weak-testing muscles marks the beginning of a new manual discipline which Goodheart named "Applied Kinesiology" (AK).

As a chiropractor, Goodheart knew that function depends upon structure; health depends upon correct posture, which is established by the natural tension inherent in muscles. From this premise he and his colleagues proceeded to use the "origin-insertion" stimulation technique on patients to restore tension in weak-testing muscles. As a result, many of their other health problems improved as well. However, not every weak-testing muscle could be strengthened by the origin-insertion technique. In order to renovate more recalcitrant tissues, Goodheart experimented with a variety of other therapeutic modalities, hoping that some of them could strengthen weak-testing muscles. The two most useful candidates turned out to be:

1. The osteopathic "lymphatic reflex" method of Frank Chapman. Treatment involved firmly massaging "neurolymphatic reflex points" which lie mostly upon the trunk and upper limbs.

2. The neurovascular method of T. J. Bennett, a chiropractor. In the 1950s Bennett developed a concept of vascular reflexes based on his observation, while holding certain reflex points under

fluoroscopy, of vascular engorgement of organs. Unfortunately, he and several of his patients are believed to have died as a result of their exposure to X-ray. For nonradiation application in AK, Goodheart developed a treatment that involved lightly holding these "neurovisceral reflex points," which impinge mostly upon critical functions of the head.

Through performing a variety of muscle tests on his patients, Goodheart noticed that those with the same organ dysfunction often had the same weak-testing muscles. When the muscles were made to test strong, visceral dysfunction also improved. He correlated these weak-testing muscles with specific glands, organs, foot and hand reflex points, disturbances of the cranial bones, and eventually with the meridian system of Traditional Chinese Medicine. His reciprocality between muscles and meridians forged a rare concrete bridge between Eastern and Western medicine. In fact, meridian theory proved so fruitful that Goodheart eventually assigned all bodily functions to one or more of the fourteen basic meridians. In AK, these are categorized as the "fourteen systems of regulation." The ancient Oriental meridian map provides not only a useful way to classify all the functions of the body but also a diagnostic and treatment compass for AK.

In his attempt to uncover the dysfunction that underlies each physical and mental symptom, Goodheart and his associates spent years developing one of the most comprehensive and systematic attempts at establishing "dialogue" with the autonomic nervous system that has ever been documented, exploring and mapping such diverse territories as:

- the relationships of muscles and organs, and the interpretation of body language;
- the relationships of musculoskeletal dysfunction, organ and lymphatic function, nutritional requirements, and emotional stress overload;
- the nature of allergies;

- right and left brain function;
- the nature and effects of stress;
- endocrine function;
- nutritional function;
- the lymphatic system;
- headaches;
- immune function;
- environmental sensitivities and syndromes of maladaptation;
- chronic fatigue syndrome;
- the multiple functions of the liver;
- the function of the heart;
- herpes simplex;
- arthritis, bursitis, and tendinitis;
- the cellular function of RNA;
- hypertension;

and a multitude of other physiological functions.

Applied Kinesiology uses standard lab tests, muscle testing, and observation of body language to evaluate functional systems of the body based on what Goodheart calls "the five factors of the intervertebral foramen": nerve, blood vessel, lymphatic vessel, acupuncture meridian, and cerebrospinal fluid. All of these are located in the intervertebral foramen, the "holes" between and to the side of the vertebrae on the back, which are near or identical to the "associated points" of the bladder meridian.

A basic tenet of AK is the concept that the organism can be "communicated with" directly, utilizing its own inherent responses to various stimuli as deduced through muscle testing.

Testing a muscle to see if it can hold strong with no other stimulus added is called testing "in the clear." AK goes further. It uses muscle testing as an indicator for almost every possible factor that could impact the human being (e.g., holding ordinary and exotic substances— from popcorn to Greek coins to different colors of thread to printed pages—over a body like dowsing rods and then testing their effects on muscle weakness). This is undertaken as a pure empirical experiment.

If a muscle tests strong, other factors (stimuli) are added one by one to the equation. If a factor makes the muscle test weak, it is considered to have a negative influence upon the person tested. If a muscle initially tests weak, factors that accompany its testing strong are considered to have a positive influence on the person. This is a radical, unique, and especially subtle method of allergy testing, for those foods, flowers, cat hairs, metals, etc., that lead a muscle to test weak are presumed to have some sort of an adverse dynamic or metabolic effect on it.

"The opportunity to use the body as an instrument of laboratory analysis," said Goodheart, "is unparalleled in modern therapeutics because the response of the body is unerring. If one approaches the problem correctly, making the proper and adequate diagnosis and treatment, the response is adequate and satisfactory both to the doctor and to the patient."[21]

If the examiner provides the stimulus (for instance, a kind of food or article of clothing) to the patient prior to or during muscle testing, the stimulus is called a "challenge." If the patient provides the stimulus by touching him- or herself, this is called "therapy localization." In localization, the person actually causes a problem area to test weak by touching it. This identifies the site of the problem and sometimes also temporarily or partially improves it. Improvement when the other hand is held on the forehead usually means the weakness has an emotional cause. Note that therapy "localization" and "challenge" are in essence both challenges and only indicate where a problem is situated, not the exact nature of the problem. Further investigation is required to elicit the source. Both methods of challenge are also diagnostically subtle and vary as the slightest and most dilute remedies are applied. Even the test may serve as a cure. AK is a parascience of energetic fluctuations.

Herein lies considerable room for error and misinterpretation of seeming muscle signs. Investigators with limited training jump to rapid (and false) conclusions as to whether or why a muscle tests weak. Multitudes of unreliable presumptions have been drawn by eager practitioners on the basis of the observed change in strength of an "indicator muscle." With no more evidence than a superficially conducted muscle test, alarmed patients have been told that their kidneys, heart, and liver are weak, or that they are allergic to spaghetti, etc. Goodheart himself has vehemently condemned such applications of muscle testing. He insists that muscle response is but one indicator of a possible need for further investigation and implores all who test muscles to correlate their findings with lab work and other indicators of different kinds.

Much to his chagrin, his warnings have gone substantially unheeded, and discredit has followed Applied Kinesiology. One hears of claimants who make their living by, for instance, determining that a subject demonstrates a need for megadoses of Vitamin E by placing a bottle of the substance on her belly and testing the deltoid muscle. One even encounters people at parties who offer, "Let me push on your arm and tell you your state of health—or your prospects for romance." Muscle testing, in these circumstances, inspires many a cartoon satirizing New Age healing. Schools of popular lay kinesiology like Touch for Health may have done much to promote the widespread awareness and popularity of muscle testing, but some of their methods such as simplified "allergy" testing have also contributed to damaging the reputation of AK itself.

ON A MORE POSITIVE NOTE the diagnostic methods of Applied Kinesiology are being successfully utilized in contexts provided by other healing systems. This has led to fusions with such fields as skeletal, cranial, and visceral manipulation, Ayurvedic taste theory, environmental medicine, and immunology (e.g., testing muscles as a guide while palpating or as an aid in prescribing herbs and drugs). In the hands of a medical doctor, the techniques of Applied Kinesiology may be used to determine the optimal pharmaceutical to prescribe. They may also furnish a physical basis for diagnosis and "substance" testing within purely vitalistic and psychic parameters, as in homeopathy, Bach Flower Remedies, and radionics. Psychological stimuli may be similarly tested in the context of psychoanalytic transference.

When combined with Applied Kinesiology, chiropractic takes on some of the features of internal medicine, becoming less dependent on skeletal adjustment alone. "Signaling errors," when liberated from an exclusively musculoskeletal terrain, can encompass biological responses to any substance in the world at large.

The diagnostic muscle-testing of Applied Kinesiology is meant theoretically to assess the effect upon an individual creature of any stimulus, animate or inanimate, in the universe that can be applied to his or her body. Thus, it is a paraphysical, vitalistic technique and the forerunner of a nonsectarian subtle cosmic medicine for assessing molecular and allergological biases across the full range of beneficial and pathological interactions between biological systems and each other and with inanimate substances. A form of it could be practiced by living entities anywhere in the universe, regardless of their body types, habitats, and stage or style of technological development. AK is simple and fundamental.

It is also the living sympathetic form of abstract mechanical sciences like spectroscopy and biochemistry, for it deals not with the mere signatures of substances but their immediate life meanings and health effects in the context of alive organisms.

Visceral Manipulation

THE WORLD-RENOWNED SCHOOL of visceral manipulation identified with French osteopaths Jean-Pierre Barral and Pierre Mercier proposes that the healthy functioning of viscera is based on their natural, unrestricted movement. From moment to moment, while providing

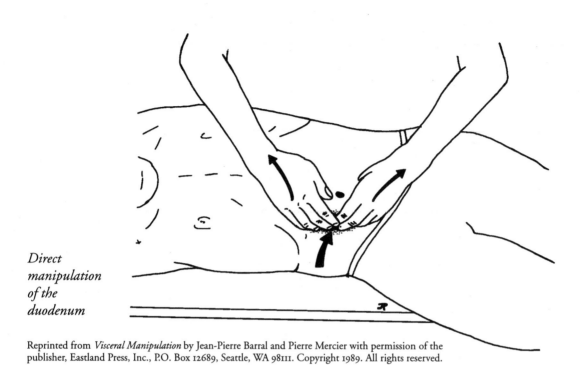

Direct manipulation of the duodenum

nutrition, oxygen, and proprioception and eliminating toxic byproducts of metabolism, the viscera are also making slight adjustments, reorienting themselves along subtly diverging vectors and axes. Thus, health does not lie solely in their functional output and contribution to the machinery and metabolism of the body but in their facility to shift continuously in involuntary search for an equilibrium the requirements of which also change from moment to moment.

These organic movements are both cyclical (following a diurnal-

---

In these next two sections (visceral manipulation and craniosacral therapy), my discussion will contain significant overlap of methods and etiologies, including virtual re-descriptions of some of the basic osteopathic principles and techniques. This is because the boundary between visceral and cranial work is artificial and overridden in most actual treatments. Both are light, guided osteopathic palpation.

MODALITIES

296

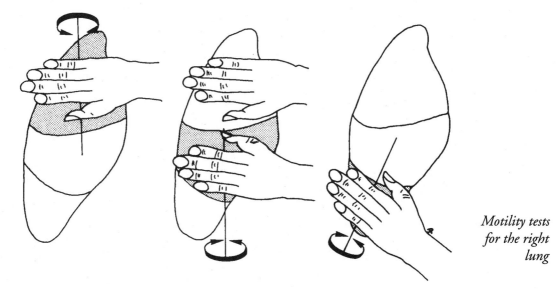

*Motility tests
for the right
lung*

nocturnal shift of energy circulation) and situational (based on a variety of extrinsic factors). This is in many ways a restatement of Traditional Chinese Medicine's hourly progression of organ activity and the relationship between, on the one hand, somatoemotional range and flexibility and, on the other, liver or kidney function.

Life is relentless compensation and reorientation to endogenous and extrinsic forces. Nothing in a body is ever static; every collision educes a semi-liquid response all the way down to cellular and subcellular levels. Tissues project energy and shape constructs into adjoining tissues, each organ struggling to glide over its neighbors but ultimately constricted by, constricting, and deforming them. Everything affixed to an organ must necessarily obey that organ's axis of movement. The orbit of a pharynx or bladder accommodates all its adhesions and attachments to adjacent organs, converting some of its shear into them, which hinders free movement of the entire structure.

The outer world intrudes into shifting, animate tissues with its own stonehard rigor, torques, whiplashes, and twinges, inflicting irrelevant

*Osteopathy
and
Chiropractic*

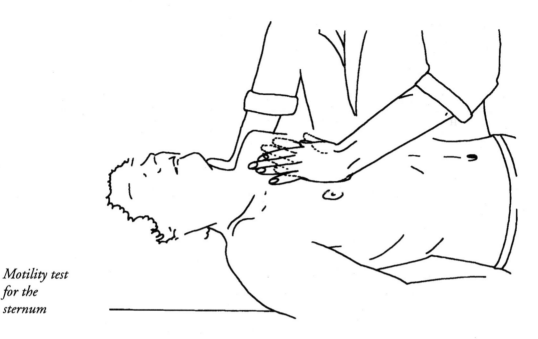

*Motility test
for the
sternum*

vectors that nonetheless circulate through concavities and burrow into
soft tissues. Visceral components absorb and project these warps, forming energetic knots and other obstructions, scarring and twisting in
ways that restrict their intrinsic motions and biological functions.

Under ceaseless traction, viscera try to discharge pressure, deflecting unwanted encroachments along all available trajectories, rotating
and side-bending, buckling and torquing, abbreviating intervals to each
others' perimeters, pushing up protuberances, taking strain off jeop-
ardized components. Fibers retaining elasticity invariably translate stress
away from their plexuses and any other compromised, vulnerable nodes.
Yet multilateral tensions irrevocably impress themselves, immobilizing
viscera.

The processing of air and food and distribution of their wastes have
the continuous potential to irritate and restrict viscera (much as inci-

MODALITIES

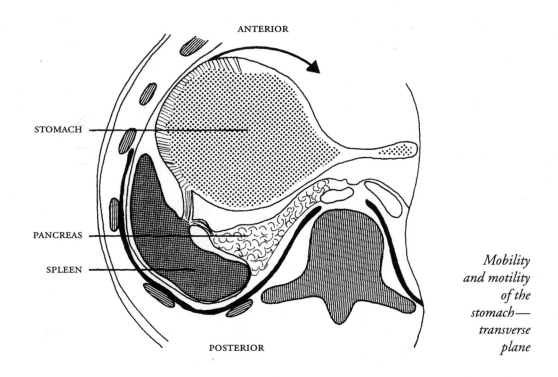

ANTERIOR

STOMACH

PANCREAS

SPLEEN

POSTERIOR

*Mobility
and motility
of the
stomach—
transverse
plane*

dental activity can knock, bump, and dislocate segments of the skeleton). Likewise, emotional changes, with their endocrinological and chemical constituents, directly impinge on visceral motility. Mechanical stresses blend with these cathexes to lock in psychosomatic patterns and deaden energy channels. Barral and Mercier write:

> A visceral restriction occurs when an organ loses part or all of its ability to move.... [V]isceral articulations are made up of sliding surfaces and means of connection. A restriction may arise either at the level of these structures or on the walls of the actual organ, and can usually be assigned to one of three categories ...: articular, ligamentous or muscular.
>
> One can also distinguish functional from positional restrictions.

*Osteopathy
and
Chiropractic*

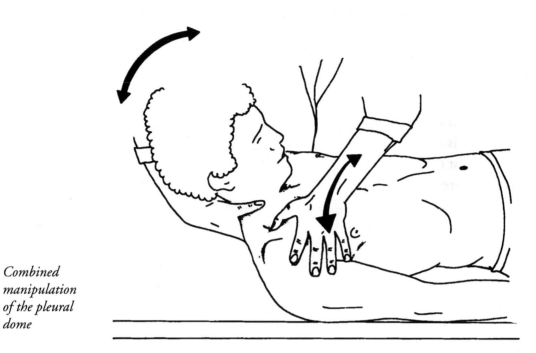

*Combined
manipulation
of the pleural
dome*

With *functional restrictions,* only the function of the related organs is affected; their positional relationships are not changed. With *positional restrictions,* the anatomical relationships of the organs are changed and their articulations are modified. For example, with a right renal ptosis, the kidney loses all contact with the liver—a veritable visceral subluxation.[22] [italics theirs]

In visceral treatment, various modes of manual assessment and palpation are used to ascertain an organ's tonicity, position, size, freedom of circulating fluids, rhythm, angle of orientation vis-à-vis other organs and their orientations, and degree of restriction. Gentle and precise, techniques of hands-on listening blend into a type of manipulation that follows each organ's tendencies and elicits its natural rhythms. According to Barral and Mercier, "Visceral manipulation is a method

MODALITIES

300

of restarting the mobility or motility of an organ utilizing specific, gentle forces. . . . We manipulate to the point where the body can take over in order to achieve self-correction, not to force a correction on the body."[23] Thus, the physician's relationship to internal organ dysfunction is not one of a surgeon or even a classical bodyworker—mechanical alteration toward a goal of what constitutes "normal" shape and function; it is at once feeling for a hidden cadence and seriality and imparting just the right stimulus in the right direction to evoke its therapeutic progression naturally. A visceral adjustment opens channels and releases blocks to allow a self-curative process. It does not (necessarily) literally repair an explicit pathology or site.

To the patient the sensation of the release may be extremely subtle, like the separation of layers within oneself that were stuck together in a background. Manipulation of the liver or colon is not painful like a "minor surgery." It is more like remembering something internally that was always there but unnoticed because it had become kinesthetically numbed. Aspects of background tissue awakening tingle and ache like layers of extremely familiar unlived or abandoned lives.

Diagnosis begins as the practitioner assesses the overall organization, relative freedom, and energetic pattern of the body of the client. This may be visual observation, hands-on assaying of seemingly blocked tissue vectors, or off-the-body temperature readings by using a hand like a sniffing dog, stirring it through a patient's energy fields and sensing for pockets of heat. Some practitioners can "see" the various oscillating fields and stress planes of the body and even the spectra of its auras; other practitioners feel these same things (even with their eyes closed—often *especially* with their eyes closed). Because tissue transmits flow, distortion, and congestion throughout an organism, while trying to release sites of somatic tension, the effects of immobilities may travel some distance to reside in a particular dysfunction or zone of pain. The toxic off-shoots of a cheap wine on the liver may initially lead to adjacent tissues trying to take tension off that organ but, as other organs continue to compensate and adjust, translating and diffusing force outward, it may end up in the left shoulder as if a muscular constriction. Of course, direct treatment of the scapula would accomplish little of a permanent nature. The method and course of palpation must reflect the pattern, depth, speed, and root of the distorting force lodged in tissue:

> For each case, you must tune into the patient and feel the rhythm, vitality and resistance of the tissue you are working with. Problems arise from insufficient understanding of the osteopathic concept. One of the big mistakes beginners make is trying to "push" the organ too quickly; the organ cannot adapt to the unnatural speed of change and the treatment is ineffective. If, after treatment, the organ goes through about ten normal cycles, you may consider the treatment to have been effective.[24]

The palpator picks a spot for entry and, meeting tissue resistance, adds about five more grams of force to mobilize not the dermis or pure musculature but the total energetic pattern issuing from that point. The touch is light because it must be durable; it must travel deep into viscera, honing toward core without attaching to intermediate structures and dissipating itself there. Too firm a touch immediately activates connective-tissue resistance; the palpation then becomes conventional massage. Even medium touch can be coopted by and fuse with an "irrelevant" tissue layer that happens to get in the way. The healer must instead gather up stress lines one by one, a vector at a time, somewhat like following ripples to a center from which they radiate, stacking them as she goes. Too light a touch merely distorts the ripples; too heavy a hand plows right through them.

The stress lines are also little beads that fall along different trajectories and in slightly different planes. Gathering them is a bit like trying to balance an increasingly higher tower of little paper boxes not resting flush atop one another, except that the skilled palpator's juggling is supported by the tissues' guiding grains, their intrinsic pliability and density, and also by almost indescribable currents of energy.

As the body responds to induction, it guides the hand along the path of the blockage to where tissue has been restricted and rigidified and "wants" to be released. It has semi-rotated, sidebent, and corkscrewed in some combination to shorten its ranges of movement and reduce the shearing and compression effects at specific nodes, and it has likely developed adhesions and barriers to motility with adjacent organs. By gently accreting lines of force and balancing multiple reciprocal axes in all three (or four) dimensions, the visceral therapist untangles and liberates restrictions and adhesions layer by layer, gathering residual energy and mass in the process and continuing inward to other nodes.

The amount of force, as noted, rarely exceeds five grams, though it may seem like more because of meeting tissue resistance before adding any quanta of pressure. Since most organs are blocked from direct therapist access by musculoskeletal structures and other organs, continued light stacking and balancing is needed to follow a vector far enough in to reach, for instance, pancreas, spleen, stomach, kidneys, ureter, structures inside the skull or behind the eyes, etc. Sometimes the therapist may raise, fold, or torque the body across the pelvis, shoulders, or chest to produce a tauter path to the proper site at the most appropriate therapeutic angle and depth. Clearly this is a method requiring great anatomical dexterity, hair-trigger sensitivity, and delicacy in stacking planes and pressures and pulling vectors.

> To perform induction, you must know the proper and precise directions of motility for each organ.... In listening, the hand passively follows the pendulum-like motion of the organ. During induction the same hand will slightly accentuate or encourage the larger motion which is that in the direction of greater excursion. Continue this process until the induced motion coincides with normal motility of the organ in terms of direction, amplitude and axes....[25]

This is a standard osteopathic mode of correction: encouraging a segment of viscera (or neuromusculature) to "go" in the direction it "wants" rather than in a normalizing trajectory. The assumption is that it can "find" its own correct orientation through enhancement of its tendency, whereas it may never stay in a position into which it is just placed. (Osteopaths tend to support and reinforce counter-energetically forced or intrinsic rhythm, even when they encounter highly erratic motions and hard blocks.)

A few examples of some basic techniques, although simplifications, give a fuller sense of this modality:

If the stomach rotates more easily toward the median axis of the body (a movement Barral named "expir"), enhance that movement by a clockwise motion in the frontal plane with a flat right hand engendering a slight suction on the skin such that, at the end of the turn, the lesser curvature under the index finger rotates posterosuperiorly and the ulnar aspect seems to retreat from the skin. Encourage the dominant expir rotation while passively tracking and supporting the rest of the cycle until the pattern releases into greater depth and range.

To release a urethral calculus, compress and rotate at the point of the stone with the heel of the hand, culminating the rotation with a light inferior stretch across the ureter. This also improves the organ's peristaltic function.

The pancreas is released by a seesaw movement in which the heel of the hand sits above the projection of the pancreatic head and is pulled posteriorly while the rest of the hand covering the body and tail of the organ induces tissue downward as the head begins to release; the fingers gradually follow. Then, as the pancreas rotates away from the median axis of the body (inspir), the same sort of induction is imparted from the fingertips to the heel. During this back-and-forth rocking, the predominant organ motion is accentuated, while its counterphase is supported more passively.

Variations, combinations, and refinements of such techniques treat areas as miniscule as the dural tube of the optic nerve, the sphincter of Oddi, and the epididymis.

THERE SHOULD ALSO BE no misunderstanding about the intended scope of this treatment. Visceral manipulation is decidedly not massage; it is meant to diagnose and treat a full range of clinical pathologies originating in the organs of the human body. It is an empirical science in the Hippocratic lineage.

Trainees are expected to study visceral geography thoroughly and, at advanced levels, to dissect cadavers to observe and feel the qualities and arrangements of actual tissue structures and their individual variations from body to body (though dead organs do not carry the energy of live ones and have begun to harden). The goal is to get the student cognizant of real structures, what they feel like and how they are attached and fused, thus not to work solely on a level of energy and sensation. Few allopathic physicians receive such rigorous education in tissue topology.

Visceral manipulation both imitates surgery and opposes it. It in fact *is* surgery insofar as it has a surgical goal, which it accomplishes by gradual inducement (without incision) over one or more extended treatments. Needless to say, it challenges surgery by achieving that goal indirectly and by a combination of intrinsic visceral movement and palpation. Health is restored by embryogenic principles of induction and organization.

Craniosacral Therapy

THERE IS NO inherent reason why cranial osteopathy should not have led directly to a fully holistic, psychological medicine long before the Human Potential Movement of the 1960s and '70s. After Sutherland discovered the movements of the cranial and sacral bones, he developed an entire system for their subtle manipulation. As a Swedenborgian mystic, he believed that he was touching the roots of the soul in the body and that his palpations were sending waves directly into spiritual consciousness. He laid the groundwork for osteopathic psychotherapy.

Craniosacral and visceral palpations, insofar as they are based on projecting intention while trusting the slightest tendency (five grams),

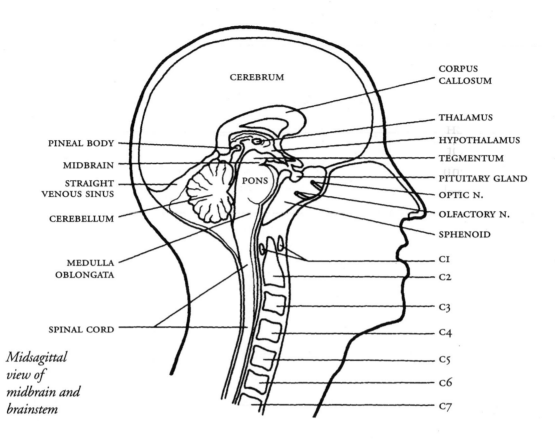

CEREBRUM

CORPUS CALLOSUM

THALAMUS

HYPOTHALAMUS

PINEAL BODY

TEGMENTUM

MIDBRAIN

PITUITARY GLAND

STRAIGHT VENOUS SINUS

PONS

OPTIC N.

OLFACTORY N.

CEREBELLUM

SPHENOID

C1

C2

MEDULLA OBLONGATA

C3

C4

SPINAL CORD

C5

Midsagittal view of midbrain and brainstem

C6

C7

are closer to Intelligence than direct applications of force. One learns to detect the glimmers of mind in motion and to track those glimmers within grosser anatomy. This suggests the realm, as noted earlier, where psychological, vitalistic, and surgical medicines meet.

A psycho-energetic trend ceased abruptly in the 1920s, as osteopaths, censored by the AMA, could no longer practice the system in which they had trained. Subsequent generations, as they became more concerned with their acceptance into the allopathic establishment, emphasized the mechanical, quasi-surgical aspects of their treatments (and

MODALITIES

even practiced standard pharmacy) to the point that cranial osteopathy almost disappeared from the medical landscape. However, in the 1980s, through a new paradigm of treatment, it was not only reborn but launched a radical new modality of healing.

ALTHOUGH MANY HAVE contributed to the revival of Sutherland's science, it was primarily a medical osteopath, John Upledger, who had the ingenuity and will to reinvent cranial osteopathy in the late 1970s and develop its model of practice. His "coming out of the closet" antagonized not only orthodox doctors but the osteopathic establishment, and he was ostracized from the profession. On his appointment to the National Institutes of Health Office of Alternative Medicine panel in 1993, however, the osteopathic journals reclaimed him as one of their own.

REINVENTING OSTEOPATHY was crucial, for a fresh perspective took it out of a sectarian domain in which it could not grow or attain legitimacy and freed it to realize its potential, as osteopaths developed listening skills and techniques in concordance with non-Western systems of massage, spirit healing, and shamanism, as well as with the movement arts and somatic psychotherapy. The Upledger Institute, with its research center in West Palm Beach, Florida, now offers a diverse and innovative curriculum in a variety of manual medicines taught throughout the world. It has become both a current locus of the secularization of traditional osteopathy and the nucleus of a new, unexplored medicine arising from osteopathy (see the Resource Guide).

A trademarked system of CranioSacral Therapy and Somato-Emotional Release was developed by Upledger and his associates at Michigan State University in the mid-1970s when they were part of an interdisciplinary team of doctors and physical and biological scientists assembled to study the relationship between energy (in various forms) and therapeutic results. At this time, cranial osteopathy was maintained mostly outside the osteopathic establishment, and even Upledger, a

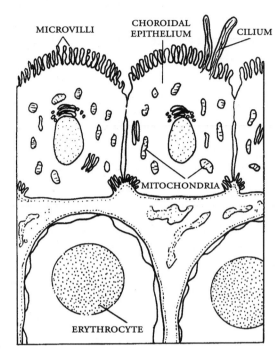

MICROVILLI · CHOROIDAL EPITHELIUM · CILIUM · MITOCHONDRIA · ERYTHROCYTE

Choroid plexus tight junctions

Reprinted from *An Introduction to Craniosacral Therapy* by Don Cohen, D.C., North Atlantic Books, 1995.

trained osteopath, was somewhat unfamiliar with its full range of principles and techniques. The disciples of Sutherland would only teach their methods to the one group least interested in learning them—AMA-sanctioned doctors. The way they upheld their school as a legitimate medical institution was by restricting their testament to a narrow professional arena. Although "following energy" has become a recognized technique in many schools of modern osteopathic medicine not associated with Upledger, and although there is a long-standing tradition within osteopathy, it was only after Upledger and his associates at Michigan State made their discoveries and systematized a protocol of techniques based on them that osteopaths (and of course craniosacral therapists of all schools) recovered the energetic aspect of their system and prioritized it then. They were then liberated to develop energetic palpation as a powerful tool and derive new techniques and make it into a science unencumbered by the osteopathic past.

Observing subtle, profound movements of dural elements during surgery, Upledger became curious about their energy and mechanics and began investigating the realm of cranial osteopathy. An initial inquiry became a life quest. Ultimately he not only liberated Sutherland's cranial model from its quarantine, he demedicalized it, both in terms of the territory it potentially could encompass and in reaction against bogus legitimacy (which had limited its application to a narrow range of treatments within physical therapy). He then used cranial fluid techniques as a path to exploring a wide range of energetic and "somatoemotional" techniques, thus became a pioneer in the development of

MODALITIES

such concepts as "your inner physician," "dialoguing with tissues," "cell talk," and even interspecies healing. In defiance of both medical and osteopathic establishments, he taught a widening compass of manual techniques to lay people in hopes of increasing the base of qualified healers and practitioners in the world (something that would not have happened had the transmission of cranial osteopathy depended on either just osteopaths or osteopaths and M.D.s). Thus, cranial osteopathy evolved into craniosacral therapy or, more precisely, Upledger adapted and transformed many aspects of Sutherland's system into a new cranial medicine, retaining techniques, reinterpreting techniques, developing new techniques, and combining elements in innovative ways based on empirical discoveries. Other cranial practitioners continued to draw on Sutherland's lineage directly and, after the success of craniosacral therapy, these initiated rival schools that often "borrowed" the more modern "craniosacral" name (see pp. 362–363).

CranioSacral Therapy has certainly given new life and status to all cranial and Sutherlandian modalities. In 1994, with the support of the

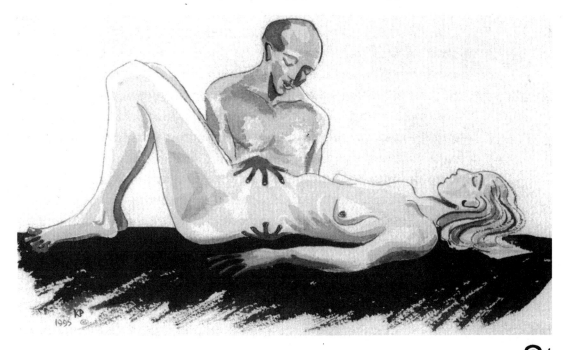

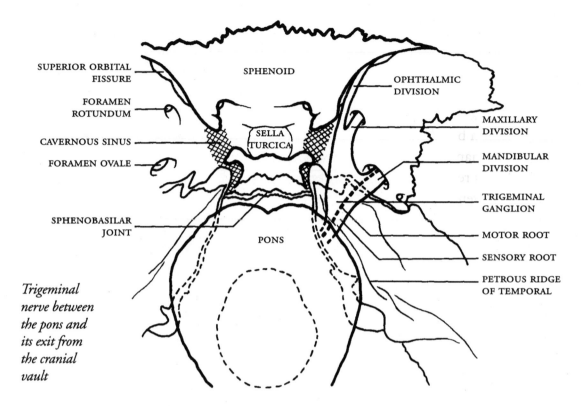

SUPERIOR ORBITAL FISSURE

FORAMEN ROTUNDUM

CAVERNOUS SINUS

FORAMEN OVALE

SPHENOBASILAR JOINT

SPHENOID

SELLA TURCICA

PONS

OPHTHALMIC DIVISION

MAXILLARY DIVISION

MANDIBULAR DIVISION

TRIGEMINAL GANGLION

MOTOR ROOT

SENSORY ROOT

PETROUS RIDGE OF TEMPORAL

Trigeminal nerve between the pons and its exit from the cranial vault

Bosnian Government and the World Health Organization, the Upledger Institute dispatched a team of its own craniosacral therapists to treat Post-Traumatic Stress Disorder in the former Yugoslavia. Cadres practicing lay volunteer healing in crisis zones clearly should be one goal of a humane "planet medicine" in the twenty-first century.

The Institute also applied equivalent methods of healing to Vietnam veterans suffering from Post-Traumatic Stress Disorder—some thirty years after battle conditions and (also) after the Veterans Administration psychotherapeutic treatments had utterly failed its patients. Their regime had become reduced to psychotropic drugs and pain-killers. As one veteran in the Upledger program commented, "I've

MODALITIES

310

learned to put my complete trust in their hands. It's like being in the hands of Rangers."[26]

IN CLASSIC CRANIOSACRAL treatments, healer and patient engage in a rhythmic interchange much like that of visceral manipulation but rooted in and tracked through the requirements and manifestations of the craniosacral (cerebrospinal) system. This realm constitutes a subtle bodywide hydraulic network driven by the pressure of the cerebrospinal fluid (as more of it is produced by the choroid plexuses within the ventricles of the brain than is reabsorbed by the arachnoid bodies). The craniosacral modality is named for the cranium and sacrum through which this current under membrane and tissue is most directly accessed. However, craniosacral therapy is bodywide and not limited to the hydraulic core. A common mistake is to assume that because Upledger focused on the craniosacral rhythm and trademarked the name "CranioSacral Therapy" to describe his work that the process has primarily to do with conditions of the cranial, spinal and sacral skeleton and the movements of its bones. The rhythm is in fact a component of and guide to events within the whole organism— viscera, psyche, and etheric fields.

Polarity founder Randolph Stone, following Sutherland, proposed that a primary energy pattern comprising the intelligence of life itself "is conveyed throughout the body by the cerebrospinal fluid. . . . [W]here this flow is impeded, then intelligence breaks down and darkness and disorder prevail...tendency to ill-health arises. . . .Where this primary and essential life force is present, there is life and healing with normal function. Where this primary and essential life force is not acting in the body, there is obstruction, spasm, or stagnation and pain, like gears which clash instead of meshing in their operation. The expansion and contraction of the cranial rhythm

Somatics

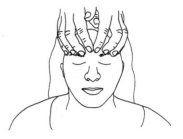

Frontal lift

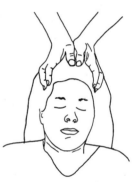

Parietal lift

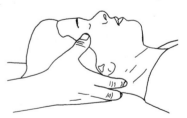

Sphenoid lift

Reprinted from *An Introduction to Craniosacral Therapy* by Don Cohen, D.C., North Atlantic Books, 1995.

... is a harmonic of the expansion and contraction of the energy system as a whole."[27]

CRANIOSACRAL METHODS FORM a larger coherent healing system with the techniques of visceral manipulation insofar as both therapies involve palpating lines of restricted motion, inducing a response through light touch, and following tissue where it wants to go, thereby stimulating a release. The bones, membranes, myofascia, blood-based fluids, and nervous system interact to form a coherent, intelligent, self-correcting cerebrospinal network that underlies all of psychic and somatic life. Through layers of this network, the neuroses and traumas defined by psychotherapists can also be addressed and treated.

Craniosacral rhythm is a fundamental pulse like breath and heartbeat, though quieter and less metabolism-driven than the rush of either blood or air. It was of course substantially known to Sutherland. In the dynamic engineering spirit of Still, Upledger rediscovered it himself, as noted above, during surgery when he observed its regularity, intensity, and centrality (he was trying to hold the dural membrane still for plaque removal by using two sets of forceps, but its pulsing movement prevailed against his mechanical pressure). He verified his findings clinically and in extensive autopsies. Subsequently, he based his mode of therapy upon accessing far-ranging domains through this previously little-understood force.

The craniosacral flexion-extension cycle extending down the dural tube to the viscera is likely generated and perpetuated because the dura-mater membrane is almost completely impermeable to the cerebrospinal fluid. Within this membrane, a homeostasis develops, regulating and rebalancing forces that build and release pressure.

The bones of the cranium, proximate to the reigning functions of the nervous system, tend to translate distortion downhill (along the spine and its dural membrane secondarily, and then through fascia, tendons, and ligaments). Cranial components like the sphenoid bone (which lies mostly behind the eyes and nose), the falxes cerebri and

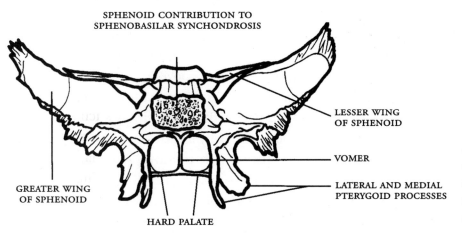

SPHENOID CONTRIBUTION TO
SPHENOBASILAR SYNCHONDROSIS

LESSER WING
OF SPHENOID

VOMER

LATERAL AND MEDIAL
PTERYGOID PROCESSES

GREATER WING
OF SPHENOID

HARD PALATE

*Posterior view
of the
sphenoid,
vomer, and
hard palate*

cerebelli, the occipital, parietal, and temporal bones, etc., function as levers, valves, and pistons of this system. The sphenoid—butterfly in shape and possibly homologous to the pelvis at the other end of the spine—is accessible to palpation only at the outer tips of the eye sockets; it is adjusted by light compression, decompression, twisting, and sliding to alter other components of the face and skull and thereby transpose freedom of movement downward. The temporal bones can be set in traction by a firm, gentle pulling of the external ear lobes. Other components of the system may be accessed from inside the mouth through the teeth or hard palate or from a remote stimulation of the dural membrane itself.

Insofar as the craniosacral system includes at its core the brain, spinal cord, and pituitary and pineal glands (hence the neuroendocrine system and its hormones as well as corresponding functions of the mind-body interface), it is highly sensitive to emotional components. The goal of the therapist is to find an access into psychosomatic homeostases through palpation, to locate zones of dysfunction and restricted function within them, and to disencumber these areas through (mostly) indirect techniques, that is, by stimulation of intrinsic rhythms or even

*Osteopathy
and
Chiropractic*

exaggeration and support of a dysfunctional pattern until it swings so far to its distortedly favored side that it returns naturally to the other (restoration by going *with* rather than fighting a distortion is familiar from visceral manipulation, described above).

In working with either viscera themselves or the craniosacral rhythm, the therapist circumscribes a part of the body with both hands, perhaps one on the lower back, one on the belly. He then adds pressure with the top hand until he feels the tissues start to move. As in visceral manipulation, the force exerted must be only slightly greater than that of tissue resistance. Once the touch becomes too heavy (generally more than the same five grams), the organism begins to respond less on the level of craniosacral or visceral sensitivity and more in terms of neuromuscular tension and stress patterns. This is not like going from good to bad; it is switching therapeutic modes (and is rarely successful). As noted before, too light a touch activates only auras or external energy fields; too heavy a touch engages muscles. Craniosacral traction like visceral manipulation falls precisely between.

Often the therapist finds the right level of force and depth by ever so subtly adding and removing increments of weight to her hand while fine-tuning the angle of entry with minute rotations at her wrist and shoulder. The former allows finer adjustments, the latter grosser ones. The tissue may lead the hand in a circular trajectory. The therapist tries to find the line of untangling, i.e., where there is a slightly greater centrifugal force, and makes a stand there. She gently stops the circle and slowly steers its orbit into the angular force, a sensation which is simultaneously like pulling taffy, attracting metal filings with a small magnet, and pulling tight a draw-string from far away. Gathering any slack remaining in the draw-string, she continues to resist the old orbit and to reign in (as she senses them) even tinier loops of slack. Cumulatively the slack represents distances within the body. As it is imaginarily drawn in, the hand is influencing either more interior organs or tissues further away. For instance, entry and steering at the level of the bladder can pull "strings" along the ureter or down to the bottom of the foot.

At the same time, the therapist tracks globally, picking up any resonance or vibration from outside her primary trajectory and allowing her touch to ride the waves of cerebrospinal fluid expressed by flexion and extension of the whole system. The larger rhythms guide the treatment to new sites or lines of entry.

The motion is followed to differing degrees with both hands until it stops (this is one form of basic release). However, if the path keeps returning to where it came from or repeats a static cycle, the therapist can gently convert (in successive rounds) the path most insisted upon by the tissue to one of release *from* this trajectory.

Variations of the process can be adapted to almost any region of the anatomy because the cranial pulse radiates from the core to the limbs in its rotatory, opening-and-closing hydraulic orbit.

Don Cohen, a chiropractor who practices CranioSacral Therapy, provides a proprioceptive description of osteopathic attention:

> ... [L]istening to the neurologic rhythms and refraining from stimulating the patient with your perceptions and remedial advice (treatment) can be a powerful therapeutic mode. The recognition of intelligence in neurologic tissue is not pathetic fallacy (in which human traits are attributed to inanimate objects). It is apparent that the nervous system is no dummy and knows when it is being listened to, and appreciates that quiet and accepting forum. I have had the experience at times of working with a patient intently, trying with all my effort to effect a real change by various means, adjusting, myofascial work, etc., and suddenly becoming aware of the tension in my own body and in the situation, and relaxing, softening my grip, and sitting down to listen to the neural rhythm. The body comes alive, pulsating, processing, revealing a mind of its own.... That this autonomic response is deliberate will be obvious to anyone who experiences it. This is the power of communication, for which all nervous systems and all people hunger.[28]

Cohen recounts the mysterious process whereby the therapist places his hands on a head or body and tunes into a rhythm that is distinct

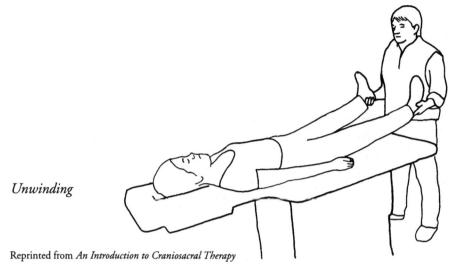

Unwinding

Reprinted from *An Introduction to Craniosacral Therapy*
by Don Cohen, D.C., North Atlantic Books, 1995.

from either his own or the patient's heart rhythms and breath.

> ... [L]et your attention float up and down the dural tube and through
> the body. It's easy to imagine. Can you feel subluxations through the
> tube? With passive proprioception, feel tension and pressure gradi-
> ents and their influence on the cranial rhythm. Trust your impres-
> sion. Then tug very gently, almost imperceptibly, on the tissues to
> gain a further impression of where the tissue is hung up. Again focus
> your attention down the body. Ask yourself: where would I place a
> push pin or a piece of tape to create this same pattern of resistance?[29]

This is likely the location of a block. Listening is often more therapeutic than adjusting because "just listening" does also adjust, very
subtly. Any time one breaks with listening to act on tissue, listening
stops and the palpation becomes shallower, as the hands cease to melt
into visceral layers and follow their torque—and the organs resist.

A WEB OF CONNECTIVE TISSUE intertwines and interpenetrates all
the viscera from the meninges of the brain, down the front and
back of the body, all the way to the bottoms of the feet. Fascia encompasses the musculature of the shoulders, chest, back of the ribs, dural

MODALITIES

tube, and pelvis as well as the wrappings of the entirety of organs and limbs (pericardium, intestines, genitals, etc.) in what is essentially a dynamically complex but single sheet. Its cohesive plait provides pathways for palpating stress lines and tracking them to impacted sites, likewise for unravelling the knots. The same energetic, yarnlike layers of fabric that a Rolfer impresses and remolds guide a craniosacral palpator through the body's shear planes, viscosity, and adhesiveness to a snarl or tangle of cysts anchoring any particular line of tension.

Pulling on fascia is like stretching and twisting a bed-sheet to find where it is snagged and get it free; it can be a simultaneous and complementary process to stack tissue to reach and recalibrate viscera and also to ride the hydraulics of the cranial pulse through cycles of flexion and extension. Successful palpation harmonizes elements of all these techniques in a single, highly sensitive but secure sequence of manual investigation and rebalancing.

T HE PRESUMPTION is that at an instant of traumatization, a negative energy matrix was injected into the patient's system and somaticized—the stronger the force or deeper the trauma, the more extensive and intransigent the "energy cyst" (in Upledger's terminology). The person holds onto the site emotionally through fear and anxiety, guilt, shame, grief, and even mourning and loyalty. In principle, it doesn't matter if the originating force was a gunshot wound from a carjacker, the collective deposits of years of junk food, or the humiliating taunts of a narcissistic parent. The psychophysiological environment continuously transmits immobilizing pathologies on both emotional and somatic levels through tissue and mind holistically.

Hand position for release of spheno-maxillary impaction

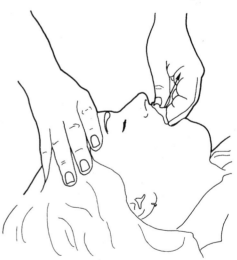

Reprinted from *CranioSacral Therapy* by John E. Upledger and Jon D. Vredevoogd with permission of the publisher, Eastland Press, Inc., P.O. Box 12689, Seattle, WA 98111. Copyright 1983. All rights reserved.

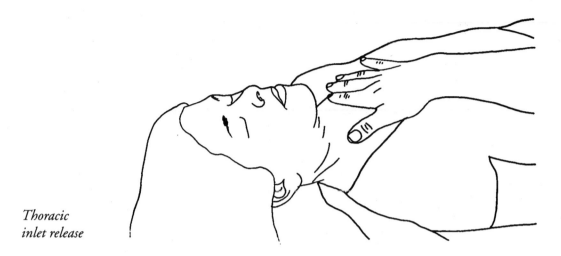

Thoracic inlet release

Reprinted from *An Introduction to Craniosacral Therapy* by Don Cohen, D.C., North Atlantic Books, 1995.

One of Upledger's earliest insights, reinforcing our characterization of the pathogenic physician (see Chapter Two), is that surgeons transfer their attitudes directly through their scalpels into the tissue layers of their patients. Their anger and disdain and, conversely, their generosity and caring are imbedded and codified in visceral memory patterns. Even the tone of the surgeon's voice while speaking idly to his assistants lodges in an anesthetized patient's tissues. Upledger found that patients could recount tales of surgical encounters with extraordinary accuracy even though they were unconscious at the time. More significantly, their bodies had somaticized the emotional tenor of the experience. "If molecularly simple recording tape has such a memory," he asks, "why not cells?"[30]

These deceptively extraneous factors determine not only the speed with which surgical wounds heal but the success of the very surgery. In fact, Upledger decided in 1994, after engaging for many years in inaugural research along diverse lines, that the primary therapeutic event he was interested in proving scientifically is the fact that *electrically measurable energies* are transmitted directly from a physician to a

MODALITIES

patient—through hands, surgical and dental tools, and attitudes—and that these energies affect healing and pathology in an explicit, quantifiable way.

By the same principle, the less physical and emotional trauma there is accompanying the formation of a cyst, the less subsequent dysfunction will arise. As one therapist remarked, "The football player who injures himself while catching the game-winning pass does not have the level of trauma of a player who gets the same injury and drops the pass." Hence, wounds and diseases originating from relatively nontraumatizing causes yield to treatment more readily because they are not as deeply encysted by emotional charge.

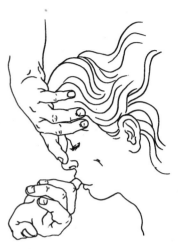

When a trauma is kept from releasing, the body has to continue to function *around* its area of entropy. It takes energy to wall off and contain a trauma and also energy to continue to function in its context. The organism twists, oscillates, displaces itself regionally to one side or another, and hammers those twists, oscillations, and sidebends inward through tissue density. Tissue structures try to protect themselves and become knotted. Not only that, but in the formation of a wound or distortion, the body is responding instantaneously to an external force while itself moving viscerally and internally, deflecting the vectors of entry so that a linear blow from an assailant, vehicle, or stationary object bumped into imbeds itself in the system at many different angles over even milliseconds of time, much like a barbed hook fashioned to catch and hold a fish. Emotional traumas have even more complex hooks of entry through the neuromusculature.

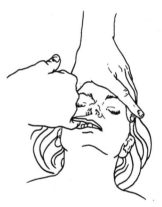

The therapist, by tracking and unwinding somatic vectors as they lead him to their source, ultimately enters the afflicted site and then can direct his or her palpations into it at matching angles. Many ailments have multiple causes and form in layers, thus must be located in layers and cured layer by layer—

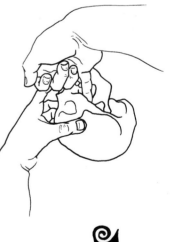

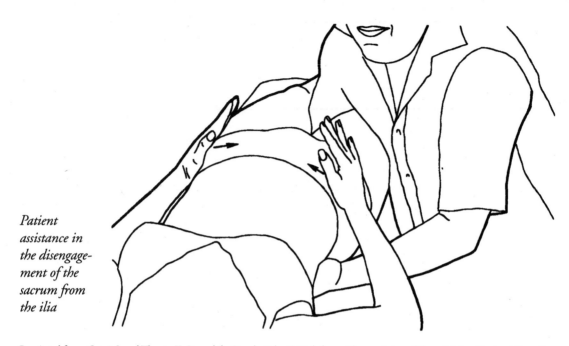

Patient assistance in the disengagement of the sacrum from the ilia

the tractions always joining at the point where the various energetic sources of the condition itself meet.

If the therapist is skilled enough to track the rhythm and fascial network to traumatized sites ("energy cysts"), then the physical forces stored at those sites may be, one by one, released. The therapist does not release such energy in a predetermined fashion; instead the patient unwinds herself in response to a sympathetic palpation that guides her to her own native rhythm and movement as it responds to the healing intention behind the touch.

In reality, there is no straightforward map either to the diagnosis of cysts or the release of them. As in other osteopathic processes, the therapist must use a combination of touch, paraphysical sensing, and intuition. Some practitioners clearly see a patient's energetic and functional breaks by looking at the body. Others don't "see" it until they close their

MODALITIES

320

eyes and stare at the after-image. Many scan it at slightly deflected angles. Some who can't see such patterns at all can feel them in their hands as they pass them above a patient's body. A fair number of people have to touch the body directly to track the flows in it. The process of using the differential ripples emitting through a semi-fluidic, visceral organism to situate the spot of a splash (cyst) is known as arcing—divining as by a living rod the nucleus of many deflected arcs.

ENERGY CYSTS AND somatoemotional traumas represent different levels of the same phenomena. The Upledger system thus distinguishes between a mechanical process of therapeutically releasing cysts and a more extensive procedure of full somatoemotional, post-traumatic release.

Cysts are treated first by arcing to their source (a process which in itself stimulates energetic dispersal) and then dissolving them, usually through indirect osteopathic techniques. Sometimes just holding and supporting the body at the correct point and angle (and then at each successively revealed point and angle) is sufficient to allow the viscera to release themselves. One Vietnam veteran concluded, "You can physically feel these energy cysts and physical events that have lodged themselves in you. You can literally feel them leaving your body."[31] Pieces of war that got frozen in tissue are melted and discharged. The organism knows what it needs and will often not only lead the therapist to appropriate sites but cue him in techniques by seeming to pull his hands in like suction or a magnet.

Following sensation is the key to treatment. One must avoid any prejudgment about what is functionally required for cure. In fact, the techniques that go straight to the core may be regarded as more invasive by the patient's system and sometimes stimulate deepening of the cyst. "Don't make the patient have to defend against you," Upledger warns, "which is not the problem he came in with."[32] If the therapist makes

Hand position for stillpoint induction

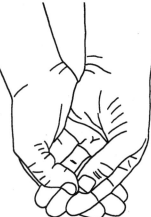

Reprinted from *An Introduction to Craniosacral Therapy* by Don Cohen, D.C., North Atlantic Books, 1995.

321

himself the problem through overzealous "fixing" and unconscious projections, then instead of release, a new layer is added to the pathology.

Full somatoemotional cure combines physical, verbal, and emotional elements. The therapist not only diagnoses and releases cysts but
guides the patient with questions about images and feelings and then,
as they are answered either verbally or somatically or (usually) both,
follows the new movements generated by the body wherever they go
(even to entirely different energy complexes). All the time, the therapist is supporting somatic and verbal expression, following patterns,
and interpolating the craniosacral rhythm as a guide.

Traditionally the process of somatoemotional release begins with
freeing the "avenue of expression": the full thoracic inlet and throat
chakra, the first and second ribs, the clavicle, all the hyoid muscles
(around the Adam's apple) and their related fascia and bony attachments, the hard palate (and through it, the vomer and palatines), and
then the tongue, gums, and teeth. Each of these areas may contain
impediments or imbedded hooks from events and circumstances in
the person's life, and these deter full expression up from the gut out
through the mouth. The teeth, for instance, have often been deeply
traumatized by dental drilling and orthodontics, with these strictures
translating inward into the vomer, sphenoid, maxilla, and affecting the
craniosacral flow itself. Each tooth can be guided and "unwound" in
the same way other parts of the body are (by following the yarn of its
intrinsic motion with a single finger or between a finger and thumb).
Such a process apparently not only releases the tooth but helps with
periodontal problems by stimulating bone and gum restoration.

The pretzel of immobilization may be so complex in its visceral,
skeletal, and emotionally cathected components that it may take as
many as five or six assistants helping the therapist support the body at
key points and following its unwindings simultaneously. Like handlers
of a giant snake, they follow the body off the table and hold it in midair
allowing it to "unwrithe" its traumas with as few restrictions as possible. Many ailments are actually a knot of such giant snakes locked in

different dimensions and symbolic systems. "I felt myself come flying off the table," an acquaintance mythologized somewhat in recounting his first craniosacral session with a group. "Suddenly I was spinning in midair and bouncing off walls."

As the craniosacral therapist steers more deeply into blocks, the patient responds by transferring the increased motility deeper. Just having his or her rhythm located and touched imparts a curative momentum both emotionally and physically in a person. The innermost tissue layers and zones are least familiar and quite profound in terms of what they contain and can release. For the deepest reaches of the body, it is like "being seen" for the first time. After all the years of functioning in not only darkness but nullity, suddenly these texture-rich movement patterns connect to the conscious mind, the numinous "self." At the moment of becoming conscious, they "exist." As they exist, they communicate how dense and vast they actually are. Their sensations are not just the momentary static of internal exercises; they arise from the cellular basis of existence. As they differentiate from the background, they envelop the person in an awareness of whom he or she actually is and gravitate toward whom he or she might be. They literally change identity.

W HEREAS ARTIFICIAL STOPPAGES of the craniosacral rhythm may be imposed therapeutically, the abrupt cessation of the craniosacral rhythm while "following" tissue patterns is always regarded as a deepening. Because the craniosacral system is a core system, it pulls the physician and patient inevitably to the right place (often marked by such a halt in the rhythm). At these junctures, the system simply does not know where to go. It puts out confusion. The therapist supports this place with his vector of palpation and waits for a change. Responsiveness here, remember, does not require cognitive knowledge of the cause of the trauma; palpation innately provides the visceral organization a protected way to reorder itself.

If the patient is verbally responsive at the time, the rhythm can be consulted, almost like a lie detector, to determine its truth. A full stoppage usually means "Yes!" If the patient is simultaneously experiencing an image or feeling during cessation, these are considered authentic reenactments of a traumatic source. Even if a reported image seems irrelevant at that moment to the therapist and patient, they must ignore their prejudice and trust the system. Whenever it says, "Stop here and wait," the therapist must hang out.

Often craniosacral cessation coincides with "memories" of being in the womb, coming out the birth canal, or in the midst of what presents itself as another lifetime. During one workshop a woman whose rhythm had stopped suddenly changed her name from Deborah to Jonathan, deepened her voice, took on an accent, began laughing uproariously, and became an elderly man committing suicide by leaping from a cliff and attempting to glide over the ocean. The moment of elation in flight was followed by intense "pain" that led her to writhe upward off the table and to reenact the jump with three people guiding her in midair. Whatever these images and sensations represent, they were crucial to the organism in exactly the form in which it chose to elicit and express them. Some people may select past-life imagery, others scenes from early childhood; some may choose episodes of racial, ethnic, or archetypal significance. There should be no attempt to assign priority or validity to one world-view or another. It is what happens energetically and somatically that is important.

Conversely, if a patient experiences graphic and revealing images, perhaps even of being murdered in another lifetime or of sexual abuse in childhood, but the craniosacral rhythm continues unimpeded, the images may be relatively discounted. They are not denied but are regarded as likely to be transitional, perhaps a form of self-conscious therapeutic melodrama guarding more truly painful events, perhaps transient portals into a larger experience.

THE CRANIOSACRAL MECHANISM no doubt has been experienced kinesthetically and medically in some fashion or other since the

Stone Age, but it was not clearly identified as a separate cerebrospinal pulse until cranial osteopathy. There is no traditional explanation for the power and range of the cerebrospinal force. That is just the way we are put together embryonically. There is also no theoretical reason why treatment of the body and psyche through interaction with and induction of the craniosacral rhythm should have such substantial somatoemotional consequences. This is pure empirical, improvisational medicine, initiated by Sutherland and practiced since by countless others. One finds cures in the act of practicing techniques.

Though one may guess at the biological or psychospiritual agency, the fact is that the craniosacral pulse and its visceral adjuncts are branches of a pathway to the core, to a first principle of life, to the holographic liquid light of the body-mind archetype, to its patterning energies and the basis of the causal, existential realm itself. We evolved that way, and we form that way anew each time in an embryo. Without necessarily any specific hand-to-pathology blueprint, the craniosacral rhythm unwinds deeper and deeper in the sense that it contacts more and more basic coherences within the organism and ultimately transmits resolutions to stressed and dysfunctional tissue. A dialogue with the craniosacral rhythm, conducted physically, psychically, and psychologically, is a dialogue with one of the deepest accessible levels of an organism's existence.

Tracking another person's cranial rhythms and visceral motilities is conducting psychoanalysis nonverbally. Foregoing strategies to unlayer resistance and decipher sublimation—sparing even words most of the time—somatoemotional release is transference without paraphernalia. The true "psychiatrist," as John Upledger proposed, is the physician within—the pulse emanating hydrostatically from the irrigation cycle of cerebrospinal fluid that autonomically goes toward points of impacted or trapped energy. In this exercise mind and body are collateral. As the sensitivity of the palpator engages the inner physician of the patient, a psychotherapeutic-like dialogue conducts itself silently, transmitting personal history solely through the contours of the pulse.

Truth is declared not by insight or cognitive interpretation but by spontaneous images and "memories" that arise when (and where) the cranial rhythm stops.

Upledger's intent, as noted, was neither to prioritize craniosacral functions nor to develop a new specialty within general osteopathy. If anything, it was to find a therapeutic locus into the extraordinarily complex system of cell and tissue layers and symbol referents that make up a human being. Because the craniosacral rhythm appears to be the closest representative of such a locus, it is studied, cultivated, and hitched upon in an often wild and bumpy passage through the range of phenomena within the organism. Subsequently it provides its own meanings.

From the standpoint of modality selection, cure, and ultimate personal freedom, it is mainly important to make people well and to give their organisms flexibility and the power to adjust to stress and other assaults on their integrity. It is not crucial to solve the riddles of the universe or know exactly whether a "voice" is an entity, an archetype, a Freudian symbol, a metaphor, or even a delusion.

If addressed in the terms in which it arises, a symptom or utterance is engaged authentically and in a venue that best serves both patient and doctor. It little matters whether we are "born again," "born again and again," or sociobiological automatons living single arbitrary lives ("Oh, Son of Man, thou canst not know…."). It is essential to give the organism the respect it requires in order for it to be willing to get itself well, which means (first and foremost) listening without interrupting.

Using techniques developed from this basic therapy, Upledger has ministered not only to victims of trauma, but autistic children, children with Down Syndrome, those paralyzed by accidents, amputees, etc., with often remarkable results. For instance, when he treated a person who had part of his clavicle removed after a motorcycle accident, Upledger put an emphasis on encouraging the bone to grow back. He saw no physical reason why bone might not be able to crystallize again, but he also had no rationale for why a method combining imaging and craniosacral therapy should have that effect. In fact, a large portion of the patient's clavicle did grow back and his mobile functions were restored, allowing him to control his cycle again.[33] It was not simple visualization but visualization in the context of craniosacral "following" and somatoemotional release, requiring multiple treatments sustained over a period of time. In cases of cancer, Upledger has prescribed imaging a golden layer of cells radiating light and, whether for this reason or another, dissipation of a tumor has sometimes followed. (See Appendix, Volume One.)

Upledger chooses always to consider the agency of cure the responsiveness of the organism, the role of the doctor being that of a helper following the guidance of the patient's own "inner physician."

ONE OF THE MOST effective craniosacral techniques is the classic "stillpoint" of Sutherland, which is a temporary, artificially imposed cessation of the craniosacral rhythm. This state can be elicited in a prone patient by the slightest outward pressure placed against the inside margins of his feet. A hand keeping the base of the patient's spine either in flexion (when the craniosacral system is at an extreme of filling with fluid) or extension (when it is emptying or emptied) also stops the rhythm. A more common method, however, is for the therapist to encourage the base of the patient's occiput to rest under its own pressure between his hands.

Inducing a stillpoint enhances fluid flow, allows hydraulic and fascial forces to accumulate shear and kinetic energy and redirect themselves, pressurizes and releases minor restrictions throughout the membranes, and relaxes the sympathetic nervous system. Stillpoint itself can be a numinous healing state, like a brief epiphany or fugue which disperses new signals, cleansing and clearing everywhere.

Although he was not referring to the stillpoint of the craniosacral pulse, in "Burnt Norton," the first of his "Four Quartets," T. S. Eliot evokes an archetypal "still point" that includes a cerebrospinal one:

At this still point of the turning world. Neither flesh nor fleshless;
Neither from nor towards; at the still point, there the dance is,
But neither arrest nor movement. And do not call it fixity,
Where past and future are gathered. Neither movement from nor towards,
Neither ascent nor decline. Except for the point, the still point,
There would be no dance, and there is only the dance....
The inner freedom from the practical desire,

The release from action and suffering, release from the inner
And the outer compulsion, yet surrounded
By a grace of sense, a white light still and moving,
Erhebung without motion, concentration
Without elimination, both a new world
And the old made explicit, understood
In the completion of its partial ecstasy,
The resolution of its partial horror.[34]

Much of this rebirth happens during a cranial-cycle stillpoint too. The feeling to the patient is a kind of waking trance in which internal landscapes blossom and flit by almost magically; mind and body go on a journey into lost zones beyond a "practical desire." Compared to other trances, stillpoint is emptier and less imagistic, more resembling a contentless dream that will be instantly forgotten. Unlike noctural dreams, cranial trances have virtually no narrative or angst and there is less grasping after loss from their terminus. They are the dreams of organs that have no agenda (in language anyway) but seek participation and recognition in the life of the organism.

CRANIOSACRAL THERAPY IS *like* psychoanalysis in its induction of an ongoing, deepening dialogue between doctor and patient. What is astonishing is that the ostensibly mute act of osteopathic "following" replicates, as it were, psychotherapeutic discourse and transference at the level of membranes and viscera. The mere engagement of the therapist with an autonomic and seemingly noncathected rhythm

appears to awaken the somatic underpinnings where emotions lodge in traumas. Guided palpation speaks to the traumas in the language of their fixations and engages them along their quanta of psychosomatic potentiation. Whereas once a louder voice (letting out "the primal scream," pounding a bed with a tennis racquet, etc.) was deemed requisite to stir the demons below, now a soft touch is preferred for inducing and placating those same demons.

There is no imperative of orgastic or deep-tissue work always to take precedence because of their seemingly greater energetic splash. A whisper alone is what awakens Sleeping Beauty or, like the princess's kiss, turns the frog into the prince. It is what converts pathological into therapeutic energy. Yes, through all the layers, the princess still feels the pea.

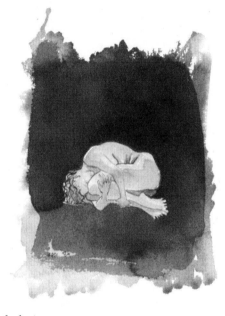

Some have objected that craniosacral work is psychodynamically and spiritually naive— that it doesn't establish or resolve transference and that it tends to infantilize patients and build dependencies on therapists unequipped to deal with projections.[35] There is a danger in osteopaths overlooking the intricate web of sublimation, projection, and transference and thus considering a case solved by one manipulation (or even worse, addicting the patient to repeated treatments without actually curing the ailment). Upledger himself has proposed that too many practitioners choose bodywork as a profession as a way to avoid psychological and psychospiritual issues while, on the surface, seeming to honor them.

Gullible practitioners making broad assumptions about traumatic memories encourage a patient in oversimplified reenactments of, for instance, childhood abuse by a parent. These turn into amateur séances supplemented with rudimentary craniosacral touch in place of candle and Ouija board. ("Oh, that must have been painful! Do you remember if she struck you?" And so on.)

Trained therapists can, however, practice a brilliant amalgam of Freudian and craniosacral work. In one instance, I was present at a demonstration session in which a psychoanalyst unwound a patient from a deep embryonic curl through an elaborate series of back-and-forth, direct and indirect maneuvers as the woman gradually recalled, image by image, sexual abuse by her father. Three assistants had to intervene to accommodate each of the vectors chosen by the woman's limbs and torso. Toward the end, the therapist encouraged the woman to find a way to "spit" (pelvicly) the intruding genital out of herself. At this point she began to improvise her own exercises and to unwind her body in spasms and shudders. Finally she stood like a titan, radiant and in full possession of her autonomy as she fired quite stunning curses toward her attacker. It was hard to reconcile this visage with her presence at the beginning of the session—tiny and self-effacing, bashful even of the request to become a demonstration subject.

What impressed me at the time was not that craniosacral work is immune to oversimplifications (it has brought its share of New Age psychobabble into the world) but that it opens avenues of recognition, self-knowledge, and release not available in psychotherapy as it is currently practiced. In so doing, it transposes the healing dialogue onto a visceral and fascial level without devaluing its essentially semantic and syntactic narrative character. Hypnotism has a similar capacity but, despite its occasionally remarkable demonstrations, the field seems stuck in feats of metaphysical riddles, to say nothing of outrageous abuses of transference.

A GENERAL AND persistent fallacy in all somatics, not just craniosacral therapy—is that of energetic literalism. Body therapists come to assume that their attention to subtle energetic sensations and charges automatically permits them to make links between physiological events and core meanings. Yet tracking traumas and dysfunctions somatically is subject to the same dynamics of therapeutic projection, distortion, character resistance, and interference as addressing them psychologically.

Often the best somatic treatment still leaves the patient's body/mind not knowing how to locate itself. While astute and well-intentioned, the therapist can introduce psychosomatic dysfunction by overlooking inertial and symbolic levels at which the patient constructs and conceals meanings. Energetic sincerity often fails to honor character. Content may be "cured," but pathology is introduced into its context.

From a psychoanalytic standpoint, all somatic systems—Western and non-Western—face limitations of their literalism, misplaced concreteness, and charismatic inflations. Substituting concepts of energies, energy fields, healing touch, and "sacred" anatomy for the dynamics of transference, they make admirable attempts to contact "core" and, through their respective definitions of "core," to heal and transform fundamental strata of body, self, and soul. Their trap is not that they are not profound; they are profound and meticulous. Their trap is that, in contexts where they do not also confer insights or conscious understanding upon ancient and primary conflicts, their literalisms and inflations provide raw material for trenchant neurosis. While deepening personality on energetic, spiritual, and visceral levels—literally creating space and texture for the self to grow—somatic therapies emotionally rigidify too.

To the degree that somatic therapies aim to heal neuromuscular and visceral restrictions, connective-tissue distortions (in Rolfing), and organic pathology through blocked digestive, cerebrospinal, hormonal, circulatory functions, etc., then all of the components of those therapies—somatic, somatoemotional, and emotional—are valid. They are not only valid, they are primal and effective (within the range and skills of the therapist). To the degree that such therapies attempt to undo the effects of trauma and developmental neuroses originating in childhood, notwithstanding language that directly addresses and proclaims such matters, they often fail at any more than superficial amelioration or fictive redirection unless they energize an entire complex which then unconsciously sinks to the source and transmutes it—and in that case the activating mechanism is the power of therapeutic touch, not concomitant psychological language. As long as that language is literal, linear, and posed in the terms of sociocultural metaphors of abuse, traumatization, low self-esteem, and past-life history, it is unlikely to enhance the treatment, and it may well serve to clutter or confuse it.

I would make one other exception—psychological language during somatic episodes does give a person a story to catalyze the personal mythology of their dysfunction from the often-powerful sensations and visceral releases of the treatment, and that synthesis has curative potential (though also the penchant to inflate). Moving an organ or neuromuscular complex while doing even simplistic psychotherapy can be a powerful act with therapeutic consequences. The next stage is whether those consequences are lasting or obviate the inflation that often attaches to moments of epiphany or sensual release. By inflation I mean the proclivity to totemize sensations and aggrandize them socially rather than to transmute them through ongoing autonomic yoga.

For a person sitting *zazen* or practicing *karate*, functional insight comes unconsciously and transforms the heart. This is professional somatics' purest form of healing. It inculcates spiritual and bodily change but not necessarily psychological change. Somatic psychotherapy still awaits a contour map of the projections, shadows, and aborted transferences cast by over-enthusiastic bodywork and the energetic metaphors it purveys.

I would apply the same yardstick to educational techniques developed by Moshe Feldenkrais and F. M. Alexander: As long as the goal of the therapist is to break psychophysical patterns and give a client freedom of movement and emotional freedom, then all the psychological components and embellishments are hygienic adjuncts to the somatic aspect of the treatment. However, when the explicit goal is to affect a generic or primary neurotic complex merely through repatterning of physiological and mental response hierarchies, the result is likely only a change in habitual physical movements, not in the emotional substratum, unless there is secondary unconscious carryover or unless the therapist is working at a nondualistic level beyond this dichotomization. Thus, a psychologically naive practitioner of these techniques is often wasting his or her time playing psychotherapist. Habit changing, greater bodily freedom, release from compulsive behavior, restoration of feeling—all of these are possible (even when psychological resistance is ignored), but resolution of ancient trauma is unlikely.

It is almost needless to say that, conversely, any psychotherapist who intends to alter physical structure and movement patterns or visceral disease by transference is doomed to failure except in the rare cases where insight catalyzes metabolically and sparks biochemical change in the organism.

Because John Upledger is one of the great independent anatomists of our time, his insights on the transpersonal, the paraphysical, and the energetic have special credibility. His claims are not those of the usual psychic healer. Originating from discoveries made during surgery and confirmed in autopsies, the craniosacral system of therapeutics is based on anatomical grids, with reference points and vector analyses more exact than anatomical loci used in most allopathy. At the same time, it relies on the transmission of extremely fine energies even to beneath the level at which they can be quantified.

In the field of energy medicine one of the most difficult feats is to remain concrete and present in the way that a patient is. Claiming to elicit and transmit rainbows, electrons, oms, miracle remissions, channeled spirits, and the like enhances a healer's reputation, so many alternative therapists engage (by name) simultaneously in *chakras,* meridians, spirits, subluxations, and energy blocks. They develop elaborate and ornate New Age styles, but they may not actually cure diseases or convert neuroses.

Conversely, the most notable thing about Upledger's practice is its utter simplicity and immediacy. While finding a patient's wavelength and meeting it, he never behaves in a self-consciously spiritual or showily energetic manner. While he gives the impression he can *feel* primacy, whatever others choose to name it, he resists adding more "stuff" in an idealized or unintentionally aggrandizing display. The moment he locates core, he goes solely where it leads him. He lets the patient determine the path and pattern of healing because only the patient can lead the way through the ellipses and labyrinths of his own condition. During this process it may occur to Upledger that one thing is the *chakra* system, another is the meridians, another is the craniosacral system, but the interpretation is incidental because he is *following* what he feels.

John Upledger perceives something so obvious it is astonishing that everyone else misses it. Everyone is looking at the same thing, and a number of healers, physicists, and parapsychologists almost get it. Now it is gradually becoming obvious to everyone.

What John Upledger sees is a world in which myriad physical, emotional, cognitive, and transpersonal factors converge to create the human sphere. These factors are rarely considered in terms of one another, at least not in a serious medical context. They include—and I want to be careful here not to simplify Dr. Upledger's position or make him seem credulous—psychic energies, subliminal and nonconscious messages, and disembodied intelligences. Upledger has explored acupuncture, the *chakra* system, Kirlian photography, psychic energy, pyramid power, and channeled spirits, and even teaches a V-spread technique in which intention is projected through a focal trough aimed by two fingers into a patient's body toward a parallel "backboard" formed by the palm of the other hand held on the opposite side of the recipient's body! At no point, however, does Upledger make paraphysical or hyper-dimensional claims *per se;* he takes the spoken (and unspoken) transmissions of the human organism in their own terms—in precisely the terms they present themselves—and follows their intrinsic wisdom. He presumes that an organism's actual signs and voices are more completely organized and deeply imbedded in the ancient network we call life than any imposed external interpretations based on mechanical and purely thermodynamic views of life (or medicine).

When bodyworkers speak of contacting the liver or the heart *chakra,*

334

this may not be an actual direct intercession between touch and cells, energetic or mechanical, but the languaging itself, which names organs and treatments and gives unconscious meanings to acts of touch. The "spleen" or "kidney" may be affected symbolically as well as physically, with the symbolic treatment being the true active one. Here the cure is channeled through a lineage of phonemes, as in Eurhythmy, rather than through the actual organs designated by them, but this lineage leads to a manifestation in tissue even as it came to represent it etymologically in the first place.

Thus, the actual viscera of visceral manipulation and the cerebrospinal pulse that ostensibly governs craniosacral therapy might not be as significant as the direct therapeutic dialogue with cells and life/mind codes that occurs when these meanings are evoked. The concreteness of somatic systems lies finally not solely in their anatomic immediacy but in the powerful metaphors they generate as well while creating and transmuting tales of energized symbols and anatomy.

Hence, telekinesis and Reiki or *chi* energy are integrated into osteopathy. As time passes, this synthesis may provide the nucleus for a whole new system as extensive as either allopathy or osteopathy. In fact, it seems to foreshadow a third-millennium medicine, permutable and "information"-based, and drawing its metaphors from holography and quantum theory.

Dr. Upledger does something so explicit and artless that it could be overlooked and yet so radical that it lies outside any contemporary paradigm—he listens to cells and tissues and tries to respond appropriately. His listening is informed medically, psychospiritually, and probably shamanically too (in the best sense). He is willing to set aside his skepticism and any preexisting belief system and respond to what is happening with the person he is helping. He does not engage in undue speculation or mythodrama. He is very "nuts and bolts." The organism tells him what's going on, and he responds as best he can. Trying out the plain and self-evident and following it non-prejudicially to its natural conclusion is, sadly, rare in the world of medicine and science.

UPLEDGER IS A former professional jazz pianist (in his youth in Detroit during the 1950s before he attended osteopathic college). His personal version of craniosacral treatment has in it creative rhythm and riffs and stretches of pure improvisation. When Upledger does hands-on work, it is as though an artist with the genius of a Charlie Parker or Miles Davis has taken as his instrument the human body. Watching Upledger perform is watching Charlie Mingus play. His whole body follows the music. Even his language is brash and jive—blues and street talk—which the organism probably respects more than the polite verbiage of a physician. He might address the heart *chakra* with "You're a hardhearted woman!" or proclaim, "Coming down into San Anton'!" or "Bright lights, big city kid!" or "Fuck that. Humor me, will you!" as he picks up and follows a resurgence of the craniosacral rhythm or addresses a stillpoint in a skeptical organism. The slightly inappropriate phrase "osteopath as superstar" has passed through my mind. Better, though, the osteopath as superstar than Eminem or Barry Bonds.

Lightness and humor are considered critical elements of treatment and cure. For one, they keep things simple and do not allow the illusion of psychospiritual complexity to cloud the concrete fact of somatoemotional existence. "Somehow," Upledger muses, "anyone who can laugh at their condition is closer to healing than another person who takes it overseriously."[36]

He tells the story of a patient repeatedly sodomized as a child by both his father and uncle. This man worked through 160 painful episodes of sexual abuse before he finally broke out laughing and declared, "Doesn't Uncle Charlie look ridiculous coming into the bathroom after me with his fly open and that stupid grin on his face."[37] It is not that the seriousness of the wound or its traumatic nature was trivialized. It is that the charge and grief associated with it, the barbs of the cyst, were released. All that was left was the somatic wound, which could be dissolved without further complication.

The epistemology of craniosacral therapy is that the body/mind provides its own methods—as ineffable as the music of Bach or a Hopi kachina dance or as implacable as the deeds of an executioner or an epileptic fit.

It is precisely this separating of layers and treating of each distinct trajectory that grounds craniosacral work in the classical precision of its osteopathic forebears. Still's pulleys and levers have transmuted as if through a black hole into a holistic psychotherapy as seminal as Freud's dreamwork.

Notes

1. A. T. Still, *Osteopathy: Research & Practice* (Seattle: Eastland Press, 1992) (originally published in 1910), p. xxii.

2. Ibid., p. 19.

3. Ibid., p. 21.

4. Ibid., p. xvi (foreword by Harold Goodman).

5. Ibid., pp. 23–24.

6. Ibid., p. 40.

7. Ibid., p. 113.

8. Ibid., p. 223.

9. Eiler H. Schiötz and James Cyriax, *Manipulation Past and Present* (London: William Heinemann Medical Books, Ltd., 1975), p. 144.

10. Still, *Osteopathy: Research & Practice*, p. 7.

11. Michael Salveson, personal communication, 1994.

12. Schiötz and Cyriax, *Manipulation Past and Present*, p. 123.

13. Ibid., p. 95.

14. Hugh Milne, *The Heart of Listening: A Visionary Approach to Craniosacral Work* (Berkeley, California: North Atlantic Books, 1995), p. 55. (This and the following three references were taken from unpublished manuscript and differ slightly from the text that was later published.)

15. Ibid.

16. Ibid.

17. Ibid.

18. Rachel E. Brooks, M.D. (editor), *The Stillness of Life: The Osteopathic Philosophy of Rollin E. Becker, D.O.* (Portland, Oregon: Stillness Press, 2000), p. 178.

19. Tom Hendrickson, www.orthopedicmassage.com.

20. Insofar as I have no direct experience of Applied Kinesiology, I have relied entirely on material provided by Don Cohen and Robert Frost, whom I gratefully acknowledge.

21. George J. Goodheart, Foreword to Robert Frost, *Applied Kinesiology* (Berkeley, California: North Atlantic Books, 2002), p. x.

22. Jean-Pierre Barral and Pierre Mercier, *Visceral Manipulation* (Seattle: Eastland Press, 1989), p. 17.

23. Ibid., p. 21.

24. Ibid., p. 23.

25. Ibid., p. 25.

26. *Post-Traumatic Stress Disorder in Vietnam Veterans: An Intensive CranioSacral Therapy Treatment Program* (Palm Beach Gardens, Florida: The Upledger Foundation, 2000), VHS video format.

27. Franklyn Sills, *The Polarity Process: Energy as a Healing Art* (Berkeley, California: North Atlantic Books, 2002), p. 127. (This quote mixes Sills' paraphrase of Stone with Stone's own words.)

28. Don Cohen, D. C., *An Introduction to Craniosacral Therapy: Anatomy, Function, and Treatment* (Berkeley, California: North Atlantic Books, 1995), p. 78.

29. Ibid., pp. 72–73.

30. John Upledger, verbal communication, seminar, San Francisco, January 1994.

31. *Post-Traumatic Stress Disorder in Vietnam Veterans: An Intensive CranioSacral Therapy Treatment Program.*

32. John Upledger, verbal communication, seminar, San Francisco, January 1994.

33. Ibid.

34. T. S. Eliot, *The Complete Poems and Plays* (New York: Harcourt, Brace and Company, Inc., 1930), p. 119.

35. Don Hanlon Johnson, verbal communication, 1994.

36. Upledger, verbal communication, seminar, San Francisco, January 1994.

37. Ibid.

For the "Osteopathy," "Cranial Osteopathy," and "Craniosacral Therapy" sections of this edition of *Modalities,* I have adapted material I wrote for the following pieces:

•The psychotherapeutic aspects of somatoemotional release in "Why Somatic Therapies Deserve As Much Attention as Psychoanalysis in *The New York Review of Books,* and Why Bodyworkers Treating Neuroses Should Study Psychoanalysis" in *The Body in Psychotherapy: Inquiries in Somatic Psychology,* edited by Don Hanlon Johnson and Ian J. Grand (Berkeley, California: North Atlantic Books, 1998).

•A discussion of John Upledger's career and medical contributions in my Foreword to *SomatoEmotional Release: Deciphering the Language of Life* by John E. Upledger (Berkeley, California: North Atlantic Books, 2002).

•The role of symbolic fields and codes in healing and the archetypal aspects of the cerebrospinal fluid in a chapter entitled "The Primordial Field" in *Embryos, Galaxies, and Sentient Beings: How the Universe Makes Life* (Berkeley, California: North Atlantic Books, 2003).

These texts may be sought for more extensive discussion of these issues. Another source on somatic psychotherapy and the relation between psychological and somatic viewpoints on mind-body states, postdating my preparation of this edition, is my essay "A Phenomenology of Panic" in Leonard J. Schmidt, M.D., and Brooke Warner (editors), *Panic: Origins, Insight, and Treatment* (Berkeley, California: North Atlantic Books, 2002).

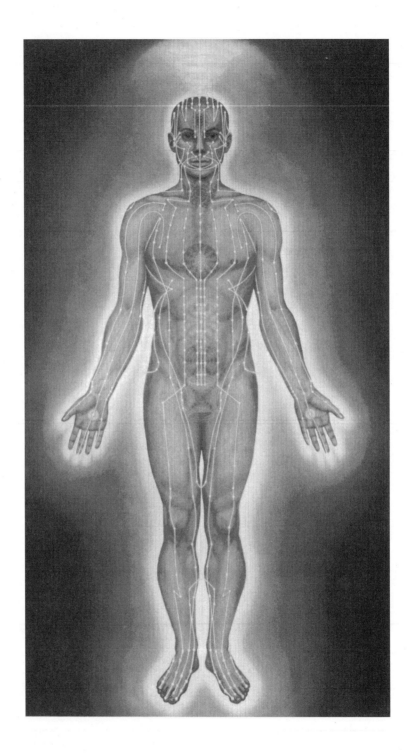

CHAPTER SIX

Non-Western Influences on Manual Medicine

Somatics from Outside the Euroamerican Orbit

THE MAJORITY OF somatic systems historically have been lay manipulative and indigenous energetic crafts that did not develop in a scientific framework or the professional context of osteopathy, Eutony, Feldenkrais, Rolfing, etc. We have discussed a number of these throughout both volumes of this book, so the goal of the present chapter is not to revisit this chronicle but to establish some basic categories.

The major domain of indigenous systems is the global spectrum of unaffiliated hands-on techniques practiced in peasant and tribal communities. These include proto-yogic stretches as well as stamping, trampling, bone-setting, brushing, massage, and other manual methods described under "Mechanical Ethnomedicine" in Volume One, Chapter Five, and "Osteopathy" in this volume. Some of these have made it into the West in refined forms that probably bear as much resemblance to ancient bodywork as Pat Boone's covers do to the originals of Little Richard. They bring together components of breath transmission, tension release, postural restructuring, New Age philosophy, energetic touch, and mechanical applications of simple anatomy, stretching, and conscious movement.

A second domain is composed of energetic systems arising from either Taoism or Ayurveda. All the Taoist energy arts developed either directly or indirectly from ancient *Nei Gung*, and Vedic energy practices are likely even older. Medicines in this category train the mind, senses, and breath to emanate vital healing power and direct it into tissues and emotional fields. Generated internally in a practitioner, *chi* or *prana* is transmitted in a disciplined, rigorous manner to a recipient (quite different from trans-anatomical faith healing). People can learn to self-heal through cultivating and applying *chi* energy internally to their own bodies.

These forms provide many elements for contemporary bodywork systems, though Eastern and Western practices have their own respective origins, views of anatomy, and courses of historical development. Traditionally, Oriental systems have been distinguished as a class from European ones by their definition of organs and the relationship of those organs to paths of energy. Even in the present syncretic world of bodywork, practitioners, training programs, and professional organizations tend to represent exclusively one body or the other (East or West) and to validate modalities within their own lineage. At the same time they may operate in ignorance of the methods and frames of reference of the other sphere. Fusions of some forms, however, began to occur in the late 1980s and continue today such that different dimensions and maps of anatomy and energy are beginning to converge. As noted, Rolfers, chiropractors, and craniosacral therapists, while applying their regular techniques, sometimes also attempt to generate and conduct *chi*.

A third set of traditions originates in the elemental aspects of Pan-Asian (Indian, Tibetan, East Asian, and Southeast Asian) sciences. It includes somatic components of Ayurvedic and Tibetan medicine, as well as constitutional modes of Chinese somatics, all described in Volume One, Chapter Nine, pp. 478–485. It also comprises Oriental massage and "pressure point" techniques such as *Shiatsu, tui na, do-in,* and *anma*. Polarity Therapy is a contemporary synthesis of principles from elemental medicines. Although systematized by a Western physician, its roots are East Indian and Amerindian.

The fourth non-Western category is that of pure mind-body-spirit.

The epitome practice of this group is meditation which, though seemingly arising in the mind rather than the body, is a disciplined form of bodywork incorporating a refined internal transmission of somatic healing (see "Buddhism" in Volume One, pp. 514–526, and "Meditation" in Chapter Eight of this volume). The bowing aspects of meditation and prayer alone make up a complex system of somatic practice resembling *Chi Gung*. The Tibetan set of *Kum Nye* comprises a similar mixture of aerobic exercises and prayers.

Yoga is a mind-body system also cultivated simultaneously for health and spiritual development. Its postures clearly involve not only stretching of muscles but focused intention and breath-directed tissue changes, probably down to a cellular level. Like *Chi Gung*, yoga works from the outside into the viscera and bones.

Ultimately, strict denominations are not useful because of the large amount of overlap among somatic systems in terms of both techniques arrived at independently in different traditions and the contemporary integration of all of these modalities and their epistemologies. Nonetheless, discrete principles and methods did arise in their own cultural and historical circumstances and took on meanings from those circumstances.

Polarity Therapy

POLARITY THERAPY IS classified here under somatic systems, but its originator, osteopath and chiropractor Randolph Stone, intended it as an eclectic planet medicine combining naturopathy, diet, exercise, massage, and faith healing. Health, he proposed, is the outcome of energy flowing unrestrictedly—while disease is solely a consequence of energy impeded. Stone says:

> In illness and disease the energy relationship in [the] River of Life and its fields is disrupted and needs to be reestablished. When the body is in good health, there is a natural balance and relationship between the breath of life and its conveyor, the blood stream as a fluid, and its rhythmic beat through the central pump called the heart.[1]

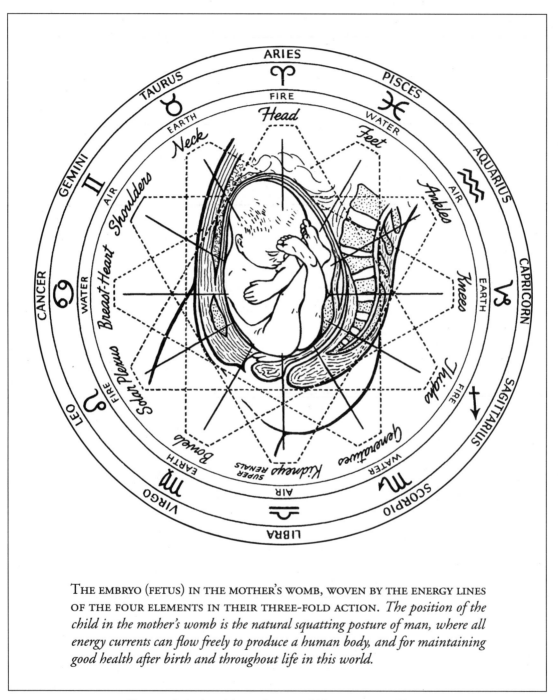

THE EMBRYO (FETUS) IN THE MOTHER'S WOMB, WOVEN BY THE ENERGY LINES OF THE FOUR ELEMENTS IN THEIR THREE-FOLD ACTION. *The position of the child in the mother's womb is the natural squatting posture of man, where all energy currents can flow freely to produce a human body, and for maintaining good health after birth and throughout life in this world.*

Illustration from Polarity Therapy *by Dr. Randolph Stone, CRCS Publications, Sebastopol, California, 1987*

Much of Polarity is simply bodywork, diet, herbalism, and astrology practiced in a context of spiritual affirmation. The cells of the body are viewed as sentient microcosms of the spirit that permeates the universe. This spirit imbues itself everywhere. We do not need to alter anything about ourselves in order to be expressions of it. Our very awareness—our tenderness, the depth of our sentience, the passion in all our acts—is spirit emanating in matter:

> [T]he potential for both health and enlightenment is present all the time, it is already within us. In times of pain and suffering it is important to focus on this truth. Even in the depths of depression, or the pain of physical illness, the potential for health is enfolded within our very being.[2]

The Polarity bodyworker regards the organism simultaneously from a karmic and energetic point of view—as an expression of transpersonal forces manifesting through organ systems. In the form of a cosmic rotating field (see Volume One, pp. 318–323), these forces incarnate simultaneously in creature bodies and the planets of the solar system. Their activity has as its goal bringing the materializing universe into harmony with the transdimensional *Sattvic* universe.

Embryogenically, a three-part creationary force differentiates as five elements (Ether, Air, Fire, Water, and Earth) which fuse in the physical realm to incubate each human being. Their electromagnetic spirals thread together yarns of molecules at the pitch of *chakra* waves. The two poles (matter and energy) radiate a creature at once dense and airy, wired and wireless. Each of us is an "etheric energy body ... created by wave circuits [and describing] a spatially oriented triaxial set of polarity relationships."[3] "Stone called this the 'Wireless Anatomy of Man,' as subtle energy does not flow in channels, or along nerve fibers, but moves in waves of expansion and contraction in interrelated and harmonic patterns."[4] From this eddy of primordial particles and secondary geometric currents emerge *chakras,* personality states, "and lifestyle habits as well as the fluids and tissues of the coarse metabolic body."[5]

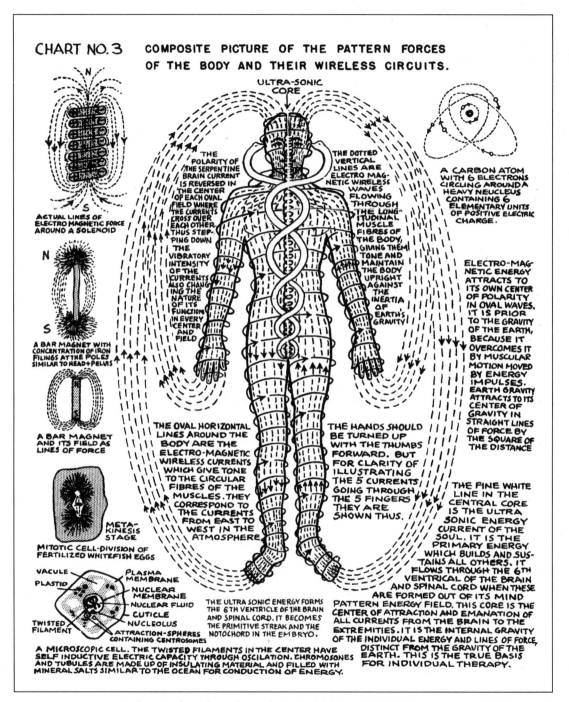

CHART NO. 3   COMPOSITE PICTURE OF THE PATTERN FORCES OF THE BODY AND THEIR WIRELESS CIRCUITS.

ULTRA-SONIC CORE

ACTUAL LINES OF ELECTRO MAGNETIC FORCE AROUND A SOLENOID

A BAR MAGNET WITH CONCENTRATION OF IRON FILINGS AT THE POLES SIMILAR TO HEAD + PELVIS

A BAR MAGNET AND ITS FIELD AS LINES OF FORCE

META-KINESIS STAGE

MITOTIC CELL-DIVISION OF FERTILIZED WHITEFISH EGGS

VACULE
PLASTID
PLASMA MEMBRANE
NUCLEAR MEMBRANE
NUCLEAR FLUID
CUTICLE
NUCLEOLUS
TWISTED FILAMENT
ATTRACTION-SPHERES CONTAINING CENTROSOMES

A MICROSCOPIC CELL. THE TWISTED FILAMENTS IN THE CENTER HAVE SELF INDUCTIVE ELECTRIC CAPACITY THROUGH OSCILATION. CHROMOSONES AND TUBULES ARE MADE UP OF INSULATING MATERIAL AND FILLED WITH MINERAL SALTS SIMILAR TO THE OCEAN FOR CONDUCTION OF ENERGY.

THE POLARITY OF THE SERPENTINE BRAIN CURRENT IS REVERSED IN THE CENTER OF EACH OVAL FIELD WHERE THE CURRENTS CROSS OVER EACH OTHER. THUS STEP-PING DOWN THE VIBRATORY INTENSITY OF THE CURRENTS ALSO CHANG ING THE NATURE OF ITS FUNCTION IN EVERY CENTER AND FIELD

THE DOTTED VERTICAL LINES ARE ELECTRO MAG-NETIC WIRELESS WAVES FLOWING THROUGH THE LONG-ITUDINAL MUSCLE FIBRES OF THE BODY, GIVING THEM TONE AND MAINTAIN THE BODY UPRIGHT AGAINST THE INERTIA OF EARTH'S GRAVITY

A CARBON ATOM WITH 6 ELECTRONS CIRCLING AROUND A HEAVY NEUCLEUS CONTAINING 6 ELEMENTARY UNITS OF POSITIVE ELECTRIC CHARGE.

ELECTRO-MAG-NETIC ENERGY ATTRACTS TO ITS OWN CENTER OF POLARITY IN OVAL WAVES. IT IS PRIOR TO THE GRAVITY OF THE EARTH, BECAUSE IT OVERCOMES IT BY MUSCULAR MOTION MOVED BY ENERGY IMPULSES. EARTH GRAVITY ATTRACTS TO ITS CENTER OF GRAVITY IN STRAIGHT LINES OF FORCE BY THE SQUARE OF THE DISTANCE

THE OVAL HORIZONTAL LINES AROUND THE BODY ARE THE ELECTRO-MAGNETIC WIRELESS CURRENTS WHICH GIVE TONE TO THE CIRCULAR FIBRES OF THE MUSCLES. THEY CORRESPOND TO THE CURRENTS FROM EAST TO WEST IN THE ATMOSPHERE.

THE HANDS SHOULD BE TURNED UP WITH THE THUMBS FORWARD. BUT FOR CLARITY OF ILLUSTRATING THE 5 CURRENTS GOING THROUGH THE 5 FINGERS THEY ARE SHOWN THUS.

THE FINE WHITE LINE IN THE CENTRAL CORE IS THE ULTRA SONIC ENERGY CURRENT OF THE SOUL. IT IS THE PRIMARY ENERGY WHICH BUILDS AND SUS-TAINS ALL OTHERS. IT FLOWS THROUGH THE 6TH VENTRICAL OF THE BRAIN AND SPINAL CORD WHEN THESE ARE FORMED OUT OF ITS MIND PATTERN ENERGY FIELD. THIS CORE IS THE CENTER OF ATTRACTION AND EMANATION OF ALL CURRENTS FROM THE BRAIN TO THE EXTREMITIES. IT IS THE INTERNAL GRAVITY OF THE INDIVIDUAL ENERGY AND LINES OF FORCE, DISTINCT FROM THE GRAVITY OF THE EARTH. THIS IS THE TRUE BASIS FOR INDIVIDUAL THERAPY.

THE ULTRA SONIC ENERGY FORMS THE 6TH VENTRICLE OF THE BRAIN AND SPINAL CORD. IT BECOMES THE PRIMITIVE STREAK AND THE NOTOCHORD IN THE EMBRYO.

Illustration from Polarity Therapy *by Dr. Randolph Stone, CRCS Publications, Sebastopol, California, 1987*

When our cells are free to resonate with their cosmic source, they express their intrinsic nature and heal us automatically. When tension, resistance, and fear impede their vibrations, they lose a degree of their attunement with the Oversoul and fall under the influence of negative and unconscious forces which germinate as diseases of body, mind, and emotions. Yet spirit, ever present, can always be tapped to heal us.

Not only can the universe get stuck, apparently we are the very sites where this happens. When we cease to be aligned with our cosmic bodies, when our own emergent consciousness threatens us, creative evolution is interrupted. Pathologies are little more than fixations of past threats, which melt immediately upon one's opening to cosmic destiny. Yet they are necessary as a way of the universe teaching us how to use our minds creatively and not as a guileful means of subverting our evolution with materialistic schemes.

Since human beings are the embodiment of an ocean of Eternal Spirit, all wounds are cosmic wounds to be healed through spiritual activity and compassion. All injuries and diseases are challenges to an expanding, evolving universe which requires density and resistance in order to grow. All healing is thus healing of spirit and is based on rebalancing the polar energy that flows through the body.

Stone drew heavily on Oriental medicines for his attribution of seasonal and diurnal cycles to phases of disease and health, stress and relaxation, despair and elation, ego death and spiritual rebirth. Polarity Therapy, in that context, is not meant to "cure" anything but to bolster the organism in its passage through inevitable manifestations of energy. Disease is primarily a stage in which one rests and gathers energies for the next transformation the universe requires.

The founder writes:

> The desire which brought us down has its latent force deep within
> the soul, which precipitates it into involution and experience. Only
> by testing our desires in the energy fields of resistance of mind, emo-
> tions and matter can we be convinced mentally; and through expe-
> rience, emotionally; and through suffering, physically. That completes

the gamut of our mental process and prowess in action and in life, as experience and proof of our own desire and folly in our cleverness.[6]

Each organ system develops its idiosyncratic mode of "thought pattern" ailments. These are imposed not by happenstance germs or other misfortunes but by susceptibility based on that organ's relationship to an individual's journey along the karmic path. Even sprains and wounds occur in tissues that need work; otherwise, they would be resilient enough to avoid injury. Accidents are viewed symbolically as ways to protect the core being from evolutionary demands for which the ego is not yet ready. When a particular set of needs confronts an individual (such as diminished capacity to feel emotions, lost autonomy, frustrated self-expression, etc.), diseases develop in areas of the body or organ resonant with each need's corresponding aspect of cosmic energy. Thus, body posture, fluidity, sickness, and health are the direct results of openness or resistance to a transcendental process which, in the end, is evolutionary and growth-oriented.

Polarity Therapy, in its simplest application, is the intention of a skilled practitioner to provide a safe, sacred space for the cells and inner intelligence of a sick person to regain their natural attunement with spirit and the universe at large. When their separate cosmic vectors of manifestation are in balance, they are capable of curing sickness at the deepest level. Techniques are intended to release energy blocks and attract divine consciousness to guiding the evolution of the individual. They are prayers expressed as palpations. Their agenda is to effect a local realignment (through the organism) of the harmonic and primordial polar fields of the universe itself.

POLARITY IS LITERALLY a medicine of the sacred anatomy (i.e., polarity grid) of the body. Insofar as all Randolph Stone's remedies and methods are based on this cosmology, they share as much with Reiki and astrology as with osteopathy. Their goal is not to fix the body/mind but to balance its cross-circuited polar energies—to awaken it to the

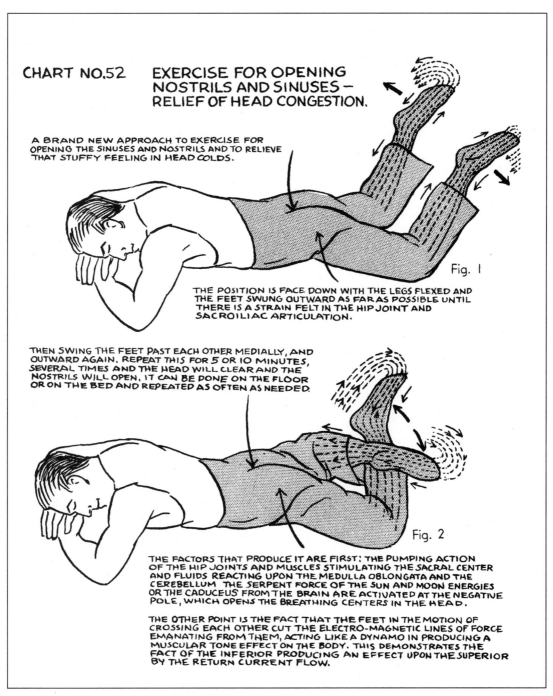

CHART NO.52 **EXERCISE FOR OPENING NOSTRILS AND SINUSES – RELIEF OF HEAD CONGESTION.**

A BRAND NEW APPROACH TO EXERCISE FOR OPENING THE SINUSES AND NOSTRILS AND TO RELIEVE THAT STUFFY FEELING IN HEAD COLDS.

Fig. 1

THE POSITION IS FACE DOWN WITH THE LEGS FLEXED AND THE FEET SWUNG OUTWARD AS FAR AS POSSIBLE UNTIL THERE IS A STRAIN FELT IN THE HIP JOINT AND SACROILIAC ARTICULATION.

THEN SWING THE FEET PAST EACH OTHER MEDIALLY, AND OUTWARD AGAIN. REPEAT THIS FOR 5 OR 10 MINUTES, SEVERAL TIMES AND THE HEAD WILL CLEAR AND THE NOSTRILS WILL OPEN. IT CAN BE DONE ON THE FLOOR OR ON THE BED AND REPEATED AS OFTEN AS NEEDED.

Fig. 2

THE FACTORS THAT PRODUCE IT ARE FIRST: THE PUMPING ACTION OF THE HIP JOINTS AND MUSCLES STIMULATING THE SACRAL CENTER AND FLUIDS REACTING UPON THE MEDULLA OBLONGATA AND THE CEREBELLUM. THE SERPENT FORCE OF THE SUN AND MOON ENERGIES OR THE CADUCEUS FROM THE BRAIN ARE ACTIVATED AT THE NEGATIVE POLE, WHICH OPENS THE BREATHING CENTERS IN THE HEAD.

THE OTHER POINT IS THE FACT THAT THE FEET IN THE MOTION OF CROSSING EACH OTHER CUT THE ELECTRO-MAGNETIC LINES OF FORCE EMANATING FROM THEM, ACTING LIKE A DYNAMO IN PRODUCING A MUSCULAR TONE EFFECT ON THE BODY. THIS DEMONSTRATES THE FACT OF THE INFERIOR PRODUCING AN EFFECT UPON THE SUPERIOR BY THE RETURN CURRENT FLOW.

Illustration from Polarity Therapy *by Dr. Randolph Stone, CRCS Publications, Sebastopol, California, 1987*

EVOLUTIONARY ENERGY SERIES

EVOLUTIONARY MIND ENERGY FLOWS FROM THE MIND PRINCIPLE OVER THE BRAIN AND THE NERVOUS SYSTEM AS PRIMARY ENERGY WAVES. SECOND, AS CONDUCTED IMPULSES OVER INSULATED NERVES LIKE WIRES FOR ALL SPECIFIC PHYSIOLOGICAL FUNCTION. THIS SERIES OF EVOLUTIONARY ENERGY CHARTS SHOW MIND AND LIFE IMPULSES FLOWING OVER THE BODY LIKE WAVES. THEY LOOK LIKE A WHEEL WITHIN A WHEEL ALMOST AS THE PROPHET EZEKIEL SAW THEM WITH LIFE ENTHRONED IN THE CENTER. THE FIERY LIFE CENTER IN THE UMBILICUS LINKS THE ENERGIES INTO PHYSICAL LIFE THROUGH THE UMBILICAL CORD FROM THE MOTHER INTO THE EMBRYO. IT IS THIS CYCLE OF NOURISHMENT AND ENERGY WHICH BUILT THE EMBRYO IN A PERFECT NEUTRAL POSITION IN THE WOMB. WHEN THE CORD IS CUT, THE BABY IS AN INDIVIDUAL AND FUNCTIONS ON THE PERPETUATION OF THIS ENERGY CYCLE BY TAKING NOURISHMENT DIRECT. THIS PRIMARY VITAL IMPULSE IS THE MOST IMPORTANT FIERY ELEMENT IN OUR LIFE FOR DIGESTION OF FOOD, ASSIMILATION, ELIMINATION AND OXIDATION. THESE ARE THE HEALING REPAIRING AND BUILDING FACULTIES IN OUR BODIES. THEY ARE UTILIZED AS A THERAPY TO KEEP THIS VITAL ENERGY FLOWING WHEN OBSTRUCTED IN ILLNESS AND BY DISEASE. IT IS TRULY A VITAL APPROACH TO RELEASE VITAL FORCES PRIOR TO CHEMISTRY AND MECHANICS.

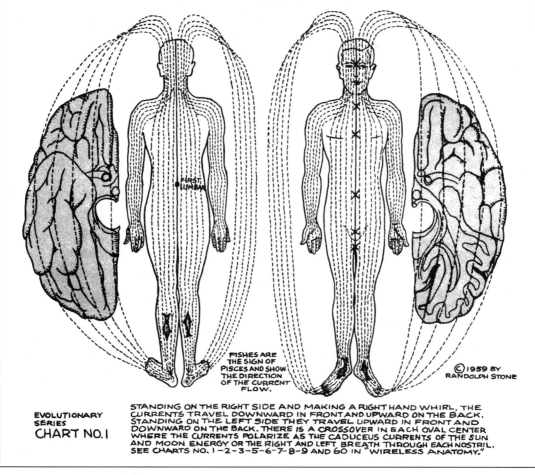

FIRST LUMBAR

FISHES ARE THE SIGN OF PISCES AND SHOW THE DIRECTION OF THE CURRENT FLOW.

©1959 BY RANDOLPH STONE

EVOLUTIONARY SERIES CHART NO. 1

STANDING ON THE RIGHT SIDE AND MAKING A RIGHT HAND WHIRL, THE CURRENTS TRAVEL DOWNWARD IN FRONT AND UPWARD ON THE BACK. STANDING ON THE LEFT SIDE THEY TRAVEL UPWARD IN FRONT AND DOWNWARD ON THE BACK. THERE IS A CROSSOVER IN EACH OVAL CENTER WHERE THE CURRENTS POLARIZE AS THE CADUCEUS CURRENTS OF THE SUN AND MOON ENERGY OR THE RIGHT AND LEFT BREATH THROUGH EACH NOSTRIL. SEE CHARTS NO. 1-2-3-5-6-7-8-9 AND 60 IN "WIRELESS ANATOMY."

Illustration from Polarity Therapy *by Dr. Randolph Stone, CRCS Publications, Sebastopol, California, 1987*

psychospiritual journey on which it has embarked by being born.

Polarity may also be summarized as a formal method for balancing organs and freeing energy channels. Calibers of balance and increments of energy come from the expression of five elements in an electromagnetic field. Inside this lodestar, positive (expansive) and negative (contracting) vibrations interact without ever quite achieving neutral (balanced) being. While the therapist may massage and adjust individual tissues and test anatomical relationships for axes of pivot, asymmetry, and "gravity of the ultrasonic core," the organizing principle of his work is always to balance the multilinear phases of energy. In the language of the system, therapeutic touch is used to conduct currents and emotions from an unchanging neutral cosmic source into a positive field of manifestation and then back to the source in a negative eliminating cycle, the hands of the therapist serving as both transmitters and resistors.

Insofar as the body's electromagnetic dissonances must be equalized, the hands function not only as modulators of energy but polar nodes with a phase dynamic between them. Their paramagnetic field is applied to knots of tension, blockages, and misalignments—all to facilitate the fluctuation of energy.

Randolph Stone conveys this electromagnetic aspect in graphic fashion:

> Death by electrocution is far from being painless, as we imagine. Electrical workmen, who have been almost killed by live wires, report otherwise. One engineer told me that a few seconds of this agony was too painful to be described. It was as if the nerves were all afire and the energy was being pulled out by the roots. This is a typical description of the forceful withdrawal or interruption of the Soul's energy, operating the body as Mind energy over the field of Prana.[7]

In an echo of other classic somatic systems, Polarity views dysfunction as the result of "a myriad of confused, contradictory, and ineffectual impulses to the musculature."[8] Like deep-tissue work, it intercedes directly in the fascial network. Like cranial osteopathy and Body Electronics, it energizes and releases traumas that have become encysted in the body.

Franklyn Sills explains this transmutative power:

> There is a change in state within the cerebrospinal fluid that allows the potency of the Breath of Life to be expressed as an ordering principle within the fluid, cellular, and tissue world. Cerebrospinal fluid [is] potentized with the Breath of Life.... Sutherland ... stressed that there is an invisible element within the cerebrospinal fluid, which is an expression of a universal Intelligence at work ... the basic biodynamic life force within the human system.[9]

AS THE GROUND OF BEING, Mind is a natural disseminator of healing energy throughout the body. It need not stay stuck in the dilemmas and repetitive problems of existence but always has the capacity to peer through the Elemental play into the heart of karma. Thus, the Polarity therapist appeals to the Mind of his client at all times. Stone repeats this formula in slightly different versions throughout his writings:

> Mind Energy is the finest form of matter.... In the human body Mind Energy flows over the brain and the nervous system and becomes animated Intelligence, Feeling, Perception, Consciousness; the root of all senses and the awareness of all sensations in and through the form of matter.... Soul is Consciousness; "Prana" is Life; Mind Energy is a neuter meeting ground between soul and matter.[10]

> The mental body as the neuter pole of action can affect the whole from any standpoint because it is the center core of all neuter fields and forces in the body and in nature. Even as the mental body blends with the physical in every cell of being, function and structure, so does the mental body, as the finest essence and phase of matter, penetrate every tissue cell of the entire body, in normal health.... Every tissue cell has a mind, as a diffused particle of the central mind.[11]

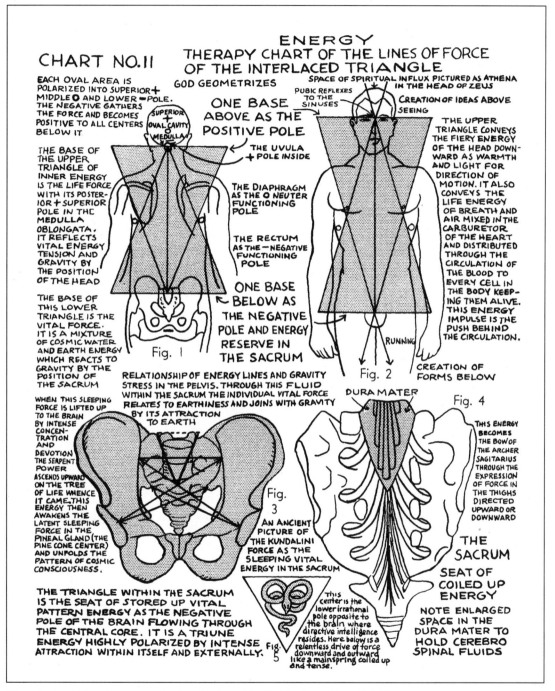

ENERGY
THERAPY CHART OF THE LINES OF FORCE
OF THE INTERLACED TRIANGLE

CHART NO. 11

GOD GEOMETRIZES

EACH OVAL AREA IS POLARIZED INTO SUPERIOR + MIDDLE O AND LOWER — POLE. THE NEGATIVE GATHERS THE FORCE AND BECOMES POSITIVE TO ALL CENTERS BELOW IT.

SPACE OF SPIRITUAL INFLUX PICTURED AS ATHENA IN THE HEAD OF ZEUS

PUBIC REFLEXES TO THE SINUSES

ONE BASE ABOVE AS THE POSITIVE POLE

CREATION OF IDEAS ABOVE SEEING

THE UPPER TRIANGLE CONVEYS THE FIERY ENERGY OF THE HEAD DOWNWARD AS WARMTH AND LIGHT FOR DIRECTION OF MOTION. IT ALSO CONVEYS THE LIFE ENERGY OF BREATH AND AIR MIXED IN THE CARBURETOR OF THE HEART AND DISTRIBUTED THROUGH THE CIRCULATION OF THE BLOOD TO EVERY CELL IN THE BODY KEEPING THEM ALIVE. THIS ENERGY IMPULSE IS THE PUSH BEHIND THE CIRCULATION.

SUPERIOR OVAL CAVITY MEDULLA

THE UVULA + POLE INSIDE

THE BASE OF THE UPPER TRIANGLE OF INNER ENERGY IS THE LIFE FORCE WITH ITS POSTERIOR + SUPERIOR POLE IN THE MEDULLA OBLONGATA. IT REFLECTS VITAL ENERGY TENSION AND GRAVITY BY THE POSITION OF THE HEAD

THE DIAPHRAGM AS THE O NEUTER FUNCTIONING POLE

THE RECTUM AS THE — NEGATIVE FUNCTIONING POLE

THE BASE OF THIS LOWER TRIANGLE IS THE VITAL FORCE. IT IS A MIXTURE OF COSMIC WATER AND EARTH ENERGY WHICH REACTS TO GRAVITY BY THE POSITION OF THE SACRUM

ONE BASE BELOW AS THE NEGATIVE POLE AND ENERGY RESERVE IN THE SACRUM

RUNNING

CREATION OF FORMS BELOW

Fig. 1

Fig. 2

WHEN THIS SLEEPING FORCE IS LIFTED UP TO THE BRAIN BY INTENSE CONCENTRATION AND DEVOTION THE SERPENT POWER ASCENDS UPWARD ON THE TREE OF LIFE WHENCE IT CAME. THIS ENERGY THEN AWAKENS THE LATENT SLEEPING FORCE IN THE PINEAL GLAND (THE PINE CONE CENTER) AND UNFOLDS THE PATTERN OF COSMIC CONSCIOUSNESS.

RELATIONSHIP OF ENERGY LINES AND GRAVITY STRESS IN THE PELVIS. THROUGH THIS FLUID WITHIN THE SACRUM THE INDIVIDUAL VITAL FORCE RELATES TO EARTHINESS AND JOINS WITH GRAVITY BY ITS ATTRACTION TO EARTH

DURA MATER

Fig. 4

THIS ENERGY BECOMES THE BOW OF THE ARCHER SAGITARIUS THROUGH THE EXPRESSION OF FORCE IN THE THIGHS DIRECTED UPWARD OR DOWNWARD

Fig. 3

AN ANCIENT PICTURE OF THE KUNDALINI FORCE AS THE SLEEPING VITAL ENERGY IN THE SACRUM

THE SACRUM

SEAT OF COILED UP ENERGY

NOTE ENLARGED SPACE IN THE DURA MATER TO HOLD CEREBRO SPINAL FLUIDS

THE TRIANGLE WITHIN THE SACRUM IS THE SEAT OF STORED UP VITAL PATTERN ENERGY AS THE NEGATIVE POLE OF THE BRAIN FLOWING THROUGH THE CENTRAL CORE. IT IS A TRIUNE ENERGY HIGHLY POLARIZED BY INTENSE ATTRACTION WITHIN ITSELF AND EXTERNALLY.

Fig. 5

This center is the lower irrational pole opposite to the brain where directive intelligence resides. Here below is a relentless drive of force downward and outward like a mainspring coiled up and tense.

Illustration from Polarity Therapy *by Dr. Randolph Stone, CRCS Publications, Sebastopol, California, 1987*

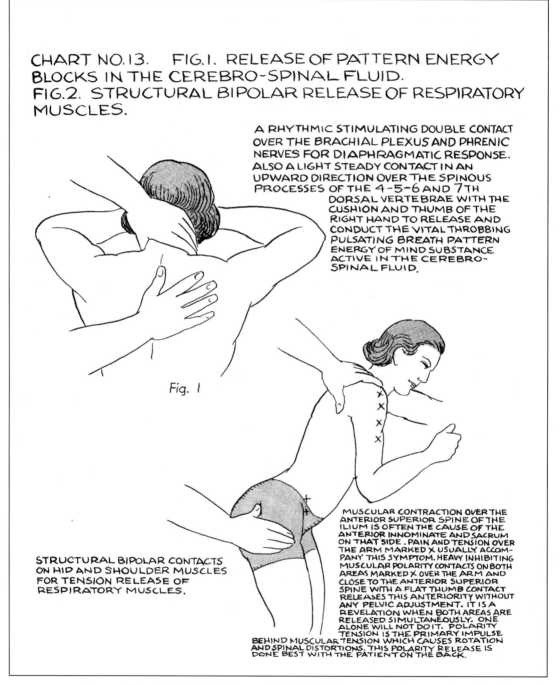

CHART NO.13. FIG.1. RELEASE OF PATTERN ENERGY
BLOCKS IN THE CEREBRO-SPINAL FLUID.
FIG.2. STRUCTURAL BIPOLAR RELEASE OF RESPIRATORY
MUSCLES.

A RHYTHMIC STIMULATING DOUBLE CONTACT
OVER THE BRACHIAL PLEXUS AND PHRENIC
NERVES FOR DIAPHRAGMATIC RESPONSE.
ALSO A LIGHT STEADY CONTACT IN AN
UPWARD DIRECTION OVER THE SPINOUS
PROCESSES OF THE 4-5-6 AND 7TH
DORSAL VERTEBRAE WITH THE
CUSHION AND THUMB OF THE
RIGHT HAND TO RELEASE AND
CONDUCT THE VITAL THROBBING
PULSATING BREATH PATTERN
ENERGY OF MIND SUBSTANCE
ACTIVE IN THE CEREBRO-
SPINAL FLUID.

Fig. 1

STRUCTURAL BIPOLAR CONTACTS
ON HIP AND SHOULDER MUSCLES
FOR TENSION RELEASE OF
RESPIRATORY MUSCLES.

MUSCULAR CONTRACTION OVER THE
ANTERIOR SUPERIOR SPINE OF THE
ILIUM IS OFTEN THE CAUSE OF THE
ANTERIOR INNOMINATE AND SACRUM
ON THAT SIDE . PAIN AND TENSION OVER
THE ARM MARKED X USUALLY ACCOM-
PANY THIS SYMPTOM. HEAVY INHIBITING
MUSCULAR POLARITY CONTACTS ON BOTH
AREAS MARKED X OVER THE ARM AND
CLOSE TO THE ANTERIOR SUPERIOR
SPINE WITH A FLAT THUMB CONTACT
RELEASES THIS ANTERIORITY WITHOUT
ANY PELVIC ADJUSTMENT. IT IS A
REVELATION WHEN BOTH AREAS ARE
RELEASED SIMULTANEOUSLY. ONE
ALONE WILL NOT DO IT. POLARITY
TENSION IS THE PRIMARY IMPULSE
BEHIND MUSCULAR TENSION WHICH CAUSES ROTATION
AND SPINAL DISTORTIONS. THIS POLARITY RELEASE IS
DONE BEST WITH THE PATIENT ON THE BACK.

Illustration from Polarity Therapy *by Dr. Randolph Stone, CRCS Publications, Sebastopol, California, 1987*

All conditions and limitations are produced by mind essence and substance.... [P]leasure and pain, health and sickness, etc., are formed by *our own thought patterns* of harmony, limitations, or discord.[12] [italics his]

Franklyn Sills puts this in more contemporary terms:

At a very basic level, we create our own world by our beliefs, judgments, and conditioned ways of perceiving. We lose touch with...the great open potential within us all.

Working with our energy system is a wonderful way to explore our conditioned relationships. All of creation is energy and it is our energetic blocks which entrap us in patterns of imbalance and ill health. Bringing awareness to this flow, whether through body-work, diet, exercise or counselling, starts to free our energies and increase our vitality. It gives us more room to maneuver in, more space to explore ourselves in ... not just as an isolated ego full of its own urges and needs, but as part of the grand interplay of energies in the universe as a whole.[13]

Stone traveled widely, especially throughout Asia, collecting useful modalities from a variety of indigenous systems. He synthesized aspects of *chakra* and *tridosha* theory, Ayurvedic dietary practices, yoga, palpation with reference to traditional Chinese meridians' acupuncture points, Sutherlandian osteopathy, native American herbal remedies and shamanic rituals, alchemical medicine, *shiatsu,* Reichian bodywork, Perls' Gestalt, various native massage techniques, chiropractic, and many other less familiar therapeutic methods. While the "polarity model" was developed fundamentally for *pranic,* spiritual work, Stone was eminently secular and pragmatic. He prescribed herbal tea blends, sprouted seeds as miracle foods, heavy dry chewing and insalivation, liver flushes, a light breakfast following the repair of mucous linings during sleep, then a large lunch.

Stone ties Polarity to diet with submolecular tropes:

The replacement of energy used in the body is sought in the whirling energy particles conveyed through food to the energy fields of the body. This is the primary factor before all other considerations! It is the attraction of POLARITY ENERGY FIELDS which is the essence of the diet problem. Food and drink must be broken down by the body energies first, and the inherent spinning electrons and protons must be liberated so they can be absorbed as building blocks and fitted into the keynote of the body and the different organs of function to which they are attracted.[14]

Stone's exercise regimens included a variety of yoga-like squats, hunkering-downs, and hanging off edges, all gently and gradually enacted.[15] Anatomically rigorous Polarity massage techniques function as *shiatsu*-like palpation in the context of breathing lessons and visualization. In this respect Polarity ironically resembles deep-tissue Rolfing more than it does any form of spiritual healing. It is quite coarse and physical because spirit has sunk so deeply into matter and shaped its own grids and conduits to matter's anatomical design. Highly specified grids of release points and organ cleansing channels release spiritual energy through meridians in tissue. Stone's therapeutic protocols have produced a nondenominational grammar for the spiritual practice of *all* systems of transpersonal and somatic psychology. That is, by using Polar energetic theory along with his or her own palpation or counselling modality, a body-oriented therapist can adjust and cleanse the body/mind along physical and mental parameters within a cosmic Etheric context.

POLARITY BALANCING CAN be similar to Reichian therapy in invoking old traumas, but in Stone's more spiritual modality, the pain of release is treated as emotional and libidinal only at one level of manifestations. Over and over the therapist reinvokes the template of a vision quest or psychospiritual initiation in which he is literally accompanying the client and interposing his own body/spirit as an electromagnetic pole to guide this passage. After all, Stone intended the

356

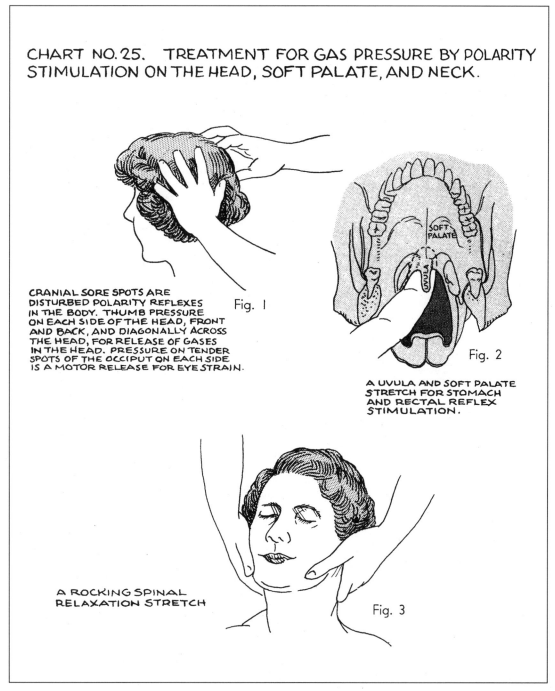

CHART NO. 25. TREATMENT FOR GAS PRESSURE BY POLARITY STIMULATION ON THE HEAD, SOFT PALATE, AND NECK.

CRANIAL SORE SPOTS ARE DISTURBED POLARITY REFLEXES IN THE BODY. THUMB PRESSURE ON EACH SIDE OF THE HEAD, FRONT AND BACK, AND DIAGONALLY ACROSS THE HEAD, FOR RELEASE OF GASES IN THE HEAD. PRESSURE ON TENDER SPOTS OF THE OCCIPUT ON EACH SIDE IS A MOTOR RELEASE FOR EYE STRAIN.

Fig. 1

SOFT PALATE

UVULA

Fig. 2

A UVULA AND SOFT PALATE STRETCH FOR STOMACH AND RECTAL REFLEX STIMULATION.

A ROCKING SPINAL RELAXATION STRETCH

Fig. 3

Illustration from Polarity Therapy *by Dr. Randolph Stone, CRCS Publications, Sebastopol, California, 1987*

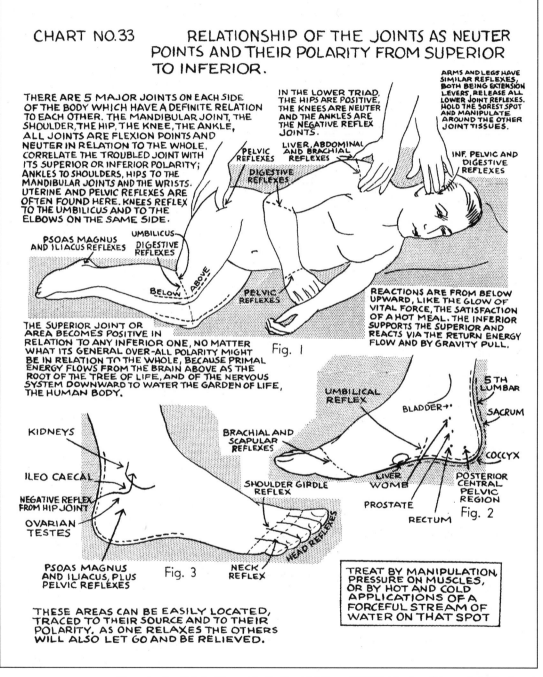

CHART NO. 33   RELATIONSHIP OF THE JOINTS AS NEUTER POINTS AND THEIR POLARITY FROM SUPERIOR TO INFERIOR.

THERE ARE 5 MAJOR JOINTS ON EACH SIDE OF THE BODY WHICH HAVE A DEFINITE RELATION TO EACH OTHER. THE MANDIBULAR JOINT, THE SHOULDER, THE HIP, THE KNEE, THE ANKLE, ALL JOINTS ARE FLEXION POINTS AND NEUTER IN RELATION TO THE WHOLE. CORRELATE THE TROUBLED JOINT WITH ITS SUPERIOR OR INFERIOR POLARITY; ANKLES TO SHOULDERS, HIPS TO THE MANDIBULAR JOINTS AND THE WRISTS. UTERINE AND PELVIC REFLEXES ARE OFTEN FOUND HERE. KNEES REFLEX TO THE UMBILICUS AND TO THE ELBOWS ON THE SAME SIDE.

IN THE LOWER TRIAD, THE HIPS ARE POSITIVE, THE KNEES ARE NEUTER AND THE ANKLES ARE THE NEGATIVE REFLEX JOINTS.

ARMS AND LEGS HAVE SIMILAR REFLEXES, BOTH BEING EXTENSION LEVERS, RELEASE ALL LOWER JOINT REFLEXES. HOLD THE SOREST SPOT AND MANIPULATE AROUND THE OTHER JOINT TISSUES.

PELVIC REFLEXES
LIVER, ABDOMINAL AND BRACHIAL REFLEXES
INF. PELVIC AND DIGESTIVE REFLEXES
DIGESTIVE REFLEXES

PSOAS MAGNUS AND ILIACUS REFLEXES
UMBILICUS — DIGESTIVE REFLEXES
BELOW ABOVE
PELVIC REFLEXES

THE SUPERIOR JOINT OR AREA BECOMES POSITIVE IN RELATION TO ANY INFERIOR ONE, NO MATTER WHAT ITS GENERAL OVER-ALL POLARITY MIGHT BE IN RELATION TO THE WHOLE, BECAUSE PRIMAL ENERGY FLOWS FROM THE BRAIN ABOVE AS THE ROOT OF THE TREE OF LIFE, AND OF THE NERVOUS SYSTEM DOWNWARD TO WATER THE GARDEN OF LIFE, THE HUMAN BODY.

REACTIONS ARE FROM BELOW UPWARD, LIKE THE GLOW OF VITAL FORCE, THE SATISFACTION OF A HOT MEAL. THE INFERIOR SUPPORTS THE SUPERIOR AND REACTS VIA THE RETURN ENERGY FLOW AND BY GRAVITY PULL.

Fig. 1

KIDNEYS
ILEO CAECAL
NEGATIVE REFLEX FROM HIP JOINT
OVARIAN TESTES
PSOAS MAGNUS AND ILIACUS, PLUS PELVIC REFLEXES

BRACHIAL AND SCAPULAR REFLEXES
SHOULDER GIRDLE REFLEX
HEAD REFLEXES
NECK REFLEX
Fig. 3

UMBILICAL REFLEX
BLADDER→
LIVER WOMB
PROSTATE
RECTUM
5TH LUMBAR
SACRUM
COCCYX
POSTERIOR CENTRAL PELVIC REGION
Fig. 2

THESE AREAS CAN BE EASILY LOCATED, TRACED TO THEIR SOURCE AND TO THEIR POLARITY. AS ONE RELAXES THE OTHERS WILL ALSO LET GO AND BE RELIEVED.

TREAT BY MANIPULATION, PRESSURE ON MUSCLES, OR BY HOT AND COLD APPLICATIONS OF A FORCEFUL STREAM OF WATER ON THAT SPOT

Illustration from Polarity Therapy by Dr. Randolph Stone, CRCS Publications, Sebastopol, California, 1987

transmission of curative love and compassion through the electro-magnetizing field of the hands.

Polarity is also a breathing system, similar to rebirthing, and likely with historic roots in the same lineage of yoga. Cycles of breath are a proximal mechanism of healing during Polarity bodywork. The therapist instructs the client to use each in-breath to put himself in touch with the radiant cosmic field, each out-breath to collapse that field and allow the dispersal and elimination of negative forces, including unreleased emotional energy and rigid mental constructs. Thus, traumas and resistance are first located by breath and flushed from the system by breathing. What is healed is not the fact of disease as much as its cellular retention. Once this bond is snapped, armor is dissolved, and the person feels attunement with higher Intelligence. Life takes on a sudden lucidity and purpose, viewed not in its meaningless terrestrial context of power, goods, and sex, but from the perspective of a higher being or deeper unity.

Polarity differs from rebirthing in its physical intercession to assist the breathing process. The therapist presides as a combination Rolfer, yogi, and shaman, alternately pressing into the perineum to release physical blocks and toxins; testing the reflex on the client's third toe; calling his attention to his higher self and to the combination of masculine and feminine characteristics within him (and the universe at large); inhibiting his psoas muscle; releasing his scapula by rocking his neck; urging him to image his moment of birth or a painful time during childhood; *shiatsu*-draining his lymphatics, neck, and nasal mucosa; balancing his sphenoid bone from the orbits of his eyes; making gentle rotary contact with the units of his upper spine and neck while evoking images of guardian angels; using the cerebrospinal rhythm to balance the pelvic and pubic regions of his body with bones in his skull, e.g., the pubic arch with the mandible; leading him in chanting mantras while releasing gas from his colon with a rocking embrace, a lift, and an expansion-stretch across his chest; stimulating the umbilical region and its myriad energy contacts; lifting and rocking opposing zones of

the anatomy; intoning sound directly into the tissues in order to deepen
the breathing; stretch-releasing the hip-shoulder connections and the
hands finger by finger; rhythmically squeezing the heart *chakra* with
the thumb; draining the prostate through ankle palpation; and embracing the client at moments of pain or important passages and encouraging him to trust in the brotherhood (and sisterhood) of all sentient
beings and to allow their spirit to move through him.

This is a hypothetical Polarity itinerary. Individual therapists develop
their sequences depending on the nature of their own practice and the
requirements of the patient.

B Y THE 1990s Stone's Polarity model had largely merged with cranial osteopathy, Breema, and other methods to produce "a mid-
dle-range theory and effective empirical technique . . . linking body,
mind, and spirit."[16] Stone had declared the primacy of the craniosacral
system as early as 1940:

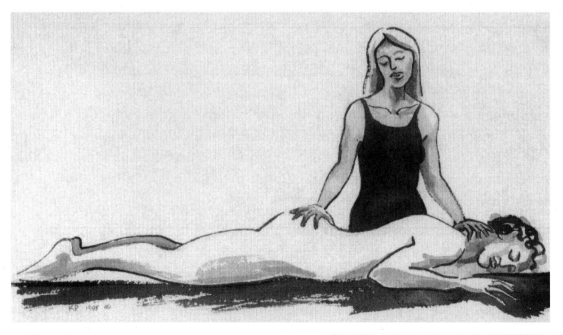

The cerebrospinal fluid seems to act as a storage field and conveyor for the ultrasonic and light energies. It bathes the spinal cord and is a reservoir for these finer essences, conducted by this fluidic media through all the fine nerve fibers as the first airy mind and life principle in the human body. . . .[17]

Stone's biodynamic work introduced new occipital holds, polar rebalances, and energetic releases into cranial osteopathy and craniosacral palpation. Establishing the cranium as the positive pole of the body, Stone reflexed its energy by Polarity principles, using it to unwind and release its own tiny bones and membranes and, as an outcome of their pivotal responses, other bones and tissues from the thorax to the toes.

Basing a negative pole at the perineum, Stone opposed its magnetic energy to neutral sites on the sacrum, upper gluteal muscles, and erector spinae; to positive sites on the shoulders, neck, and occiput; and to reflex sites on the ankles, thereby balancing the entire parasympathetic nervous system. Mechanically this palpation enhanced the innate expansion and contraction of the brain (its cranial rhythm), the capacity of skull sutures to flex in relation to one another, and the reciprocal tension (stretching and relaxing) of the brain's dural membranes under the biodynamics of the cranial rhythm and the skeleton and viscera of the whole organism.

For the sympathetic nervous system he used the coccyx as a negative pole and harmonized it with a reflex at the heel, positive poles at the sphenoid bone and foramen magnum, and various tender points at the shoulders and along the spinous processes and gluteal muscles of the buttocks. Deep-pressure massage along these axes reinforced the energetic pulse of the cerebrospinal fluid, increasing its capacity to imprint the Breath of Life in cells while transferring cranial movement via the sacrum to the pelvis and lower limbs.

Thus, Stone derived an aspect of Polarity from cranial osteopathy while transforming osteopathy in the process.

Non-Western Influences on Manual Medicine

Franklyn Sills places this in the largest imaginable context:

Each cranial rhythmic impulse is an expression of the groundswell
generated by the Breath of Life, and each tide [Long Tide, Mid-Tide]
is holographically enfolded in the other. Each tidal unfoldment is
thus implicate in the other. Each rhythm is a holographic shift in
state from an implicit Stillness into explicate form....

Think of the Long Tide as an expression of an intention generated by the Breath of Life as a discrete organizing force, or form,
within the wider play of the universe ... a tidal phenomenon that
carries the Intelligence and organizing intentions of the Breath of
Life into form.... The Long Tide seems to come from "somewhere
else" as it manifests within the human system. Like a tornado, it
seems to arise out of "nowhere" and return to "nowhere."[18]

Not surprisingly, many Polarity therapists practice "craniosacral"
therapy, and a version of the Upledger protocol has been claimed by
their guild as an offshoot of the esoteric branch of their own heritage.
Craniosacral work is currently being formally integrated into Polarity
Therapy by its board members. One group of syncretic therapists has
blended Polarity with Sutherland's modality to produce a new and
powerful alliance of osteopathic and psychospiritual techniques. Associated with Rollin E. Becker and Sills and sometimes called Craniosacral
Biodynamics, this unique synthesis is often confused with Upledger's
CranioSacral Therapy, but is of different lineage and etiology. This has
led to a series of professional disputes regarding which tradition developed which specific cranial technique and which training is truly "craniosacral."

In fact, the problem is more nomenclatural than substantial, for
Upledger specifically and intentionally called his work "CranioSacral
Therapy" to distinguish it as a modality from other applications of cranial osteopathy. He wanted to emphasize a fresh start to palpation, basing it more on following energy and implicit tissue bias than imposing
structural modifications. On this basis he and his associates and students developed a whole new system and set a precedent of improvis-

ing techniques to match what the practitioner actually felt under his or her hands. CranioSacral Therapy was rooted in osteopathy but intentionally distanced from it. It essentially developed its own repertoire of "osteopathic" procedures. Thus, the use of that precise terminology by Polarity-oriented cranial osteopaths might be viewed as disingenuously trading upon the reputation of the Upledger Institute in order to promote a different innovative modality, albeit one profound and authentic in its own right. That many non-Upledger cranial workers feel that Sutherland and Stone give them prior dibs on the term is no excuse to fool the public. Upledger's CranioSacral Therapy is distinct, with its own training, core techniques, and license. Any Polarity-based, Sutherlandian synthesis is most accurately called Craniosacral Biodynamics or something else entirely.

Chi Gung Tui Na

CHI GUNG TUI NA (literally, "energy-power-push-pull") is an Oriental bodywork science, a system of great antiquity which, over generations, has come to include a complex, empirical set of exercises and treatments for carrying out medical procedures. Its frame of reference lies not in a Western view of anatomy but Chinese cosmology (see Volume One, pp. 359–367). Kumar Frantzis, as one of the few *Chi Gung Tui Na* practitioners with an experiential knowledge of both Eastern and Western anatomical systems, not unexpectedly comes down heavily in favor of Taoist bodywork as a uniquely complete system in relationship to which Western bodywork is just beginning to develop rudimentary prerequisites. For instance, Frantzis proposes that Western craniosacral therapies rely on the attributes of only one of the three cerebrospinal rhythms familiar to the Chinese traditional practitioner (this critique is disputed in Polarity and craniosacral communities). Recommending that Chinese approaches can "save the West hundreds of years by simply not reinventing the wheel in terms of somatic bodywork,"[19] he gives the following examples:

Readjusting a vertebra that is out of alignment is a relatively straight-forward procedure. The difficulty lies in how quickly the vertebra goes out again. Sometimes simply stretching the tissue around the misaligned vertebra is sufficient, but often in chronic cases this is not enough. The Chi Gung Tui Na therapist will trace the Chi from the offending one or more vertebrae to everywhere else in the body that is either being imbalanced or disconnected by the problem in the vertebrae, or is generating energy that is causing the Chi in the vertebrae to go awry and become physically misaligned. The body-worker will then do appropriate corrections to relieve the stress on the vertebrae from both directions. This will relieve the negative cause-and-effect relationships throughout the whole body.

[In the case of a broken ankle,]

... the Chi Gung bodyworker will want to go into more detail [than a Western therapist] using twisting techniques, acupressure, and anti-inflammatory medicine to reduce swelling. He/she will want to check energetically if the damage has extended up the client's Chi lines to their hip, spine, internal organs, neck and arms. The therapist will then use both physical and energetic techniques to correct the bro-ken Chi connections, to prevent the client from in time developing problems in the hip, spine, liver, kidney, shoulder, neck, etc. By doing work at the level of Chi, the Chi Gung bodyworker ensures that a cascading effect does not issue from a minor ailment and become a severe problem later on....[20]

As noted earlier, all bodywork systems, even bone-setting and Rolf-ing, have an energetic component. However, *"chi"* bodywork is carried out on either an energetic plane or inside the imaginal replica of an energetic plane; thus, its physical and neuromuscular aspects are deemed either secondary or artifactual. The goal is the generation of *chi* energy from its reservoirs in the body and the skilled transfer of that by intrin-sic and intricate movements designed expressly for the purpose of arous-ing *chi* and distributing it to cells and organs.

On the surface, *Chi Gung* exercises are distinctly non-Western and non-medical, resembling exotic dances or martial-arts sets. The practitioner simulates a combination warrior/necromancer. Arms move up and down and in circles; fingers float and flick; the foot kicks in swift tiny arcs; the torso twists and rotates. The sets have graphic names like "Swimming Dragon," "Painting a Rainbow," "Separating the Clouds," and "Flying Wild Goose." (Demonstrating the "actual" sound of a movement that looked like a mere outward fling of his arm and hand, Frantzis let out such a roar that his arm suddenly seemed a fire hose releasing an invisible gas.)

> The Chi Gung Tui Na therapist at work will sometimes look very strange. While the left hand is working on the physical tissue of a client's damaged shoulder, simultaneously, the right hand can be on his/her belly, knee, foot or head, correcting a Chi imbalance. The right hand may stay on one spot, or in the course of a few minutes move ten or twenty times to different body points, to make Chi balancing adjustments. The hands may even leave the patient's body to clear out connected Chi imbalances in the person's external etheric body aura. The therapist will move back and forth between physical tissue manipulations, acupressure points and other Chi balancing interventions. His/her hands will move over the client's body like a piano player's over a keyboard.[21]

This split between Eastern and Western somatics reflects both a real divergence of etiology and orientation and a superficial scissure for present lack of a Rosetta Stone to link the two. For instance, whereas *Chi Gung* is considered an energy system based on *chi* flow, Occidental body medicines are usually defined as manipulative or, at most, neuroelectric. Even those Western systems that are explicitly and self-declared "energetic" do not situate or attempt to move energy in the same manner as most Oriental systems. So, is *chi* the same substance or Etheric fluid as that released by chiropractic bone adjustment or Ilse Middendorf's perceptible breath? Or is it a unique current of *Nei Gung*?

There is, of course, ultimately no *real* barrier between Oriental and Western "bodies"; any "field theory" of somatics requires that they trade

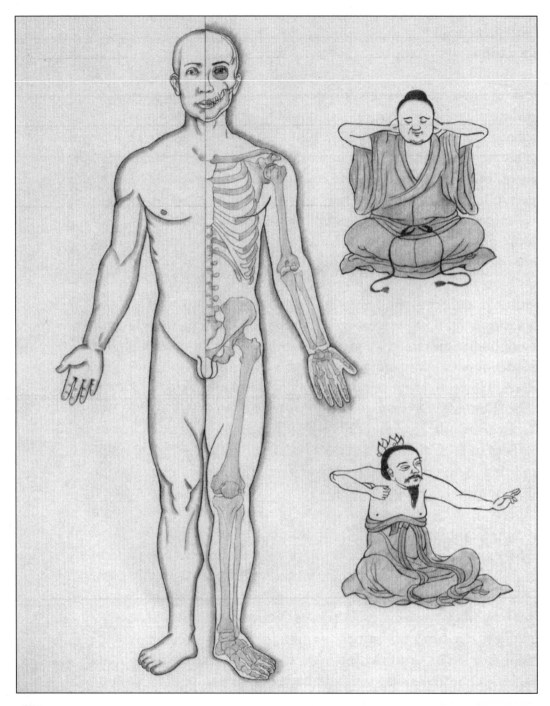

in the same currency, for they arise from the same morphogenetic process. There is no distinct Asian anatomy and no realm of bodily experience in the East or the West that could not match a corresponding realm in the bones, blood, fascia, auras, and organs of actual bodies in the other. Thus, there is no reason to assume that craniosacral touch and Rolfing do not stimulate *"chi"* flow, whatever it is.

The multiple, dense levels of complexity we intuit inside us are real, even if they cannot always be anatomically specified. By approaching the composite energy body from different angles, at varying layers of depth, and with their own idiosyncratic emphases, particular somatic systems activate discrete properties, currents, and meanings which manifest in the physical body in unique ways.

In the context of its own culture the *chi* body is a complete body, an esoteric body made of finer and more seminal stuff than the visceral body. It is the energetic template for the elemental body and its discrete organ systems. In the therapeutic sense also, it is a superior body. When harmonizing adjustments are made in the *chi* body, these translate instantaneously and exponentially to tissues and organ complexes. Likewise, when the integrity of protective *chi* is violated, the organs are more susceptible to diseases.

The various different forms of medical *Chi Gung* are precisely different patterns of *chi* generation and transmission based on traditional geographies of *chi* in the body. Yet if *chi* were not real and empirically confirmable, these network grids would be little more than curiosities or antiquities.

Frantzis attributes the Oriental discrimination of *chi* to different principles of education:

> The first year or two of Chi Gung Tui Na are spent learning how to make the hands sensitive to the flesh and Chi they are feeling in the body. Without "the hands" no form of bodywork will be totally effective. Often people spend months or years learning various somatic bodywork techniques to no avail. Although they have the intellectual knowledge of anatomy or acupressure/trigger points, they are

not accurately able to feel the body's reaction to their touch. Many techniques in Chi Gung Tui Na are devoted in the first two years of training to simply learning to accurately feel the body. For example, when touching the surface of the belly one can accurately discern how flesh is moving all the way down to the spine. This becomes critical in knowing how to vary pressure and when one is forcing the body (which can cause resistance or damage) or when the body is giving its permission for the safe bodywork procedure to continue. It also allows the therapist to gather critical information which a pair of dead hands cannot. The training also shows the therapist how to project energy accurately and with precision over long distances in the body—so that, for example, by working on a client's foot the therapist can tell how the Chi is changing in the patient's head, hands, spine, or even closer, their ankles or knees. Without this sensitivity it becomes impossible to track the Chi in a patient's body and to change one's technique appropriately and instantaneously based on the most effective possible therapeutic intervention.[22]

Chi Gung Tui Na is based on feeling and conducting energy, and Frantzis believes that a relative absence of manual sensitivity severely limits Western bodyworkers, though he adds that he is encouraged by recent developments in craniosacral therapy, visceral manipulation, Rolfing, and myofascial work because of their emphasis on energetic palpation. Of course, this is the view from within the *chi* model, and Western practitioners usually assume that they have arrived at similar or equivalent modes by their own intuitive and empirical techniques. Certainly there have been many quite sensitive practitioners of palpation and other modes of touch in the West. What Frantzis in fact may be noting is that the particular form of self-deceit that allows one to practice bodywork mechanically with dead hands in the West is less common in traditional China.

In Taoist and Buddhist cultures (as probably once in ancient Ayurvedic cultures), boys and girls are trained young to recognize their own *chi* and to cultivate it. They cup balls of *chi* energy in their hands and carry, roll, and juggle them in versions of calisthenics. *Chi* is considered a real substance from the day of one's birth and is established experientially, not philosophically or mythologically—for instance, by the practice of *t'ai chi ch'uan.* Young *chi* athletes are as fancy, dexterous, and shifty with their various-sized energy balls as American basketball players are with their concrete, externalized ball. An inner referential image of the *chi* body matures with the individual. By contrast, Western youth are rarely trained in what is meant physically and energetically by the experience of *chi* or *prana,* so they must develop their apperception of these realms later in life and in the contexts of other modes of knowing. (When I was in high school in the 1960s, a precocious friend attempted a version of *prana* practice during gym warm-ups; the coach called him a fag and dismissed him to the locker room!)

INSOFAR AS THE *chi* body exists beyond its metaphor of vital energy, Western healers have likely interacted with it under different names. Not only may it have been inherited in a protean version by separate guilds from a Eurasian base culture, but it may have been rediscovered empirically and even lost again many times over the last two millennia.

There seems little question that systems like osteopathy, Rolfing, and Eutony each affect a *chi* body in their own ways. It is merely that none of their movements or acts are *defined* in terms of direct *chi* experience or *chi* channeling; thus, they may have effects upon *chi* not necessarily accounted for in traditional Oriental systems. But they *do* influence elemental energetic flow, and if it were not for such flow (i.e., if we were only mechanical and electrical), these Western systems would not have the extraordinary power they do. In truth, they do not have to reify *chi* in order to locate a general energy field in the body. That energy field likely contains dozens, if not hundreds or thousands, of subtly distinguishable waves, layers, phases, and manifestations which collectively provide the basis for a heterogeneity of therapeutic modalities.

The variety of *Chi Gung* sets may be itself an empirical reflection of the abundance of patterning through which *chi* can be activated.

Cultural context plays a critical role in rendering systems both practicable and meaningful. It should never be a case of which system is more sophisticated or traditional but which system brings the practitioner to a functional therapeutic level. In the end, cure is system-blind, while effective practice of any technique must account for (and sometimes discount) its own idiosyncratic application of cultural metaphors. Once this is done, Rolfing, *Chi Gung,* Feldenkrais, Eurhythmy, and all sorts of other systems may be used independently or interdependently with success and yet with no map that depicts where they overlap or even what is happening.

To this degree, *Chi Gung* is a somatic system in the same way and to the same degree that various Western systems are. It is based on internal discriminations and extraordinarily fine distinctions between degrees of visceral sensation. The *Chi Gung* practitioner must *feel* where nodes and energy gates are located in order to move energy and must then track that energy through grids that become recognizable only by his paying attention to hair's-breadth sensations and boundary transitions cultivated through practice.

Feldenkrais Method, by contrast, as a relatively new system, is based more on scientifically defined neuromuscular discriminations chronic losses of function originating from the habits of technological civilization. It defines motility in a manner that is logical to Western anatomy, and, as noted in Chapter Four, the discriminations it makes are usually far more accessible to Western practitioners for awakening to all bodily energies, including *chi,* because they arise from familiar and habitual modes of perception and build from those by gradual heuristic procedures. However, there should be no illusion that Feldenkrais (or any other European technique) can provide anything more than first steps (by Taoist standards) toward functional techniques for medically generating and utilizing *chi.* They may be necessary first steps for some, to bring them even to the threshold of experiencing enough sensation to be able to search for a *chi* layer, but finding *chi* means discriminating a particular mode within that sensation. This is true whether *chi* exists as a concrete substance or not. Quite apart from the reality of *"chi"* is the *"chi"* experience and culturally specific activities centering around a dance of *"chi"*—the sense of the arms suddenly elevating and of energy rising and sinking within the body—these exist as existential facts. The issue is then how to cultivate and enhance that experience, not how to categorize it in Eastern or Western nomenclature.

The thousands of distinct *Chi Gung* sets are letters of a therapeutic alphabet (see Eurhythmy, pp. 98–99). These represent highly practical maneuvers for gathering and clearing *chi*—nothing more (no decorative add-ons) and nothing less. In application, *Chi Gung* movements are repeated again and again and again with variations only of expanding sensation and discrimination. The seemingly external aspects of motions replicate and reinforce an internal process of contacting, gathering, and moving *chi* and at the same time literally palpate the *chi* field, which is vaster and more charged than the physical body. The practitioner sweeps up and accumulates his own *chi,* disperses stale and stagnant energy, pushes energy into the ground, and, by the principle of Yin and Yang, circulates fresh energy into the organs (*chi* fluctuates like water, swelling up to balance any dispersal downward). The movements pass through exactly those zones around the body where *chi* is thickest and at orientations to the body which most efficiently condense *chi* and instigate its flow.

THERE IS A distinction between Buddhist medical *Chi Gung,* which pretty much matches the series of exercises described above, and Taoist *Chi Gung* based in *Nei Gung,* which has its own repertoire of external forms but prioritizes another, purely interior protocol of visioning, making palpable, and dissolving blocks. In one of its many techniques, the practitioner closes his eyes and starts perceiving inwardly, beginning at the energy field above his head. Working his way slowly down his body on the outside and inside, he tracks sensations. He passes through the crown of the cranium, the temples, the third eye, the eyeballs, the neck, the shoulder girdle, the shoulder blades, armpits, vertebrae, sternum, solar plexus, belly, liver, kidneys, genitals, anal passage, perineum, pelvic bone, thighs, ankles, feet, bottoms of the feet, right through the energy field in the earth beneath his feet. Of course, there are many other possible locations to visit. Any tissue or organ is a candidate for penetration and dissolution. It is a matter of sensitivity to flow and density, patience, and capacity.

A beginner tracks the body close to its surface (because that is what he is capable of). It may not be feasible at first for him to get through his eyeballs to their interface with the brain, so the surface of the eyes is felt and energized. By degrees he goes deeper. Merely to locate the pelvis internally is difficult for most people. Later the goal is to send attention right through its bone. Likewise, as a cancer preventative, one learns to work his or her mind gradually up the anal canal. The overall process is one of continually gathering and sweeping all excess energy downward, paying particular attention to contractions, areas of tension and hardness, and any other sensations, "especially," Frantzis emphasizes, "if you do not know what they are." During these sweeps, one softens and releases blockages, turning "ice to water, water to gas."[23] The mutation from ice to water is a relatively straightforward one of sensing and relaxing already-liquidic tissue. From water to gas is a sophisticated alchemy that follows and enhances the true introduction of *chi*.

Standing erect in a balanced, open posture, a trained practitioner can complete a cycle of the body in ten minutes, an hour, or many hours, depending on the speed and depth of awareness. One can move a millimeter at a time or an inch at a time. Subsequent passes over months and years can go more slowly and deeper until one is cleansing not only the surface meridians, but the blood, the marrow of the bones, and the inside of the brain. (The objection of the post-Maoist communist government in China to these exercises in their form as *Falun Gong* is paranoid to the point of ludicrous, but then Confucian tyrants have always feared Taoist magicians.)

As should be clear from prior discussions of internal methods, this

is not a visualization technique. It is a process of actually tracing proprioception from the dense physiography of the body into its *chi* fields and thereby activating it. The question of whether honoring every subtle sensation leads unerringly to the *chi* field is irrelevant because *there is no other way to find it.* A practitioner cannot guide a person into his own *chi* field road sign by road sign or even prove its existence; he can only give him a set of clues through which he ultimately intuitively arrives at it himself. If he picks up other sensations along the way, these can be sorted out as the awareness of the *chi* field is confirmed by repeated sweeps, over long periods of time. Eventually the movement of *chi* becomes clear and other sensations also become clear as what *they* are.

Initially the *chi* feeling may be so fragile as to seem like nothing, but it is this minute sensation that attention must follow until something more gritty and rubbery is apprehended. Many people feel *chi* most readily in the field formed by opposing the rounded palms of both hands to each other. This "ball" of energy is also, as noted, the *t'ai chi* ball that is rolled through the postures of the martial arts set. A more subtle trace of *chi* can be picked up in equivalent "bubbling well" points at the base of the feet. Both of these areas are critical gates for the medical movement of *chi.*

A next stage of development might be sequential forays pulling *chi* from the inner surface of the arms into the palms of each hand and then pushing it back in. Later, *chi* is sent along one arm into the body, through the heart, and out the other arm without the aid of the palm.

Once again, this is not a mere exercise routine or gymnastics. The purpose of Taoist *Chi Gung* is to heal chronic tension, tumors, and broken bones, and to repair the damage of strokes, radiation exposure, and viral infection—major medical ambitions. None of this would happen if there were not a *chi* body to contact and if such a template body were not accessible in a manner that alters fascia and viscera in the physical body. Frantzis used Taoist *Chi Gung* on himself after his back was broken in a car accident in New Mexico. Told he would never walk again, he summoned up his *pranic* strength and began working his way down

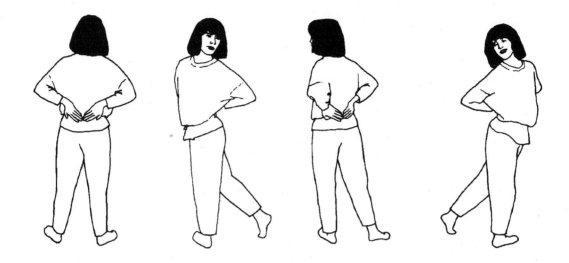

Dancing on the Grapes

from the top of his head, encountering and dissolving immense resistances, especially at the damaged points.[24] Because he already knew *Chi Gung,* he was adept in internal tracking and was able to attain the level of depth required for such a drastic treatment. Not only did he walk, but he regained his prowess as a highly mobile and effective martial artist.

Breema

TAUGHT AS A combination of massage and spiritual exercise, Breema was introduced to the West by Manocher Movlai, a Kurdish rug merchant in Oakland, California. It is unclear how much of his system is native Kurdish and how much was adapted and improvised by Movlai. He cites his great-grandfather as his original teacher:

> He would do a lot to make us view the body not as an anatomic object. This alive, dynamic phenomenon is in constant change. This energy system is connected to the totality of existence on all levels.... He would say, to touch a human being, another body of [a] human being, is as mystical as touching the stars.[25]

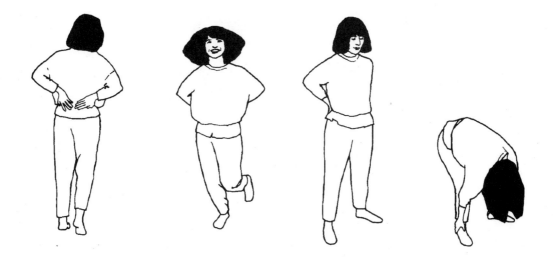

Breema can be performed as a one-person cycle of movements and breathing exercises which, from the outside, appear combinations of ceremonies and exercises. Their names are evocative of their movements: "Grinding the Wheat," "Chasing the Arrow," and "Dropping the Load." Self-Breema includes breathing cycles, hops, stretches, foot and head rubs, and facial and bodily brushes ("Erasing the Page") plus combinations of these (such as holding one's hands on the kidneys and hopping in such a way as to pull and twist the torso and points of contact in "Dancing on the Grapes"). The emphasis is on letting natural movements and weight shifts stretch and massage parts of the body (including viscera) by the simple operation of posture and gravity.

More commonly Breema is practiced by two people in a bodywork session. The same use is made of natural movements and weight shifts, but posture and gravity are now the effects not just of one body moving in space but two bodies acting on each other as fulcra, ballasts, pulleys, wedges, gears, etc., in complex sequences of shifting positions. Movlai emphasizes that during such treatments, both participants are equally the givers and the receivers. The exchange is based solely on their

Non-Western Influences on Manual Medicine

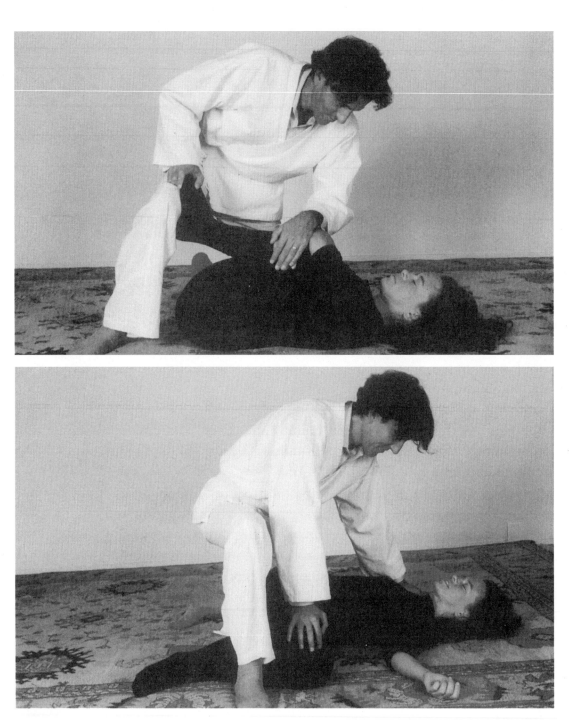

mutual and simultaneous presence and permission, their breathing in unison, and the reciprocal weights of their bodies. He explains this in his inimitable English (somewhat sanitized with my bracketed inserts):

> My mind receives [an] impression of [your] body, [your] body receives [an] impression of [my] mind. While [my] mind [is] receiving [an] impression, [my] body is active. While [your] body receives [an] impression, my mind is active. If this active/receptive principle is understood within myself, then this gentleman who is lying down here becomes . . . who is body, who is mind? He is body while I am mind. I am the body while he is the mind.
>
> [The] division—I am me and you are you—which is falsity and [which] I created all of my life, disappears. . . . In the principle of active/receptive, there is only me or there is only you. . . . In that non-verbal understanding, that which you do is in harmony with yourself, with the person you're working with, with the whole universe.[26]

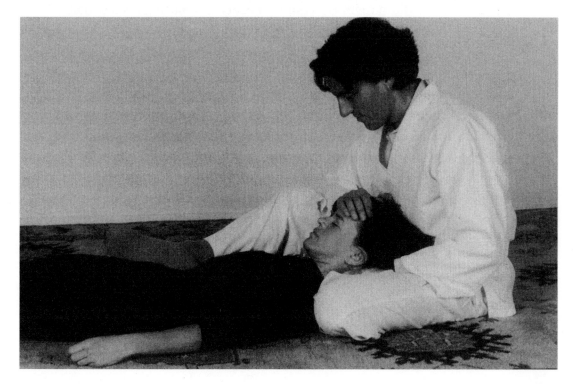

The pair doing Breema is engaged in a process, partly choreographed, partly improvisational, of mutual aid and support, of recognition of each other's bodily presence, each other's gravity and breath. Breema is a kind of two-person yoga involving a subtle energetic and emotional transfer between the bodies that enlarges and heals both of them without diagnosis.

THE BREEMA PRACTITIONER makes contact with the other person's body by first taking into account the location and relative ease of her own body. After settling into a comfortable position and internally acknowledging her own breath and weight, she puts a hand or foot on her partner and then follows intuition. Although there are standardized sets, the placement may be anywhere, and in some cases the knees, elbows, or belly become the massaging "limb." Simply stepping on the insoles of the feet of a prone partner and then slowly transferring one's own weight to them is a common beneficial starting point. Many moves involve taking a strategic position contiguous to one's partner and then leaning in such a way that one's weight is transferred to the other person's body. Sometimes the weight transfer is direct and linear. Sometimes it curls along an edge of the body, giving a deep-tissue massage. Sometimes it turns into a lift or displacement so that the two bodies acrobatically support each other in a stretching position.

In the most linear sequences, each of these leaning transfers bears the relationship of a dot in a dotted line to a complete continuum, with an arm or leg or path along the torso of the partner representing the vector. The shift and its cessation follow a pattern of "press, hold, release": the press is merely the weight transfer, the hold is the duration of the breath, and the release is the transfer back.

A lean involves a gentle but firm transfer of weight from the practitioner's body to the recipient's. Equal time is given to the lean toward the recipient, to the "hold" at the deepest point of the lean, and to the release of the hold, as the practitioner's weight shifts away from the recipient and back toward her own body. Leans often take on a rhythmic quality of their own and can have a deeply soothing effect.[27]

The dotted line can go anywhere. One of the simplest such sequences involves a single hand on a partner's leg, then pressing, holding, and releasing consecutive points, traveling the length of the thigh, down the calf, along the ankle, foot, toes, and aura beyond the toes. After a parallel track down the other side, the practitioner closes the sequence with three light brushes back over both paths simultaneously.

> … Gentle nurturing brushes which strengthen and deepen the effects of the treatment … can be done with the feet, but more commonly the hands are used. Brushes are done with a relaxed hand; again, the movement comes not from the arm and hand but from the body's center. …
>
> After a particular series of leans, the practitioner might change the recipient's position by, for example, standing up and carrying the recipient's leg up and along with her, then gently placing it on the other side of the recipient's body, causing a twisting action in the spine.[28]

One such succession of moves involves stretches in which one transfers weight to a partner by holding onto one or both of their limbs like a vine and then extending the person by gradually leaning backward oneself, supporting the other body each degree of the way.

In a compressive sequence, one places a partner's feet on one's own belly and then very slowly, with long pauses at each degree of arc, raises and folds his legs and brings one's own weight to bear down through the partner's feet, rolling his knees toward his head a fraction of an inch at a time.

Other moves involve rocking and cradling the partner in postures ranging from hands cupped on his ears to a full therapeutic embrace, rapping or drumming on his forehead or chest, and raising his limbs and dropping them suddenly in a sequence of tosses around his prone body. Movlai says:

Everything we do in Breema, we do it with all of the whole body. So, we don't have "brush with the hand." We have body, body. Body, body. And then something magnificent happens.

That which is the total emanation of this entity [the practitioner] and that which is the total emanation of this entity [the other person], they create a new emanation of this entity [makes a gesture encircling both people]. This new emanation has the power to bring everything into harmony.[29]

An elbow on the partner's shoulder blade is another favored position or, most exotically, a belly resting on the belly of a partner (Movlai uses the Japanese designation—the *hara* on the *hara*—in place of the more obscure Kurdish *delegen* on *delegen*). Movlai points out that as a result of their location closer to the brain, the hands are far more detrimentally judgmental than the feet or *hara*. When the feet are used instead, on a very deep level the partner experiences the absence of critical probing.

All of these activities are consensual and collaborative. The parties are equal healers, applying complementary weight and breath, which has a mutual stretching and expanding quality for both:

In Breema, we don't have lift. . . . I want to do that, I lift. The word "lift" mind understands [as] one thing: order the body to LIFT. But, I lean and I lean. I lean and I lean.

Also, in Breema we don't have the word "pull." Pull, pull. Mind understands pull as force. Pull. Breema is no force. No force ever is used in Breema. The weight of the body is used as a carrier of energy, that's all. So, instead of having pull and push, we have lean forward, lean backward. Lean forward, lean backward.[30]

The effect is almost of a person exercising alone, doing stretches and leans, and seemingly by accident drawing along a partner. At the same time, this indirect attention is transposed into the recipient's body as if it is the practitioner's own.

Transferred between bodies is a subtle energy, a sense of presence, plus the continual element of surprise. This "startle" is crucial to keeping the mind of the receiver open and in a state of wonderment: 'What will she do next?' is an endless silent question until there is no question and everything that happens is instantaneously received. Each range of unlikely juxtapositions projects its own new reality and new mind-body template.

Because of the regular interchange of the practitioner's feet and hands as primary treating agents, the person being touched loses basic orientation vis-à-vis a simple hands-on massage. The sense is instead of being touched by more than one person or by a person so nimble as to be in many places at once. The treatment feels most like spiritual or animal company—the innocent curiosity and comfort of another creature.

The first time I received a treatment I slid into a trance state in which I experienced a closed-eye movie of luminous, rapid-fire archetypal

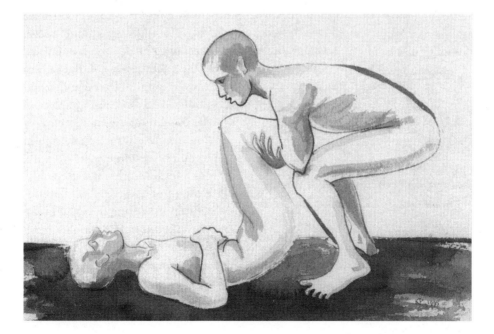

images that seemed right out of a Jungian opticon—temples, mandalas, sphinxes, buddhas, tapestries of the Flower of Life, spinning geometric forms, one replacing another in silent drumbeats. It was as though my mind had nothing to do with the procession. As the demonstration flipped by, I felt obscure emotions and a sensation of wholeness. Was this medicine?

Movlai remarks:

Breema is the only method I know of [that] has nothing to do whatsoever with diagnosis, does not diagnose, does not even look, does not even study, doesn't have anything to do with the client or patient or whatever you wish to call it.

In order to have this non-judgmental activity, the mind, which by nature is judgmental and classifies, has to be occupied in such a way that it does not have any energy left to go through the root of the habit of judgmentality.

Therefore, this mind has to be constantly like a recording machine. Always, [its] job is to record body having a weight, body breathes. As soon as I want to look to see how she [the client] is, my mind is incapable [of recording] these two things together: weight of the body and breathing of the body....

Then why is it Breema doesn't want to diagnose? [It] is really [a] magnificent thing why this is so. Because, you see, Breema does not believe there is such a thing as an illness or sickness. Now you may say, half of this planet or ninety percent of this planet, people are ill and sick. How come Breema can say such a thing; it's absurd. I agree with you.

But...Breema does not believe in sickness, although we experience it. But, we experience it in the absence of vitality. [It is] the same way Breema doesn't believe in darkness. But we experience it in the absence of light. Light carries the substance, darkness does not. Vitality carries substance, sickness does not!

So, where do you put emphasis? Where there is substance? Or where there is not? You go to the dark room and fight with the darkness. In a few minutes, all your energy drains because you have to hit [an] imaginary, non-existent something.[31]

If you merely go toward disease with the intention of diagnosing it or fixing something, your mind and intention will become imbued with the contagious limitation of disease. You will always be sick. In Breema terms, if you go toward pure energy, you will become energy. By that definition, all our systems of healing derive and provide the diseases we then bring to our medicine women and men to treat. Meanwhile, Breema-like systems will provide spontaneous cures for some of these diseases without ever a diagnosis or a name.

We cannot fix each other, Movlai is saying, and he is in keeping with general holistic etiology. Only the "architect" within the body has true knowledge of what is happening; only it can heal. But "you can support and give guidance and help one another." You can lead another person to "his own essential nature."[32]

Notes

1. Dr. Randolph Stone, D.C., D.O., *Polarity Therapy, Volume One* (Sebastopol, California: CRCS Publications, 1987), p. 2.

2. Franklyn Sills, *The Polarity Process: Energy as a Healing Art* (Berkeley, California: North Atlantic Books, 2002), p. 159.

3. Bruce Burger, from his journal notes on professional Polarity documents, 1994.

4. Franklyn Sills, *The Polarity Process,* p. xii.

5. Bruce Burger, from his journal notes on professional Polarity documents, 1994.

6. Randolph Stone, quoted in Franklyn Sills, *The Polarity Process,* p. 161.

7. Dr. Randolph Stone, D.C., D.O., *Polarity Therapy, Volume One,* p. 68.

8. Bruce Burger, *Esoteric Anatomy: The Body as Consciousness* (Berkeley, California: North Atlantic Books, 1998), p. 297.

9. Franklyn Sills, *Craniosacral Biodynamics: The Breath of Life, Biodynamics, and Fundamental Skills, Volume One* (Berkeley, California: North Atlantic Books, 2001), p. 13.

10. Dr. Randolph Stone, *Polarity Therapy, Volume One,* pp. 18–20. This and the succeeding two quotes were adapted by Bruce Burger for use in *Planet Medicine.*

11. Ibid., pp. 55, 8.

12. Ibid., p. 5.

13. Franklyn Sills, *The Polarity Process,* p. 162.

14. Dr. Randolph Stone, D.C., D.O., *Polarity Therapy, Volume One,* p. 106.

15. Alexander Binik, "The Polarity System," in Edward Bauman, Armand Ian Brint, Lorin Piper, and Pamela Amelia Wright (editors), *The Holistic Health Handbook* (Berkeley, California: And/Or Press, 1978), pp. 99–107.

16. Bruce Burger, personal communication, 1994.

17. Franklyn Sills, *The Polarity Process,* p. 126.

18. Franklyn Sills, *Craniosacral Biodynamics,* pp. 54–55.

19. Bruce Kumar Frantzis, *The Tao in Action: The Personal Practice of the I Ching and Taoism in Daily Life,* unpublished manuscript.

20. Ibid.

21. Ibid.

22. Ibid.

23. Bruce Kumar Frantzis, verbal instructions during a class, November 1993.

24. Bruce Kumar Frantzis, *Opening the Energy Gates of Your Body* (Berkeley, California: North Atlantic Books, 1993), pp. xxviii–xxix.

25. Manocher Movlai, transcribed from a class at the Breema Institute, Oakland, California, November 30, 1992.

26. Manocher Movlai, transcribed from a class at the Breema Institute, May 18, 1992.

27. Cybèle Tomlinson, "Breema Bodywork," *Yoga Journal* (November/December, 1994), p. 97.

28. Ibid., pp. 97–98.

29. Manocher Movlai, transcribed from a class at the Breema Institute, June 2, 1988.

30. Ibid.

31. Ibid.

32. Manocher Movlai, transcribed from a recorded talk at the Breema Institute, no date given.

MODALITIES

CHAPTER SEVEN

Contemporary Systems

Zero Balancing

Zero Balancing is a system of somatics developed by Fritz Smith.[1] The son of a prominent chiropractor, Smith trained as an M.D. and osteopath in the 1950s, and subsequently became a certified acupuncturist, a student of Shakti Yoga as taught by Swami Muktananda, and a Rolfer. Out of these varied experiences, he formulated his own distinctive set of ideas and techniques, though he did not initially give them their own title of Zero Balancing (a student would later do that).

Smith defines Zero Balancing as hands-on body balancing and integration which aligns energy fields with skeletal structures. Zero Balancing has its taproots in osteopathy but is distinct in that it is a nonmedical approach to health and wholeness, which uses "energy" as its guiding metaphor. Alignment through Zero Balancing attempts to atomize stress by vibrations flowing through the person, releasing compensatory resonances within the nervous system. Zero Balancing tends to be a complementary health system to craniosacral therapy, Polarity, acupressure, acupuncture, and Body-Mind Centering.

Although Bonnie Bainbridge Cohen, the founder of Body-Mind Centering, had no prior contact with Zero Balancing, she did experience its work at the source when she arrived at Esalen a few days early for a 1989 seminar and found Fritz Smith teaching. Joining the class, she discovered a strong affinity to her own system as well as a range of useful techniques. Later she wrote: "Dr. Fritz Smith, osteopath, acupuncturist, and the founder of Zero Balancing, transmitted to me the dynamic and mutable life of bone."[2]

Like Polarity, Zero Balancing is a practical, empirically derived technique and the reflection of a spiritual philosophy. Smith conceived the 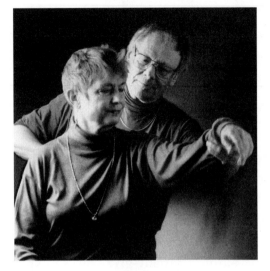 relationship between energy and matter much as Rudolf Steiner did in his development of anthroposophical medicine. Insofar as the skeleton is the densest state of incarnating tissue, Smith was attracted to the bones and their junctures as fulcra of the physical and vibrational body. The deepest strongest currents of energy in the body flow through them.

The Zero Balancer assesses skeletal energy by sensing and evaluating currents within bones. He feels each bone, working his way down the body from the neck and spine to the hips, legs, and metatarsals, paying specific attention to the skeleton. He tests every rib, vertebra, and each of a specific class of joints known as foundation and semi-foundation joints. The sacroiliac joint, the intervertebral, costovertebral, and costosternal joints, and the tarsal and carpal joints of the feet and hands in Smith's terrms have more to do with the transmission of energetic and mechanical forces than they do with providing locomotion for the body. The Zero Balancer weighs the end range of motion and the supporting ligament tension of each of these joints as a gauge of its energetic integrity. He holds the bones and joints in stillness and, lifting slightly with his fingertips into an area of tension or stasis, waits there for a few seconds or so, altering the geometric equation forming the skeletal nexus and thus providing it with an energetic as well as a mechanical basis for reorganization. Once establishing a fulcrum (or balance point), he pauses until the client's energy releases or fills the zone.

Zero Balancing involves learning positions of holding which transmit "balance" to the organism—not those positions which are precisely symmetrical but which mean "balance" in organismic terms. "A fulcrum," Smith says, "is a balance point or lever around which movement occurs and by means of which energy and forces are brought to bear."[3] He has portrayed these as three-dimensional grids of pressure in relation to which systems within the body start to oscillate and reorient themselves. The power of such grids is in the transmission of their shapes inward and outward, large and small ripples which give off multiple replicas of themselves, both larger and smaller, each replica then casting out countless more. Complicated geometric forms enter the body/mind at different levels. By repeated use of fulcra, a skilled practitioner can balance the body's entire field of energy.

Smith explains:

> Of fundamental importance is the fact that if the foundation and semi-foundation joints become imbalanced, the body tends to compensate around the imbalance rather than to resolve it directly. This results in the formation of subclinical patterns of stress and imbalance which not only limit a person's full function but can eventually lead to gross and symptomatic pathology.
>
> For instance, the small tarsal bones of the feet are designed to absorb the impact of walking and the tremendous pounding they receive every time a step is taken. If they become energetically out of balance, then every time a person walks, the stress of impact goes deeper into their body because it is not being absorbed by the first line of defense located in the feet. Zero Balancing helps to recalibrate these joints to absorb stress and thereby lessen stress patterns elsewhere in the body.[4]

Smith defines his cosmology by a familiar metaphor from contemporary physics: that light exists as both a particle and a wave, and so, in a sense, we represent "entrapped light." Physical or structural bodywork attends to our particle nature, and vibrational or meridian flow contacts our wave. Zero Balancing addresses both aspects of creation—

structure and energy. The hand holding the bone feels the body simultaneously as wave and as particle. By creating a balance point, a fulcrum, and maintaining this in stillness, the therapist guides the particle and wave to the point of zero where they vibrate equally, wave as particle, particle as wave.

Smith adds,

> Another analogy I make is to a sailboat: we have the sail as the structure and the wind as the energy. Somewhere the wind hits the sail; somewhere in the body energy and structure meet. They have an interrelationship. Zero Balancing looks at that relationship, the interface of energy and structure. The pure energy systems, like acupuncture and homeopathy, or *Chi Gung* and Reiki, work with one side of the equation; the pure body handling systems, like osteopathy, chiropractic or Rolfing, work on the other side of the equation. Zero Balancing does both by bringing energy and structure into one working piece.[5]

After establishing his method, Smith reflected that Ida Rolf was probably working with both energy and structure while teaching from the perspective that she was reshaping things only structurally:

> When I was studying Rolfing I was fortunate to be Ida's model for seven sessions.... In those days "energy" had not yet been "discovered" by the West, and there was no "energy vocabulary" by which Ida could describe or teach exactly what she was doing. It was only years later, after I knew that vocabulary and had learned to control energy through touch, that I surmised that Ida was actually working with energy as well as structure and thereby didn't create hurtful pain. As she'd go through my fascia, a bolus of energy developed in front of her thumb or elbow which opened up my field, so that when she got there with her own structure, my physical body was already in motion.[6]

ZERO BALANCING MAY be *chi*-based, though in ways different from *Chi Gung*. It resembles Reiki in its "holding in relationship to energy."

Smith distinguishes it from pure spirit healing as "structure-holding energy."

Zero Balancing and craniosacral therapy are both osteopathic and rely on palpation of the body. The Zero Balancer works directly with the vibration of bone itself. He does not necessarily read the craniosacral rhythm or blend his own energy with that of a client. He tracks precisely where his energy ends and another field begins, and then he maintains that demarcation consciously. Although there is no equivalent to somatoemotional release, Zero Balancing offers a profound unwinding of its own, quite visceral and with a grounding impact. As one Zero Balancer told me, "Craniosacral work can feel like a trance. In fact, many people have the sense that nothing is happening and discount it for that reason. In Zero Balancing, there is a very clear sense of boundary and that something is happening. There is a profound way in which the simple holding of the bones touches a person at the core, often relieving intense chronic conditions in just a session or two."[7]

EACH ZERO BALANCING treatment takes about a half hour. The patient lies on his back. The holding is done through clothing. The entire body is touched during a session, though the arms, for being off the central axis, are usually paid less attention.

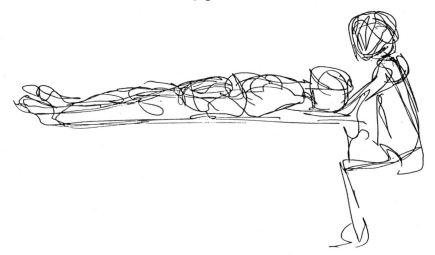

The impact of adding Zero Balancing to his repertoire for any somatic practitioner will depend on prior training. For the clinician with little or no experience in hands-on bodywork, it presents an integrated body-handling approach. For an acupuncturist or skilled energy worker it shows the body side of the body/energy equation and offers new ways of opening structural blocks which may impede the energy therapy. For the spiritual bodyworker it supplies the energy side of the body/energy equation and opens a new dimension of hands-on touch. For the psychologically oriented therapist it is a way to enter into dialogue with expanded states of consciousness induced through touch.

Body-Mind Centering

BONNIE BAINBRIDGE COHEN has been a participant in many of the somatic systems thus far described, as well as in other dance, movement-related, and neuro-developmental systems. She is a modernist in the sense that her work defies systemization and crosses traditional boundaries—between, on the one hand, dance, performance, song, and sports, and, on the other, occupational therapy and classical bodywork; likewise, she shifts from ceremonies to treatments, from improv sessions to classes. Bainbridge Cohen is evocative and seminal, but she is not (nor does she intend to be) systematic in a conventional or academic fashion. Thus, her training opens up areas that would not ordinarily be accessible or even definable. Like Gerda Alexander, she developed a medicinal system within an artistic and aesthetic framework and then enlarged it within a broader therapeutic context.

A student of hers, a former classical ballet dancer who became a Rolfer, gives an appreciation of her range and depth:

> Bonnie's work allows you to go, through attention, from your body as an organism, to a particular organ, to the actual cells that make up the organ. Once you get to that depth, you can decide what tissues you'd like to access. Then you allow those cells to initiate the movement.[8]

Bainbridge Cohen proposes to contract, energize, and transform tissues and cells —not by palpable shape, moduli, or anatomical intercession, but by tuning (somehow) inside their own discrete sentiences and experiences and communicating with them. Choreographer Phoebe Neville notes:

> Instead of learning about the colon from a book, we learned what it feels like to mobilize it, to move from it. It can be very intense because the innervation of the organs goes up to the limbic system in the brain, the center of emotion and memory. When one starts exploring different organs, memories and emotions come up—old accidents, eating disorders.[These connections recall] the Chinese medical model, where organs are associated with different emotions.[9]

Bainbridge Cohen explains:

> Though we use the Western anatomical terminology and mapping, we are adding meaning to these terms through our experience. When we are talking about blood or lymph or any physical substances, we are not only talking about substances but about states of consciousness and processes inherent within them. . . .
>
> The study of [Body-Mind Centering] includes both the cognitive and experiential learning of the body systems—skeleton, ligaments, muscles, fascia, fat, skin, organs, endocrine glands, nerves, fluids; breathing and vocalization; the senses and the dynamics of perception; developmental movement (both human infant development and the evolutionary progression through the animal kingdom); and the art of touch and repatterning.[10]

Skilled at intuiting novel pathways to proprioception, Bainbridge Cohen guides her students as they extend their minds into certain zones of the body, such as the thoracic cavity, and feel the distinctive oddities there. Each area discovered expands a deepening awareness of other areas. She instructs them on moving in ingenious ways that awaken dormant sensations of organ presence. She is always working toward more interiorized apperceptions and away from mere skeletomuscular

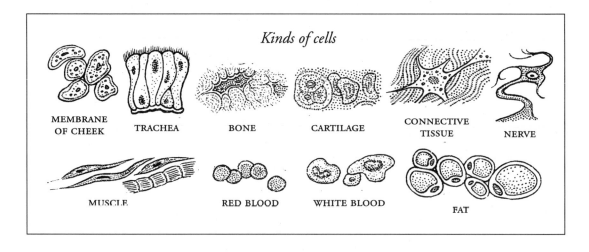

Kinds of cells

MEMBRANE OF CHEEK TRACHEA BONE CARTILAGE CONNECTIVE TISSUE NERVE

MUSCLE RED BLOOD WHITE BLOOD FAT

perceptions (though these are part of overall awareness). Whether intentional movement and internally directed attention can make physical, molecular changes in organs or merely affects the cultural totems assigned to them is not really critical to the practice of Body-Mind Centering. Bainbridge Cohen guides awareness ultimately down to a cellular level from the rationale that cells, as the foci of autonomous life, are the entities most primitively responsive to intention. This means "cells" as units of mind, "cells" as metaphors for mores of life, actions, and, at the same time, the billions of actual independent entities making up our bodies.

Cell contact requires extraordinarily refined internalization and precise trajectory. One is reminded of the Sun which took the breadth of a sci-fi novel (Frank Herbert's *Whipping Star*) to slow down its perception and find a narrow enough wave-band on which to send a critical message to the tiny human beings on one of the worlds that circled it.[11] Bainbridge Cohen probably has not even given up on atoms, molecules, and, for that matter, quarks, or whatever exists underneath those. If these are there, they contribute in some way to the overall kinesthesia of mind and existence and thus are phenomenological. Put differently, if they were not there, how would we feel? Don Hanlon Johnson recounts the early stages of awakening organ sensation with Bainbridge Cohen:

MODALITIES

She once worked with me lying on my back, while she sat behind me, hands cradling the occipital region of my head. She said, "Now I am in my bones moving your bones." I experienced unusually clear feelings of my cranial bones and the articulations of my skull and the vertebrae of my neck. I told her of my arid spinal sense. She continued, "I will go into my fluids. Now I am in my fluids." As she gently cradled my head and rocked it, I felt the gushing of fluids contained in my head and neck, followed by vibrant pulsings inside my spinal column. It felt like oil flowing deeply through my bones, so unfamiliar that my mind went blank for a moment, and I felt an ecstatic pleasure.[12]

If Bainbridge Cohen's practices sound fantastic, her childhood prepared her for wonders. She was born in 1942 into "the Ringling Brothers and Barnum & Bailey Circus, where her father sold tickets and her mother was a trapeze and high-balance artist and Roman racer; who rode two horses with one foot on each."[13]

"Ordinary reality consisted of acrobats risking their lives on the highwire, the bearded lady and the snake lady. The structure of her everyday experience reflected the polymorphous quality of three rings filled with horses, elephants, clowns, acrobats and fire-eaters, all performing simultaneously."[14]

"I grew up," she says, "with the extraordinary being natural, and therefore things other people considered miraculous or impossible never were impossible for me. . . . It took me two years to figure out how to get into my blood, to differentiate it from lymph. That's where the circus influence came in—it gave me the sense of possibility."[15]

In her youth Bainbridge Cohen was an occupational therapist, enlarging her repertoire by learning various forms of dance therapy and neuro-muscular reeducation. In 1968 she "went to Europe, where she taught movement and bodywork at the Psychiatric Research Clinic of the University of Amsterdam and worked with injured dancers at the Pauline de Groot dance studio . . . During her year abroad, she also trained in England with Karl and Berta Bobath, originators of neuro-developmental therapy, a method of restoring developmental movement patterns in children with brain injuries."[16] After she married Leonard P. Cohen in New York, she moved to Japan at the end of the 1960s so that he could continue his study of aikido. While there she began teaching at the Tokyo government's new rehabilitation school for the training of occupational and physical therapists and at another established training program under the auspices of the Japanese national government. This required her (with a smattering of Japanese language) to treat and educate physically disabled Japanese students who had limited ability to converse in English. She studied with a Japanese healer, Haruchika Noguchi. One description of his mass training conjures up images of both a riot and a giant worm. Noguchi instructed an entire stadium: "The people got up from their seats and went down to the center of the stadium—waves of people, all exercising in the stadium floor. They did what he called *katsu-gen-undo,* a vitalizing movement wherein people move in any way that the body makes them move. It is supposed to become an unconscious way of moving, and it gains a certain momentum.... [People] would begin to move, and their body movements would get bigger and bigger. Some would continue moving in this way. Others would be jumping up and down, crawling, sitting, standing—whatever they wanted to do."[17]

During this time, unknowingly Bainbridge Cohen was laying the groundwork for Body-Mind Centering. Soon thereafter, like Sutherland and Matthias Alexander, she began to conduct experiments on herself in order to learn to discern the separate states of consciousness within the different tissue complexes of the body. She did this by projecting her increasingly refined attention into what she imagined as bones, tissues, and organs. She first put her focus on the major bones and viscera and then worked her way down into tiny bones, deep visceral textures, and the boundaries between organs, dwelling in each place in order to experience its intrinsic feeling of itself. She traveled through this Underworld with the faith of a *Chi Gung* master, to feel what is there to feel, to nurture it and follow it inward as far as there is confirming sensation.

After reading the above description of her initiation, Bainbridge Cohen elaborated:

> Exploring movement and consciousness has always been at the root of my being. It is my inherent language—my primary perception and mode of existence. My mother always said that I began dancing in the womb. The challenge of translating movement consciousness into the exact science of Western anatomy, however, began in 1973, but I did not realize that it would entail all tissues until 1976, when I had the insight into the organ and endocrine systems. It then took me until 1982 to "break the code" and embody all of my systems.[18]

Bainbridge Cohen emphasizes that BMC *is* a highly systematic approach to transmitting embodiment of all of one's body tissues within the context of one's history and developmental process, but the transmission also occurs improvisationally according to the dynamics of the moment, the relationship of the people involved in the process, and the environment.[19] Bainbridge Cohen, after all, is a performance artist who developed some of her concepts while collaborating with Contact Improvisation master Nancy Stark Smith, so her lessons are as much organ and tissue dances as exercises. She tries to incite spontaneous, authentic visceral performance from deep bodily sensations and the topokinesis of desire.

The natural enactments of feeling states and emotions manifest the hidden life of tissues. The arms, legs, neural ganglia, and skin are constantly being charged and recharged by the animal personae of the viscera. Organs and fluids strive to express themselves through the varied poses, gestures, and styles of daily life but are suppressed by requirements (or imagined requirements) of etiquette and by limited views of the self. That is why new modes of organ expression need to be developed and trained. The latent body, unminded (or primitively minded like a jellyfish or newt), cries out for the motions it needs. Neuromuscular elongations and unwindings provide avenues of performance for inner nodes and epithelia—those which are usually squelched by higher ganglionic functions of the nervous system. If freed by radical movement, these forms satisfy the nonverbal cravings and expressions of the deep organs and also usher us along the same whorls to their substance and core. A great movement is not only appreciated by the conscious minds of those watching its performance but their livers, hearts, lungs, and kidneys.

The hoisting of partners in modern dance, our everyday chattering in rivers of consonants and vowels, the turning of a double-play in baseball, a girl's flirting at a party, a seal's dive —all of these are direct expressions of lungs, heart, spleen, gonads, lymph, blood, and ultimately cells. The precise feeling of each of them provides a vestibule into more discrete and subtle levels of tissue.

From her history of dance notation, Bainbridge Cohen proposes mapping the exact vectors of each neurovisceral gesture, be it the strike of a polar bear's paw or a baby struggling to walk. She draws her charts of the underlying origins of these movements in order to capture the spirit at their core. In her book *Sensing, Feeling, and Action* she similarly explores the organs and circulatory flows of the interior body through photographs of individual human "street" poses ranging from spleen and gonad intensity to liver exaltation and relaxation, pancreas-and-gall-bladder sweetness, and shameless open-heartedness. These snapshots come from different milieus and cultures and each represents the unconscious abandonment of a man or woman to a desire or will originating in an organ substratum. Bainbridge Cohen tells us: "Notice the outward radiating of this woman's heart and the drawing in of her gonads . . . reflected in the crossing of her legs, the holding in her ankles, and the expression of modesty. . . . Notice the woodcutter's active, assertive intent through the energy emanating outward from his liver. Visual clues are the expandedness of his liver area and outward widening of his elbows."[20]

We are always acting out the desires and also the fears of our organs. "They" reembody each of the stances, activities, and "artifacts" of contemporary life. Our ordinary motions and gestures yield deep-acting

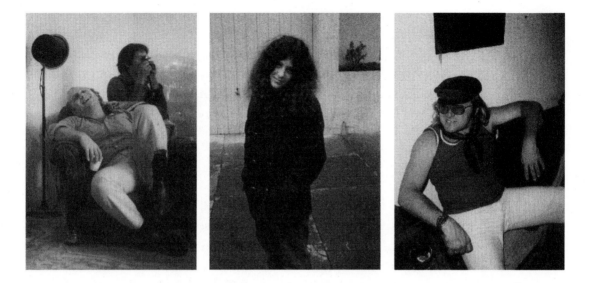

LIVER: *In the man on the left, notice the release of his liver as he relaxes in his chair. Visual clues are the soft expansion through his liver area and the relaxed widening through his elbows.* GONADS: *In the woman, notice her energy drawing in through her heart and gonads, creating a seductive pos-* turing. GONADS: *In the man on the right, notice his energy emanating outward through his gonads, contained in his liver, neutral in his heart, and emanating outward through the lower lobes and inward through the upper lobes of his lungs.*

Captions by Bonnie Bainbridge Cohen. Photos by Bill Arnold.

medicines. How much more powerful and curative would these become if they didn't have to cut wood or act coy but were permitted unrestrained expression in boundless ritual space!

Bainbridge Cohen seeks the same range of uninhibited somatic play from clients in sessions:

> As important as knowing the name of the reaction/response, and as important as doing the patterns, is to understand what the reflexes, righting reactions and equilibrium patterns have to do with expression. For example, in this little girl I'm working with, on her right side which is fine, she's really bloodful and she waves her hand up and down. Yet she never waves the other hand up and down. She might *reach* for something, she'll use it *mechanically*, but it's like it

Contemporary Systems

doesn't *belong* to her, it doesn't have the bloodfulness. She's stuck in her nerves. I feel that it's the reflexes that carry it to the blood level.

Without the reflex, there isn't expression and without the expression there isn't the reflex. So one of the things I'm trying to do is help get emotion into the movement of her arm. . . .

Anything, anything. Stroking her mother's hair, grabbing her daddy's beard, slapping her hand on the table to make rhythm, playing, flailing her arm in anger.[21]

Idiosyncratic and subtle, Bainbridge Cohen's instructions to her trainees come from privileging her own (and their own) internal odysseys and the creative modes of action that these generate through immediate experience. She will not give up authenticity and potential in order to bottom out in a simplified version of a discovery of motion (however interesting), as she leads students from one fully inhabited domain to another to get eventually to either one she originally targeted or another that is novel and unknown even to her. In an ocular exercise, she tells the class, "When you go to look, don't *try* to move your muscle or your bones, but let the eye respond to the light that's being reflected. Once you become receptive to that phenomenon, let *go* of the reception as your purpose and let that become the *support* for seeing."[22]

Then she asks them to embody each specific muscle of the eye and to perceive how the activation of each muscle alone and in various combinations affects one's vision, consciousness, and movement.[23]

Like craniosacral and Polarity practitioners, she places great value on internally experiencing the unique water generated by the embryonic neural tube sealed within the meninges and arachnoid membrane.

"The CSF (cerebrospinal fluid) is a rarefied fluid," Bainbridge Cohen tells a class; "it gives the feeling of being suspended between heaven and earth. Find the internal fluid and let it travel; it goes into lightness—not because I push up but because I rarefy through the CSF." As she says this, she rolls over on the floor, then rises on her toes with arms floating upward. For those less able to experience the CSF quality kinesthetically, she suggests, "Play with images, like a leaf falling." Around the room the students resemble an introductory modern dance class—waving, dipping, rolling....

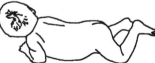

"There's something so luscious about fat, and so powerful," she remarks. "But in our culture, this soft power has been repressed."[24]

The healing effect of this work arises from the transmission of unconscious messages and a combination of touch, intrinsic movement, and the therapist responding naturally to her clients and providing them with new matrices of behavior.

"The nervous system has the potential for innumerable patterns," Bainbridge Cohen says, "but the patterns are not accessible to us until they are actually stimulated into existence, until we actually do them."[25]

She specializes in applying BMC in the treatment of infants and young children who have mild to severe developmental difficulties (the younger the better), at least in part because they put her at the gateway to the orientation and organization of the psychosomatic domain and also because children are moldable and receptive to techniques in unexpected ways. Bainbridge Cohen continues, "The children have been my mentors. They teach me constancy of presence, immediacy of response, direct perception and love."[26]

Homolateral movement

Homologous movement

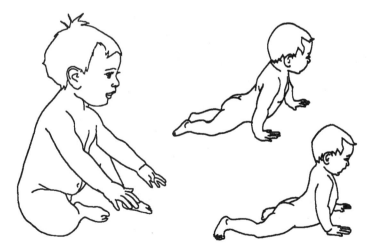

Spinal movement

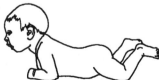

399

After reading an earlier version of this section and then looking at the book as a whole, Bainbridge Cohen offered this clarification of her own development:

> I am a daughter of the matriarchal lineage and not a synthesis of the male heritage you have so carefully scribed. . . .
>
> The following are excerpts from a journal I kept for an individualized science research class while a senior in high school (age 16 years). There were 12 students in this class, each exploring a research project of our own for the year.
>
> (dated October 6, 1958)
>
> I have chosen to study the muscular and skeletal systems of the cat. . . . Besides knowing the names of the muscles and bones, I want to know what they do, how they work, and if possible, if something happens to them if they can be cured, and if so, how.[27]

Subsequent journal notes record her after-school visit to a Cerebral Palsy Home concurrent with a wish to study dance therapy (though her high school counselors had no knowledge of such a field) plus a description of coloring in the parts of a cat on a drawing. A "Prospectus for Possible Research," written at the age of twenty-one while an occupational therapist at Bird S. Coler hospital in New York, shows how early the substantial roots of Body-Mind Centering were in place.

Bainbridge Cohen then adds that many of the somatic modalities I put in her lineage are incidental to the formulation of Body-Mind Centering, the curriculum for which was substantially in place by 1982. She recalled having three or four early Feldenkrais sessions and "observing one or two classes of Moshe . . . and him working with a client the last year he taught (about 1983?)." She also received some Alexander sessions in the mid-1970s, "the first three Rolfing sessions in 1980 and the other seven in 1989. . . . While I am very grateful for the help these practitioners and approaches provided me, they are not the roots of BMC. However, I am extremely indebted to them for the environment they have created in the culture, so that the development of BMC has flourished."[28]

She continues:

I describe the following of movement in terms of the cerebrospinal fluid because it is the basis of effortless movement, which I have been exploring with consciousness since 1965 and teaching as a distinct fluid since 1982. What John Upledger and Dick McDonald gave to me was the awareness of the rhythmic flow of the CSF when the body isn't moving and the knowledge of its flexion/extension pendular rhythm.[29]

In place of the above masters, Bainbridge Cohen lists dozens of teachers, all of whom have provided her with some essential link in her chain and who demonstrate just how many possible somatic lineages there are. Among these just from the 1960s:

> Dr. Adolf Haas, my professor of psychiatry, showed me the existential nature of being, the blessing of suffering, and the limitless range of compassion. He taught me about "the shadow," I and Thou, and the reality of the imagination.... He also taught me never to introduce a person into a world in which he or she cannot live.[30]

Would that mainstream psychiatry still had such integrity of compassion!

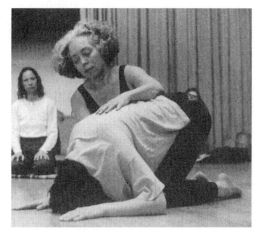

Erick Hawkins, one of the giants of modern dance, gave me a technique that allowed me to embody my philosophy of life and to extend it into moment-by-moment awareness. He showed me effortless movement and the art of doing without doing.

Yogi Ramira, an Indian yogi and physical therapist from Madras, introduced me to the techniques of yoga, its power in the healing of organic imbalances, and the effect it has upon one's state of mind.

Berta Bobath, a physical therapist, and Dr. Karl Bobath, world leaders in the treatment of persons who have brain dysfunction, taught me that if a person doesn't change directly under my hands each moment, then I should do something else. They showed me how the developmental process underlies all movement and how to repattern the nervous system based on that process, regardless of the manifested problems.[31]

Then from the 1970s:

Professor Cheng Man-ch'ing, a master of t'ai chi, Chinese medicine, poetry, and art, gave me a glimpse of the enormous power of effortless strength, in the guise of a laughing old man. . . .

Haruchika Noguchi . . . showed me the reality and power of magnetic energy as experienced through off-the-body touching. . . .

Irmgard Bartenieff, dancer, physical therapist, and student of Rudolf Laban (founder of the Labanonotation and Laban Movement Analysis), stimulated in me unfathomable questions of how the body moves. These questions led me to an expanded view of how muscles move, the dynamics of flow and quality within movement, and the phenomenon of spatial tension and harmony. . . .

Eido Roshi, Zen teacher, showed me how to sit. He along with Chögyam Trungpa, Rinpoche, Dr. Yeshe Donden, and other Buddhist teachers show me that presence both transmits and is transitory. . . .

From aikido, the martial art, I learned how following, harmonizing, and blending with the ki of others forms the basis of repatterning.[32]

She concludes:

Being a nonlinear processor, Richard, I feel I can now say what I mean. The development of Body-Mind Centering has many roots and yet it has always existed inside of me. It has been transmitted through my blood—through the experience of all my mothers. Its blueprint is contained homeopathically in my bodily fluids. All others have helped me to clarify, elaborate and articulate it.[33]

Dancers, wizards, guardians, and angels play hide-and-seek with us our whole lives. Their origins scattered through time and space are mysterious and transcendental. We are flooded with their insignias and microdoses from within and without, from archetypal as well as cultural (and perhaps also ethereal and astrological) sources, codes that travel as long and far as meteor-seeds through an empty universe and then choose us for their expression. New forms burst into bloom everywhere from a latency which, though invisible, is as ripe as the arras of pomegranates behind the High Priestess in the second trump of the tarot. We imagine the falling fruits on linear vines, the stems of which we trace to the ground into which they disappear. But there is also a nonlinear process that extends on so many other branches, into dimensions that go beyond branches. In that sense, there is no history; there is only life and matter. And there are myriad arcane voices and intelligences, human and otherwise.

Body-Mind Centering is a benchmark of the innovative forms now emerging, systems which phenomenologically, improvisationally usher in new modes of perception while rooted in the techniques and tools developed by their forebears.

Continuum

EMILIE CONRAD grew up in New York in the 1930s and '40s, training from her youth to become a professional dancer. Her specialties were classical ballet and primitive dance. In 1955, longing to experience the primal rhythm at the roots of so many dance forms, she traveled to the West Indies. Entranced by the music and the culture, she ended up staying five years, immersed in Haitian dance and religion and finally organizing her own dance troupe.

"Once she was back in New York ... the dissonance between the liquid, organic rhythms of Haiti and the frantic, manufactured pace of Manhattan grew to such a pitch that Conrad thought she would go mad.... In the midst of her inner chaos [she] began to realize that what we call our body is, to a large extent, a cultural construction. The disparity between how New Yorkers and people in the West Indies move and view their bodies convinced her that each culture 'imposes on its members a definition of the human form.' Beneath this construct, Conrad sensed only movement."[34]

It was that original movement, preceding culture, preceding any form of cognitive knowledge, to which Conrad would address her future inquiries.

During the formative years of being caught between cultures, she modeled, taught primitive dance, and recruited another dance troupe. "On occasion, she and her troupe did performances in nightclubs based on voodoo rituals. She has recounted . . . the night during an ecstatic solo fire dance, when she suddenly felt she had 'crossed over, beyond the possibility of ever coming back.' That 'crossing over' meant for her the breakdown of her culture, with all of the categories of meaning and bodily experience."[35]

In 1967, after a move to Los Angeles and a serious automobile accident—in a state she experienced as a "black hole," constantly dizzy and blandished by voices and visions from ancient cultures—she decided to yield entirely and let what was happening guide her. After all, those voices and visions intimated what she had been seeking ever since she had embarked on her study of dance almost thirty years earlier—an inherent form of movement.

> I had to give up everything I believed. . . . I saw that what I called "my body"—how I moved, talked, even how I thought—was a cultural imprint. With all my training, I had been teaching "my body" to dance. But deep inside there was already a dance going on, if I would perceive it—a dance of myriad movement forms beyond anything I could think of. I had to feel it. . . .[36]

This boundless reservoir of energy Conrad likened to pure love. Automatic as breathing, it imbued every cell and molecule of her organism. From an intuition of this state she began to explore what she later called "micromovements," initially while lying in bed at night. She understood these inklings as glimmerings of motion-sensation trickling from her absolute nature. She distinguished them from the externally visible and culturally recognized movements of most choreography and somatic work. "The result [was] Continuum, an approach to the body based on intrinsic felt movement rather than imposed patterned movement."[37]

Once again, somatic phenomenology led to a new ontology of human existence.

Later, after Conard began working with people suffering from severe neuromuscular afflictions, she saw that such primal oscillations manifested even in paralyzed persons.

In the case of one twenty-three-year-old woman partially paralyzed by polio since age one, "Emilie simply stayed present with her hands on the young woman's body. She sat like this for hours at a stretch, giving no instructions, not even guiding her in visualizations. At first, Susan felt only heat. Then one of her legs began to shudder and move in strange ways that were similar to the ways that Emilie had found herself moving in her bed. Over a four-year period of weekly four-hour sessions, many of which were observed and subjected to electromyographical analysis in the UCLA kinesiology laboratory, Susan manifested a range of subtle and finely articulated movements.... 'Paralyzed people,' [Conrad] writes, 'can feel movement inside their bodies, but because our culture does not value this kind of movement, they think they cannot move. Helping Susan get in touch with the movement within her atrophied leg allowed the inner movement to surface and ripple across the skin and eventually enabled Susan to lift her leg.'"[38]

Continuum movements are unlike any other somatic form. Conrad emphasizes their unconscious, unpredictable, nonserial motility. Her patterns arise as certainly in paraplegics as in athletes. She has referred to them as "liquid smoke" or "singing the body electric." The flesh undulates as if an anemone in water. Its solid parts ripple. Ribs become waves. The spine reverts to a soft notochord. As pulses of energy flow radially outward, front and back are indistinguishable. Fishlike, eaglelike, spongelike, and zebra-like, these vestigial animal motions emerge from deep in visceral space. When chairs are present, the torso may writhe up one or an adjacent pair like a snail, either legs first or arms first, and either frontally or dorsally, and then wrap over and around them like a snake.

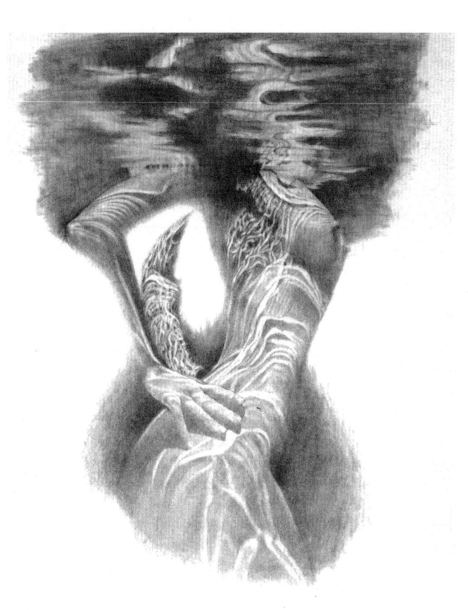

F OR A PERIOD of thirty years Conrad built a practice based on these
discoveries, teaching workshops of micromovements and treating
a diversity of ailments by eliciting people's natural forms of motility.

"I want you to move," Conrad tells people, "but not with your space
probes, not with your arms and legs. I want you to feel the movement

in your body. Start anywhere, with your ribs or with your ass." She begins to demonstrate. Her buttocks move, almost imperceptibly at first. The movement spreads to her back. "Suddenly aliveness happens," she continues, now in a droning voice. Her eyes are slits. Her right shoulder begins to twitch. "Pay attention to how the movement wants to go. It takes strange pathways." Her left leg is lifting off the floor, her right arm twisting forward. Her elbow bends, her fingers curl and twist, her torso undulates in slow waves. "I am an unpredictable thing."[39]

At one Continuum workshop a woman with the intestinal disorder known as Crohn's disease (who had just been diagnosed as having only a few months left to live) began moving in an utterly strange but fluid manner. The next day her doctor could find no evidence of the illness. In several instances of people with major spinal cord damage, Conrad has been able to track alternative pathways to their central nervous systems.

She encourages paralyzed people to crawl on their hands and knees across the floor and then follow their own unexpected micromovements. Some clients she instructs to intone "wo," "sth," or other unfamiliar sounds from far back in their throats or by vibrating their tongues against their palates. Other exercises involve moving one part of the body, like the ring finger, slowly for fifteen minutes. Each instruction consists of eliciting innate motion and letting it expand multidimensionally into space.

The breathing and movement forms of Continuum are based on creating pathways into visceral and cellular space. Their goal is to break with entrained neocortical rhythm and invoke deeper creature rhythms inside the organism. Conrad teaches several breaths, the initial one being "hu," a rapid panting during which the jaw, lips, throat, and neck muscles constantly morph, fluctuating in depths and textures of a "hu" sound while deriving it uniquely from different parts of the anatomy. The "hu" alphabet keeps the breath from imposing any regularized pattern, thus is meant to elicit the natural rhythms of visceral and cell life.

Continuum's lunar breath is slow passage of air from deep in the throat and thoracic cavity. It replicates a breeze rustling through leaves or how the Moon would sound if a real object were sailing through clouds.

The theta breath is created as the tongue is pressed behind the upper palate, causing a split release of air. Conrad's long exploration and development of this breath has led her to believe that it sends a scalar wave into the body's electromagnetic field, which serves as a directional path into many viscera and tissue complexes. Because the split of the tongue marks the origination point of the neural-crest cells and the seal of the embryonic primitive streak at the upper palate, her intuition is that the neural tube might dispatch theta signals into the regions of the body where migrating cells originally implanted sensory pathways.

To use Continuum to enter the meninges around the brain, Conrad recommends starting with a theta breath, whistling it smoothly out the palate while stroking the cranial temple at its single available contact points with the sphenoid bone (the corners of the eyes), one finger per hand on each point. As "theta" launches her signal into the brain, a rich lunar breath should follow, its exhalation so vast and diffuse as to seem to be passing through every pore of the body. The backs of the eyes, including the outwardly blind pineal "eye," should scan inwardly for the brain. They travel down the neural tube, as the mind pictures the head separating from the spine. The "aw" breath, which Conrad associates with spinal fluid, comes next. The head falls back, presenting the Adam's apple as if a wolf were about to wail. Instead, the outbreath makes tiny froglike yawps, each one a slight recoil at the start of the exhale, releasing itself semi-voluntarily afterward. Ordinary lunar breathing ensues; attention goes to the seam between the back of the ear and the head and squiggles from there into the soft, spidery membrane of the arachnoid.

Conrad has created a syllabary of such breaths for visiting different regions inside the body. Since all tissues have vestigial consciousness and since all are part of our kinesthesia and sense of being, they are all enterable. Unconscious mind is ceaselessly traveling through a cellular domain anyway, bringing its intelligence to the organs and functioning as an inner physician. In contacting and penetrating them intentionally, in resonating our breath and mind with their emergent consciousnesses, we can try to repattern and change them.

The cells apparently respond in some fashion to our respectful journeys into their domains; if they have disharmonies, these are transduced into different configurations. Perhaps embryogenic healing is activated: a change in movement and breath becomes a change in thought and structure; new proteins and collagen molecules self-assemble. Perhaps even DNA transcription is altered. Of course, this may all be a grandiose fantasy, but it is one closer to our biological reality than the giant machineries whose houses, cities, and vehicles we inhabit. A modality like Continuum has a chance of putting us in touch with the avatar inside each of us. If intentional self-healing is possible, this is one of the places it could begin.

For us in the West, the internal science of breath-mind medicine is at its bare beginning. Its potential is limitless.

When shamanic healing dawns in our own culture, it will likely replicate thousands—if not millions—of such instances prehistorically and among tribal cultures. Micromovements presided at the birth of speech, magic, and ritual courtship, and inform the guiles of hunting strategy. It is no wonder they emerge fresh in the sensory expression of each person's true somatic being.

The Return to Autonomous Movement

AMIDST THE DIVERSITY of somatic strategies and disciplines, a rather simple theme stands out—freeing movement, dispatching unconscious mind into viscera, signalling cellular mechanisms, and releasing somatoemotional tension. The majority among the human species have lost this basic inheritance—core autonomous function. If unstifled, cells and organs perform sympathetically and do not require our abstract homilies for them. From the silence of their sheer evolutionary depth and embryogenic layering, they establish and maintain inherent metabolic substantiality, and inform behavior. They energize stagnations and knots of disease.

In our striving for intentional behavior and controlled performance we have forgotten that we embody these natural sympathetic movements and automatic motions, not only at a neuromuscular level but at differentials of cells, organelles, and molecules. "'We do not move. We are movement,' Emilie Conrad tells her students."[40]

While creating a techno-superculture, we have ignored that our survival and well-being rest on a substratum of tissue and fascia vibrating in a harmonic cacophony of cell nuclei calling like thousands of different species of birds, all of it sustained by an interior realm of water, oxygen, and chlorophyll. We clabber this milieu by not inhabiting it fully.

Just as we are heartless when we cannot feel our hearts, we are mindless when we do not experience mind in our tissues. In place of somatic mind, we derive pretentious and egoistic substitutes for creature existence—we who are homeostatic fields right from seed.

Embodiment occurs as global and regional waves responding to the topokinetic exigencies of prior waves, all moving from a germinal template of two cells to billions of separate epithelia and domains of tissue making up a functional life-form. This process displays exquisite algebraic and complexity-field properties: rhythm, quantum uncertainty, seriality, counterpoint, melody, commutability, phase transition. It is because we *are* music that we respond to its vibration so profoundly.

The mind also has natural movements and organic patterns. Aspects of these jell as insights, emotions, modes of proprioception, and bliss. "If Martians were looking at us through some interstellar resonating device," says Emilie Conrad, "I am sure they would marvel at how our planet has arranged us.

"'Look, look,' they would say. 'Their bodies are mostly water and yet they move about the earth in this apparently solid way.'

"'Just look at how each organ is maintaining its link with all of its undulating strands.'

" 'They are like fish out of water, but they carry it with them.'
" 'How amazing these humans are!' "[41]

Animals nearly always move and think autonomously. Aboriginal primates were likely more "flowing" than their socialized descendants.

Stone Age people were probably aware of *chi* and knew how to stimulate it from the feedback of daily experience; they were also doubtless attuned to the rhythm of the pulse and the white light of cerebrospinal fluid. They recognized their own capacity to direct energy outward; hence, were masters of voodoo, Reiki, *t'ai chi* and the "evil eye."

It is a reasonable presumption that powers of self-healing and healing—and perhaps even telekinesis and telepathy —occurred immediately and uncritically among Cro-Magnons and their kin. That is, they didn't even know that there was such a thing as *chi* or psychic energy; yet they experienced them as absolutely as wind, prairie, and their own being. We have transferred all of these functions, in whole or in part, to intellectual categories and machines.

Whether telekinetic abilities were once generally accessible or always elite, it is clear that we have a great deal of difficulty inculcating them today, even at the highest levels of our own practice—Dzogchen, Kriya Yoga, *Chi Gung,* cybernetics. In fact, we are not sure they even exist. This leaves us in a state of schizophrenia. Seeking to generate power extrinsically while denying it intrinsically, we become virtually powerless. At the same time, we continue to erect and surround ourselves with the most super-powerful machinery imaginable.

F OR ALL ITS other avocations, somatics is the cutting edge of our urgency to confront the crisis of faith in ourselves and restore autonomous function. It would be an oversimplification to claim that somatic systems seek mainly to break down millennial habits of cortical overfunction and resistance in order to restore natural movement and homeostasis to the human body and psyche, but to overlook this component would be to miss an archetypal theme.

The craniosacral rhythm is apparently a reliable intrinsic compass of well-being and organismic truth. When the flow of cerebrospinal fluid is uniform and the flexion-extension of organs unimpeded, a person is more at peace and healthier, more capable of compassion and creativity. Thus, cranial osteopathy and craniosacral therapy seek to restore a primordial state of fluidity and cohesion.

Systems like the Feldenkrais Method, Alexander Technique, Eutony, Body-Mind Centering, Continuum, and various forms of dance and movement therapy all provide the organism with means of getting around conscious overdrive, past the cerebral cortex into autonomous flow. Their lessons are intended to trick or guide the body into more basic, less artificial functioning. In that sense they are the precise opposite of most educational practices, which seek to compound layers of structure and gain full cognitive control over emotions and spontaneity.

All somatic, sensory-motor modalities tell us that the habits of repression whereby we have subjugated our animal selves lead to poor health—neurosis, dysfunction, and skeletal and neuromuscular blocks in which tissue pathologies attach. Their protocols prompt the bones and tissues back to their own dances.

Western science, as noted, has no discrete definition of *chi*. *Chi* is not blood, lymph, cerebrospinal fluid, or even electricity and magnetism. At times it is proposed as a concurrence of these things. But is *chi* not also simply a fusion of autonomous and subcellular movements, all working together as one movement with the virtues of all of them uniting in a single elixir-like sensation of a healing current? Although *"chi"* training is a lesson in feeling a specific thing called *"chi* energy," that may mostly be a custom of historical Chinese nomenclature. *Chi* may also be the ground state of autonomous movement; its therapeutic and shamanic virtues may be the sum benefaction of natural body-mind flow. A practitioner may claim to be raising *chi,* but there may not be a concrete substance to raise like water in a well. There may

only be the multidimensional coherence of living tissue and its creative, synergistic capacity—and this may represent all its modes of cosmic as well as psychic energy.

"What we call 'body'," says Conrad, "is not 'matter' but movement. The body is a profound orchestration of many qualities and textures of movement, interpenetrating tones of fertile play, waiting to be incubated. What I see as body is the urging of creative flux, waves of fertility. The cosmic play that we enter this atmosphere with still goes on at an intrinsic level—we are mostly not aware of the world we carry.

"It is *there* in this cosmic soup disguised as organs and cartilage and tissue that the universe is moving in its creative flux like a giant egg waiting to be fertilized. The amniotic matrix moves with the same undulations that started the cosmic swirl that we call Earth in the first place.

"Our intrinsic world *is* our cosmic connection, it is our legacy of love and wonder—it is where God plays at midnight, it is the big bang, the splitting of atoms, and the message of Jesus."[42]

THE GOAL OF this discussion is not to reduce all somatic systems to one denominator or to suggest that a return to cell talk or the wild is the goal of somatic epistemology. Animals, though in a state of freedom, are in prisons so diabolical we should be glad to entertain only our own self-made demons. The fact is that men and women live in society, in bodies conditioned by society, and minds shaped by cultural concepts. Natural man became tribal man; and tribal woman became a farmer, an artisan, a merchant, and a politician. If natural man and woman had sustained a state of perfect grace, none of these symbolic realms would have arisen. In fact, "s/he" would have happily remained a lizard and a tiger for the duration.

Animals do not encounter the riddles and existential dilemmas that men and women do. Men and women require the realm of symbols and artifacts to mediate the exigencies of their exquisite condition. But men and women also need their animal roots, their animal powers. They must become animals to become humans. That was the collective perception of shamans and medicine teachers worldwide at the dawn of history. That is now our injunction—to become animals while remaining simultaneously capable of self-awareness and reverie.

The complications and responsibilities of our phenomenological and totemized world portend myriad subtleties of psychological and philosophical transformation. Even as some sort of accreting force is driving us toward global society, transnational economy, and a purely metaphysical realm of experience, the original dissipative force is still attempting to restore to us (and restore us to) our birthright as living organisms, as waves.

We are not ideas, and we will never be machines. We are creatures. All our joys, grievings, and resolutions are based in the density, limitations, boundaries, and kinetic charge of tissue. We cannot transcend this condition cybernetically or prosthetically. We can never become true cyborgs or inhabit virtual realities. Despite New Age fantasies, the flesh is not merely a vehicle to deliver a spirit seed to a higher dimension. The biosphere is an extremely powerful manifestation of spirit seeking identity and experience in holograms of becoming-sentient matter. The goal is thus not to glissade or bootleg out of bodies but to transform bodies into Shaolin temples and vehicles of healing. Bodies are the ultimate test (in this realm anyway) for spirits on a vision quest. They are spirit's choice, its grail. They are likewise what it needs (and has always needed) in order to become whole.

Somatics is thus a contemporary healing art and at the same time the primary metaphor for a healing imperative we have yet to develop. On a planet beleaguered by environmental despoliation, denial, duplicity, and the ceaseless false promises of politicians and gurus, bodywork systems represent one of the few signs of renewal.

We do not know why we are so unreliable and unfaithful. But at least these systems do not judge us, they emanate from us. They assume the good will of every man and woman. They teach us how to be who we are at our best. Wilhelm Reich was on target when he said that no revolution is possible until its requirements of mental and physical hygiene have been met.

Somatic systems train us to act on behalf of the planet because this is what we do naturally when we don't interfere or are not bought off by artificial and substitute pleasures. When we honor the flesh, we honor the biosphere.

If bodies are the spirits of the universe in crisis, somatic systems address their spiritual nature directly and with dignity. Body-oriented therapy is spiritual therapy because, as Ida Rolf proposed, there is no other way to go to the house of the spirit. The body is the only part of spirit we feel from within. Thus, unless we learn to live in bodies in a biosphere, we cannot contact our spirits. They told us precisely this by becoming bodies and by making that brazen act into the implacable and inescapable density of the world and ourselves.

We can no longer contact spirits as religious abstractions or pieties and ghosts. For all the translucent specters and high radiant forms presented by world religions and the New Age for both worship and transmutation, we have ended up with startlingly few usable replicas of spirit.

This time we chose not to be able to escape. We vowed to see this one through.

We are cosmic beings having a human experience. Yet we are still pretending through elaborate ceremonies to be somewhere else.

Somatic modalities are as kaleidoscopic, contradictory, ambiguous, and embattled as we are. The individual systems seek to restore us to our visceral natures, but never by a miracle from on high. Each leads us to encounter some essential aspect of freedom and well-being that is embodied in shear planes of tissue and blocked by a once necessary but now extraneous habit or affectation of cultural process.

Notes

1. I am grateful to Fritz Smith, M.D., for his help in completing this section.

2. Bonnie Bainbridge Cohen, *Sensing, Feeling, and Action: The Experiential Anatomy of Body-Mind Centering* (Northampton, Massachusetts: Con-

tact Editions, 1993), p. 159.

3. Fritz Smith, note on the text of *Planet Medicine*, 1994.

4. Ibid.

5. Ibid.

6. Ibid.

7. Wazir Peller, personal communication, San Carlos, California, 1994.

8. Stephanie Golden, "Body-Mind Centering," *Yoga Journal* (September/October 1993), p. 126 (quote from Don Van Vleet).

9. Quoted in Golden, "Body-Mind Centering," pp. 90, 126.

10. Bainbridge Cohen, *Sensing, Feeling, and Action*, p. 2.

11. Frank Herbert, *Whipping Star* (New York: Berkley, 1977).

12. Don Hanlon Johnson, *Body, Spirit and Democracy* (Berkeley, California: North Atlantic Books, 1993), pp. 212–213.

13. Golden, "Body-Mind Centering," p. 89.

14. Johnson, *Body, Spirit and Democracy*, p. 209.

15. Bainbridge Cohen quoted in Golden, "Body-Mind Centering," p. 89.

16. Golden, "Body-Mind Centering," p. 89.

17. Mia Segal, interview in *Somatics* (Autumn/Winter, 1985–86), p. 16.

18. Bonnie Bainbridge Cohen, notes on the text of *Planet Medicine*, 1994.

19. Ibid.

20. Bainbridge Cohen, *Sensing, Feeling, and Action*, pp. 46–51.

21. Ibid., p. 148.

22. Ibid., p. 20.

23. Bainbridge Cohen, notes on the text of *Planet Medicine*, 1994.

24. Golden, "Body-Mind Centering," p. 87.

25. Ibid., p. 99.

26. Bainbridge Cohen, notes on the text of *Planet Medicine*, 1994.

27. Ibid.

28. Ibid.

29. Ibid.

30. Bainbridge Cohen, *Sensing, Feeling, and Action*, p. 158.

31. Ibid., p. 159.

32. Ibid.

33. Bainbridge Cohen, notes on the text of *Planet Medicine*, 1994.

34. Carolyn Schaffer, "An Interview with Emilie Conrad-Da'oud," *Yoga Journal*, no. 77 (November/December 1987), p. 52.

35. Johnson, *Body, Spirit and Democracy,* p. 115.

36. ibid., p. 116.

37. Schaffer, "An Interview with Emilie Conrad Da'oud," pp. 52–53.

38. Johnson, *Body, Spirit and Democracy,* p. 117.

39. Schaffer, "An Interview with Emilie Conrad Da'oud," p. 54.

40. Ibid., p. 52.

41. Emilie Conrad-Da'oud, "Life on Land," in Don Hanlon Johnson (ed.), *Bone, Breath and Gesture: Practices of Embodiment* (Berkeley, California: North Atlantic Books, 1996), p. 297.

42. Ibid, pp. 311–312.

PART III

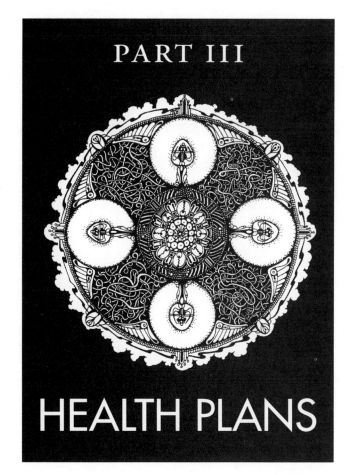

HEALTH PLANS

CHAPTER EIGHT

The Spectrum of Healing

Internalizing and Externalizing Medicines

ALL MEDICINES CAN be viewed in relation to one another on a spectrum from Internalizing/Active to Externalizing/Passive. That is, every medicine is either anatomicopharmacological (changing structure or chemistry, hence external and linear) or energetic/stimulating (hence internal and resonant). Most holistic and indigenous medicines are based on the internalization, transduction, and integration of rituals and substances. The icons placed by the medicine man in his sand painting; the darts, sigils, and swords of the shaman in his *mesa;* the letters fed to the patient in the Eurhythmic alphabet; the touch of fascial integration and muscle energy; the breaths of meditation; and, on another level, the subtle and molecular qualities of palpations, foods, and herbs—all are meant to be taken into the deep being, absorbed and assimilated. Their true power is long-term and secondary. They work mostly after an active systemic response from the recipient—and likely stimulate such a response—and because they act according to laws of cure, from the inside out, from the past forward, their shocks and subcurrents give rise to levels of healing often quite removed from the initial physiological effect. Scents, microdoses, sounds, visualizations, breath, prayer, etc., are potentized, thus affect the body primarily on a meta-cellular, perhaps even a subatomic, telekinetic level.

Conventional medicines are generally external, direct, and work *on* the recipient, preferably at once. Medical doctors perform on the physical/mechanical plane. It would be useless for them to try subtle palpation or praying over patients. In fact, it is dangerous when external healers are attracted by holistic energetic fads. Unless they transform their whole experiential base, they simply turn other modalities into metaphors of mechanical medicine. They do not stimulate a secondary curative response, or if they do, it is diffuse and random.

By the laws of nature, no medicines are purely internal or external. Just as medicines of internalization progress from discrete material substances and events, so medicines of externalization internalize, though usually the remedy has a different systemic meaning from its proposed external intent—and even from its external biophysical effect. Often their secondary response is pathological (iatrogenic) in that palliative or superficial cure dampens the immune system and stagnates the vital force. The long-range consequence of an antibiotic in the latency and potentiality of the body/mind is often more profound and "medicinal" (even if deleteriously so) than its initial, intended effect on the disease or than the disease itself (despite the fact that the medicine's physiological activity may be successful in reversing the symptomatic phase of a disease).

Iatrogenic pathology has become a major health hazard in the West; liver damage, change in blood chemistry, kidney dysfunction, impotence, neurosis, slurred speech, and fungal infestation are all recognized by-products of popular antibiotics. However, the real problem is since these medicines are not chosen according to any laws of cure (homeopathic, Ayurvedic, shamanic), they can be internalized ultimately only in a way that weakens the system and makes it susceptible to future disease. After successful surgery removing his spleen a patient may have no further physical symptoms, but the field of his meridians, his emotional balance, and kinesthesia may be so altered as to incubate a psychosis or tumor over time.

	Internalizing/Active Pole
First Level:	Meditation, Prayer, Self-Reflection (Taoist *Chi Gung,* Reiki)
Second Level:	Activity (*Dō-in, T'ai Chi Ch'uan,* Chanting, medical *Chi Gung,* yoga, some Feldenkrais exercises)
Third Level:	Healing by the Senses (touch, vision, hearing, dreams), Craniosacral Therapy, Zero Balancing, Bates Method, homeopathy
Fourth Level:	Diet and Herbs (Body Electronics, much of Ayurveda)
Fifth Level:	Bodywork (*shiatsu,* chiropractic, Rolfing), Sensory Stimulants (aromatherapy)
Sixth Level:	Acupuncture, Psychotherapy
Seventh Level:	Surgery, Radiation, Drugs (allopathy)
	Externalizing/Passive Pole

In a complex world, there is no easy or linear solution to the dilemma of how direct and external or long-term and internal a treatment should be. In general, a person should choose the most internalizing medicine of which he or she is capable at the time and which the stranglehold of the disease allows, while cultivating other more internalizing methods preventatively and for future use. This way healing can plumb to the deepest safe level. Holistic bravado should not encourage risking one's health or life trying to heal at a more internal, active level than one is presently capable of. The chart above offers a hypothetical spectrum.

The lower the number, the more active the person treated has to be—the more he or she has to cure himself or herself. Cures represented by the higher numbers are, by degree, relatively quicker and more direct and mechanical. A symptom in the seventh category is dealt with in a matter of months or even minutes. The first level requires years (though spontaneous cures of faith—quantum leaps— are also possible).

As one moves up the scale and treatments allow more sluggishness and inactivity by the patient, the physician can substitute mechanical techniques and technologies for systemic vitality.

The chart is very malleable; it is an intuitive guide, not a taxonomy. Although the medicines of the first and seventh levels are extremes, those in between differ by only minute degrees and can overlap even across five or six levels depending on how they are practiced. Drugs, radiation, and surgery *(note!)* are not outside of the spectrum but at the opposite pole from meditation. "There are no wrong medicines," says Paul Pitchford, acupuncturist and Chinese herbalist who devised the chart on which this one is based. "People choose the medicine they need."[1]

The examples are likewise rough approximations. Most medicines are multilayered and combinatorial, and include elements of self-reflection, activity, diet, and healing by the senses within their explicit modality. For instance, craniosacral palpation can be carried out as subtly as chanting or as musculoskeletally as Palmer's chiropractic; chiropractic itself can be equally subtle or coarse. Acupuncture can mellow to *dō-in* or be highly electric. Madame Ou likes to shoot her *chi* through the needles, the source of her nickname "Madame Ow," and she is very effective. ("Does it hurt?" she asks. "No? How about now?") By contrast, Robert Zeiger does a very quiet, zen acupuncture, a carefully considered needle at a time, trying to harmonize with the body's sensitivity. His method works just as well. (See Resource Guide.) Taoist *Chi Gung* resembles meditation; Buddhist medical *Chi Gung,* exercise. Kumar Frantzis compares the grosser external movements of medical *Chi Gung* to upping the wattage in a light bulb from maybe 40 to 100 but the internal movements of Taoist *Chi Gung* to changing to a whole different order of light.[2] Even crude factory drugs have internalizing herbal properties in them, for they are based on herbs historically and pharmaceutically.

Although in this discussion I take a critical view of passive externalizing medicine, the hierarchy is not ideological; it represents a range of potentiation. Potentiation can remain static or evolve.

Purely vitalist medicines could be considered at any level depending on interpretation. They are herbs if one chooses a metaphor with pills and infusions, and they are prayers if one thinks of them by analogy with the "rays" of faith healing.

We cannot assess doctors for holism even as we cannot rate them according to the technologies to which they have access. There is no "healing authority" that declares which treatments are therapeutic and which ones are iatrogenic or secondarily pathological. The critique of all mainstream doctors as benighted hacks is a New Age cartoon. Most are well-trained, able to heal, and use good judgment for the plane on which they work. Almost any of them are capable of extending lives and relieving painful and debilitating ailments. Some paths to healing necessarily include radiation and chemotherapy.

ONE CANNOT DO everything, so it is hard to know where to begin. All around us are various holistic orthodoxies proclaiming: eat macrobiotic food ... take out mercury fillings ... animals in nature don't cook ... primal therapy (or rebirthing or somatoemotional release) to clear trauma ... yet only a homeopath can dissolve inherited miasms ... vaccinate to prevent disease ... antidote your vaccinations to prevent even worse disease ... filter fluoridated water to protect your immune system (because fluoride suffocates healthy cells) ... replace milk with whey to avoid heart disease ... drink trace minerals ... sun your eyes ... stay out of the sun.

It becomes crazy-making because healing cannot be *instead of* living. One freelance editor at North Atlantic Books joked that she should get hazard pay for working on radical healing and "food as medicine" books. "I've already thrown out my microwave, stashed my aluminum cookware, stopped eating sushi (which I love, but too bad, it has parasites)," she orated one day. "I go out of my way to avoid Safeway and buy organic fruits and vegetables, at considerably higher prices I might add. I read all cans, boxes, and jars for additives, I got a brand-new reverse-osmosis water filter, but not a Grander Technology Living Water System or its energy rods. I take enzymes before every meal (I have to remember to bring them to restaurants). But I'm still freaked out about my mercury fillings and root canals, parasites from my cats, the fluoride that reverse osmosis doesn't remove, and the pesticides in restaurant wine. I'm glad I know about all this stuff now, but it sure does strain my relationship with my family and make my daily life pretty complicated."

Recently I forewarned the assistant to a former dentist, about to visit our office with a prospective book, that I had very visible mercury fillings in my teeth. I wanted to get any hex from him out of the way.

"Don't worry," he laughed. "Harold will bring along his drill."

F OR MOST PEOPLE in the West today, medicine practiced at the seventh level is perfectly acceptable; even its failings are acceptable. People demand concrete, immediate change at any cost, and this is what they tend to get. They are like sponsors laying out hundreds of thousands of dollars for the seconds of prime-time, which happen to be their lives. Often they win an extra ten, twenty, or thirty years compared to, say, a character in a Jane Austen or Willa Cather novel— which is like winning the lottery.

Mechanistic medicine may be linear and algorithmic, but it is the same linearity and algorithm that gave us the combustion engine, MRI, and the computer chip, without which we would live quite different, dramatically shorter lives.

Those who prefer the seventh level reach nervously for a cigarette, a cup of coffee, or the symptomatic relief of their jobs or social lives.

Heart surgery is another commodity for the home-improvement, standard-of-living, SUV, DVD junkie, and he dwells in all of us to some degree. We go on amassing artifacts of externalization. This is the way we live, some of us for a very long time.

Carton-a-day smokers, recipients of transplanted organs, and workers in carcinogenic factories sometimes outlive faith healers and lamas who die of stomach cancer or leukemia at relatively young ages. Genetic and karmic factors are imponderable. Pure longevity is not the major criterion anyway for integrity or depth of life experience. Because a particular monk fasted and meditated regularly and then died at forty does not mean that we should not practice yoga or manage our diets according to therapeutic principles. We do not know all the factors in his case or ours. Because a *t'ai chi* master succumbed suddenly to liver toxicity in middle age does not mean that *t'ai chi* is not curative. Whatever keeps people alive and well does so for unique and individual reasons, and for different reasons with different people. If George Burns, after smoking all those cigars, survives to sing at ninety: "I wish I were eighteen again, going where I've never been," then something keeps him alive, perhaps the original vaudeville elixir. Something else keeps Bob Hope and Strom Thurmond alive in this same parable.

An ocean of creature experience and biological process, by definition unexamined and beyond remediation, underlies any life and medical directive. Simply living energetically and creatively is far more critical than attempting to cover all bases. If one tracks one's own process, he or she may be drawn from muscle testing to psychotherapy to diet to meditation, or, in other instances, in a near opposite cycle. As a condition changes, so must one's attention and the direction of treatment. "Listening" is the key to both life and healing—staying with the pattern a particular event (or act of attempted cure) initiates and following its effect to the next level of diagnosis or insight.

Holistic medicine may be understood as an attempt to practice our disease crises as crucibles of transformation; it is also an attempt to get us well at a core level without making us sicker in the process. It is not a guarantee of freedom from disease or of longevity.

The Most Internalizing Medicines:
Prayer, Meditation, Self-Reflection, and Activity

MEDITATION, INCLUDING FORMS such as Zen and Vipassana, is a conscious method for entering unconscious being and transforming it through concentration. For the practitioner of meditation, thoughts are a slipstream of breath, organs, and mind, a thoughtless mind that penetrates the mindedness of the whole body. When the so-called "drunken monkey" mind is tamed and stops reeling from distraction to distraction, worry to worry, the breath and stopped thought settle in a deeper, prior self that is calm, profound, and capable of projecting attention and healing energy into organs.

One Sri Lankan master writes: "[The] method of allowing the simple facts of observation to speak and make their impact on the mind will be more wholesome and efficacious than a method of introspection that enters into inner arguments of self-justifications and self-accusations, or into an elaborate search for 'hidden motives.'"[3] To work on an illness, meditation must cut deeper than the illness and skirt being trapped in the intrinsic arguments of that illness at any level of body/mind. That is, to cure the most deep-seated physical illness would require *thinking* the cure and conducting those thoughts to the seat of the pathology. Mind is the most acute, efficient healer.

Of course, we have trouble clearing our minds sufficiently to think *cures* rather than *about* cures, and we are not comfortable enough with our sensations and breath or cognizant enough of their exquisitely minute impulses to direct them at the core of a disease. Disease might even be defined as the absence of clear mind and natural breath.

The pain of a disease is a form of awakening mindfulness and setting in motion a cure; if at all possible, it should not be anesthetized. It is the most direct connection (i.e., path) to not only the ailing organ but the principle of reintegration. It leads through organized sensation to a compromised source.

Meditation also allows one to penetrate neurosis—first, by perceiving it as a thought-form; second, by detaching oneself from subservience to its patterning; third, by getting beneath the character structure of one's invention of personal reality; and finally, by discovering the emptiness beneath the roots of all thought-forms and dissolving them into lucidity.

A few terrestrials who fully grasp this situation devote long periods to living in caves meditating. Through the piety of their intentional suffering, they intend to cure, in one super-intense dose of practice, conditions which otherwise would deepen and spread over a lifetime and become quite difficult to root out piecemeal among the distractions of the world. The Burmese teacher Goenka offers more accessible, ten-day versions of such retreats throughout the world in the simple Vipassana tradition of Sayagi U Ba Khin. At sites, for instance in Washington state and California, ordinary people from all walks of life gather to sit and meditate. There is no financial charge, and nothing else happens but instruction, meals, walking, and sleep. Even reading and writing are not allowed. (See Resource Guide.)

Most diseases for most people fall beyond the realm where the meditation of which they are capable can unravel them. Yet the commitment to meditation, even in the first halting try to listen to a thought, is a step along a pilgrimage whose fruition is the realm where mind and disease converge.

In *Chi Gung* the activated and internalized mind operates via the subtle medium of the *chi* itself. This is different from even the most contemplative version of cognitive mind. If the *chi* is not immediately perceptible—as it is not for most people—then the mind tracks what *is* perceptible until that reveals what it is, then the next most barely perceptible thing, and so on through the layers. Remember Mikao Usui and his discovery of Reiki.

P RAYER IS A different sort of medicine from meditation. Whereas meditation arises from breathing and emptying the mind, prayer emanates from faith and ritual. When Jesus says, "Your faith has healed you," he means not an obedient act of acknowledgment but a spontaneous meditation that changes one's nature, cells, and in a sense, the universe too. For prayer to heal, one must have faith in God or the gods inside oneself or in the forces of the cosmos to which they correspond. Submission (bowing) is an instantaneous act, but developing the capacity to submit in an emptying manner takes most of a lifetime.

Prayer and meditation combine in mantras and chants. Chanting can expand its range in a community context, as during Navaho sandpainting rituals and Christian and Muslim faith healings. A group of people collaborate on a common field in which individuals can be touched and changed. The field may include supernatural beings and mythological events; it accesses the cultural identity of the tribe, where many illnesses originate. The following invocation, part of the Navaho Beautyway Ceremony, retains its primal power even in translation:

Prayer to Big Snake Man at Dropped-out Mountain

Young man this day I gave you my tobacco, at Dropped-out
    Mountain, Young Man Big Snake Man, Head Man!
Today I have given you my tobacco, today you must make my feet
    and legs well, my body, my mind, my sound, the evil power
    you have put it into me, you must take it out of me, away, far
    away from me!
Today you must make me well, all the things that have harmed
    me will leave me
I will walk with a cool body after they have left me.
Inside of me today will be well, all fever will have come out of me,
    and go away from me, and leave my head cool!
I will hear today, I will see today, I will be in my right mind today!
Today I will walk out, today everything evil will leave me, I will be
    as I was before, I will have a cool breeze over my body,
    I will walk with a light body.
    I will be happy forever, nothing will hinder me!
I walk in front of me beautiful, I walk behind me beautiful, under
    me beautiful, on top of me beautiful, around me beautiful, my
    words will be beautiful!

I will be everlasting one, everything is beautiful![4]

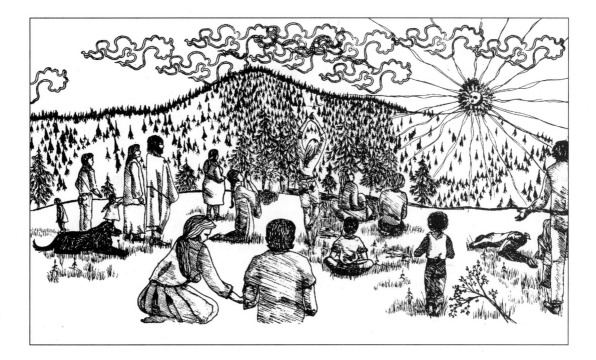

In the right context, prayer can change exactly what it proposes to change—the relation of time and space, mind and matter, and the role of destiny. The best way to escape an undesired fate is simply to petition the universe with dignity, humility, and naive and utter faith. Perfunctory and situational prayer, by contrast, are decorative and usually of less efficacy.

Self-reflection (witnessing) might be defined as the continuous act of noting and internalizing events—not narcissistically but as a token of one's objective presence in the world. True self-reflection is continuous prayer.

Witnessing life alters one's frame of knowing and being and thus rethreads the matrix within which health and disease occur. The potential to carry out this process selflessly will differ from person to person. Some will substitute clever insights for true self-reflection. Gurdjieff claimed that, despite the strong desires of individuals, it was impossible

The Spectrum of Healing

to cultivate true intention without a specific shock to break with the abstract lethargy imposed on life. Only such a jolt could separate a "third force" and release us from our dualism and trance/mirage. His dances and exercises were to prepare and cultivate this awakening. They were to jar mind from imbuing itself with habitual, collective existence and its numbing effects.

A mode of self-reflection leading to emptiness lies at the core tantra of Buddhist Dzogchen practices, a source of energy for both healing and clarity of mind:

> When we observe a thought and it disappears, immediately afterwards another thought arises, that might be: "I am seeking the origin of thought and I find nothing!" This too is a thought.... It is a thought that thinks about the origin of thought. In this way many thoughts can arise continuously. Even though we may be convinced that their essence is emptiness, nevertheless they manifest ceaselessly. The same applies to our senses: all the objects we perceive are the ceaseless appearing of our karmic vision. This, then, is the nature of clarity....
>
> All of this evinces the function of energy in the aspects of its continuity and its capacity to produce something. Through our energy there arise all the manifestations at the level of subject and object, that can be pure or impure, beautiful or ugly....[5]

These acts, practiced daily, ultimately heal mind through body and body through mind.

ACTIVITY IS THE somatic counterpart of self-reflection, or in the plexus of mind/body, it is "reflection in movement." This includes regular activities such as walking, standing, breathing, talking, tensing, relaxing, eating. Are we grounded in our true selves or do we graze symptomatically, moving anxiously, and adrenalizing our emotions?

The role of lifestyle in disease etiology broke into public consciousness through 1980s studies linking inactive and stress-based patterns to heart disease, strokes, and cancer. A growing awareness of the importance of aerobics and exercise spawned industries of new activities from jogging to gym workouts, to more hi-tech Pilates regimens, fitness parlors, and "jazzercise." These represent degrees of recreational self-reflection. Our actual pathology, however, is more than just a lack of action; it is a formulaic misuse of body/mind based on recruitments of it for cultural tasks and empty poses. When spurts of activity are encouraged without internalization, prior imbalances are merely displaced. It is preferable to move slowly and consciously through awkward spaces rather than to labor in an attempt to make up for everything at once. Hiking, *Chi Gung*, yoga, riding a bike, rock climbing, and simple stretches can have substantial long-term therapeutic effects. In fact, in emphasizing internalization of conscious micromovements, Continuum is so the opposite of Pilates that Emilie Conrad refers to the latter as "the p word."

In an exercise based on Feldenkrais principles, one is instructed to move a part of his or her body in a circle like the hand of a clock. The part may be the chin (lower jaw), eye, whole head, foot, a single toe, shoulder, pelvis, etc. Where the circle gets cut off, e.g. from the hours between 2 and 4 or between 8 and 11 (or any other arc) being skipped, then there is the possibility for learning how to scan through that missing zone and regain its sensation awareness and mobility. This is not accomplished through force, prior agility, or speed. Ballet dancers and gymnasts who can twist in remarkable ways may totally lack the skill. In fact, they are often quite paralyzed by the "clock." The only way to fill in arcs is to execute a gradually smoother circle and "experientialize" the components that are missing. Likely they were known once and lost through fear, rigidity, and postures based on lack of self-esteem and reinforced repetitively through the years.

Every abandoned section represents a loss of something for the whole being. All of life experience, in one way or another, is an opportunity to restore degrees of arc. Our tissues ultimately seek such wholes rather than isolated "hits" of feeling or bursts of movement. We exist only synergistically, as wholes. In rounding out the circle, one restores an aborted series of autonomic movements in oneself. Jaw and foot circles may be minute and peripheral to core viscera, but they transfuse their circularity throughout the body. Toe and eye circles are incredibly powerful, for they require the mind to find and inhabit remote and finely discrete sections of arc and all the cellular oscillations and tissue fields leading to them.

D*ō-in* is an Oriental form of self-massage and daily exercise. A practitioner familiarizes himself daily with his body by interacting with its integuments, bones, and organs, draining waste, removing calluses and surface deposits, breathing, chanting, intoning. The entire physiology is included: the spirals of the ears, every joint of every finger and toe and the space between them, every orifice and wart. The connections of all the organs and meridians are massaged at the ears, at the eyes, on the feet, sometimes the tongue, and at numerous other points. These can be used for diagnosis, stimulated, or sedated.[6]

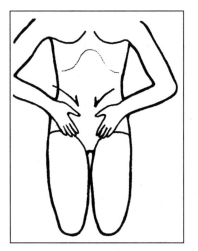

Some of the separate exercises resemble mantras; others are primal calisthenics and adjustments. In one set of movements, eyes look into the infinite distance while the person kneels with hands clasped at the level of the heart. Sounds are sensed in the spiral of the ears' vestibules, but no particular sound is listened to. The hands are clapped clearly and sharply. Then the body is twisted around. The teeth are beaten together.

In a related sequence, the tongue is used to collect and taste saliva from the upper region of the palate. In another, each finger is rotated tautly at the point where it connects to the hand. The fists are drummed on the back with the spine held straight: this is meant to relieve not only sciatic nerve pains but throat congestion and hemorrhoids.[7]

The point of each exercise is not to strengthen any particular muscle or capacity but to redistribute attention and vital energy. *Dō-in* is

physical movement directed toward visceral resonance—to clear the mind and to move fear, anger, and negative tendencies while stuck deposits are loosened, blocks eased, and wastes drained from the body.

Health Plans

Healing by the Senses

A CERTAIN PORTION OF any cure is mediated by complex nonalgorithmic feedback between the individual sensoria and the organism. Primal information is assimilated from this process, no matter the external modality or originating mechanism. An untold number of people develop illnesses, even potentially fatal ones, then heal them endogenously through their immune system or tissue reprogramming without ever knowing they had such a disease. The choices people make in their daily activities, seemingly based on other issues, often turn out to be, synchronistically, the correct medical decisions.

The senses play direct roles. They are pathways into and out of the viscera, active channels that contact all parts of us through our substance and the aspect of us that is sentient. In healing through the senses, we are altering not only consciousness and memory but the elemental forces and polar field of the body.

Autogenically, the daily senses are catalysts of *any* healing process. Active at all times, digesting, absorbing, discriminating, eliminating, exchanging functions and information, they may also be cultivated through meditation, sensory modes of Ayurveda, palpation, or innumerable other practices.

Images go directly into the brain. Chanting transmits pure vibrations. Taste and smell are catalysts in diet, flower essences, and herbs. Ayurveda distinguishes bitter, sour, sweet, pungent, astringent, and salty as healing modalities all by themselves. Touch is a component in virtually every cure. It marks the seam of tangency between any herb or palpation and the body—on visceral, cellular, molecular, and atomic levels. Touch also generates an array of primary and secondary effects, including sensations of kinesthesia, body balance, and magnetic fields.

The primordial substances that make us up proliferate in the envi-

The Spectrum
of Healing

435

ronment. Air is a metabolic agent. Rain is a tea even when absorbed from the atmosphere without drinking, so are redwood groves and plants and mineral waters. Heat and cold pass through pores into the body, too. Everything in the environment is potentially drawn and assimilated into our organisms—sounds, images, tastes, impressions. Every motif—colored thimbles at a market, a stray image of a building on a side street, a smell of a factory—is reexperienced silently for its richness and context, its psychosomatic background and passage into body/mind. Even washing dishes is a therapeutic exercise. How we take substances, coarse and fine, into mind, stomach, and lungs (and how we keep them out) determines to a large degree who we are.

Some of the flavors and elixirs sought traditionally by aromatherapists and herbalists reside innately in scent-bearing nimbi and invisible dust percolating within simple landscapes. Even without a formal aromatherapy we pass along streets and trails (in sun and in rain) and are transformed in mood by elusive fumes and fragrances—why not in metabolism and health too? Gardens, glens, ponds, shifts in wind, nearness to a beach, even stale office buildings carry both pathogens and medicines. This subtle, ever-shifting play of scent won't necessarily cure an existing disease, but it continuously juggles the matrix from which either vitality or lethargy develops.

Conversely, a particular external substance or mechanism may be intentionally *directed* into the organism through the senses. Either modality can be effective, but autogenic sensory healing and mechanical sensory treatments fall at opposite poles of the curative spectrum. Healing by the use of music and electronically generated sound or in a biofeedback machine is at least as passive and externalizing as deep-tissue bodywork, whereas natural sounds, scents, and dreams are often extensions of self-reflection and awareness.

MEMORY IS ANOTHER collective sense: even someone with Alzheimer's "remembers" that he or she exists. Through our recall we are suffused with layers of sensations and cognitive fields that incite new impulses and cells as they occur. Psychoanalysis, from that perspective, is a medicine of memory, for it changes people by changing their histories, by translating their stories into other stories.

The senses also provide nodes of focus and startle (or recoil) in healing. Noncognitive surprise within the organism initiates psychosomatic processes. A faith healer dislodges a mind/body set of lameness (or deafness); a healing shaman presents the shockingly visible form of the disease; an emetic "vomits," leading to spontaneous cleansing; a visceral therapist suddenly removes the weight of his hand from the thoracic cavity. *Curandero* Eduardo Calderón shoots a spray of holy water from his mouth into moonlight. The psychotherapist remanifests the moment of trauma. These are bolts of energy, allopathic and homeopathic shocks. Surgery and drugs offer such "shocks" too, but (as in ironically named shock treatment) they usually deaden the senses, away from information; they *remove* a symptom without kinesthetic and elemental activation. In a material age, which is correspondingly an age of anesthesia and painkillers, the doctor who does not arouse the senses (cause pain) is a hero!

A healing process begun by a jolt or an evocative image or an essence must be integrated over time. The more intensely the initial surprise is able to penetrate overall systemic stasis and get into the viscera, usually the deeper its impact and the more primal the healing processes it activates.

Dream Healing

DREAMS ARE A complex form of spontaneous healing incorporating the senses and the memory. Physiologists now propound an ancient parable: nightly dreaming heals organs. It little matters whether images of sleep inspire auto-medicines or catalysts themselves ride on dreams; images and chemistry are linked in a psychosomatic equilibrium. In our discussion of Freud in Volume One, we explored the curative basis of dream in terms of sublimation, transformation of negatively cathected elements, and the biodynamics of wish fulfillment. Here we will examine dreams as phenomenological events that spontaneously energize cures.

Curative dreamwork can be cultivated and refined, whether through focusing on the dream's iconography and itinerary after waking or by actually trying to wake within the dream (as shamans and lucid dreamers do from the metaphor that life is another dream in which we must train subtle awareness). In either case, the dream images are considered a symbolic and archetypal transfiguration of sleep itself. They provide a narrative stage for the inner physician. Whether the "physician" could also heal subliminally without a wake of images we will never know, but dreams appear to generate a deep rejuvenation and transition of viscera and fluids. It is latency becoming blatancy, projection becoming energetic landscape.

A series of transfigurations rules our inner lives or we wouldn't exist; our cells and tissues wouldn't cohere. One thing becomes another, as we ceaselessly project symbol through symbol, form through form, body through layers of mindedness, mind through holograms of organic structure. Different medicines and therapies apparently express their variant harmonies within a deeper resonance represented at a level of visualization and trance by dreaming. An herb may be a magician, a magician turns into a chiropractor, the chiropractor moves a rock that represents the sick organ, but the rock later is the sign of a homeopathic remedy—and all this is still a shadow play for deeper waveforms of mind, matter, and energy concretized in waking life by visits to actual practitioners.

Dream beings do not issue or respond to direct commands like: "Pay attention to this problem!" or "Heal this!" Core resistance is stronger than any mere cognitive suggestion of change. The dilemma of the hypnotherapist is that superficial and false responses, either of compliance or resistance, or both, replace authentic links. Insofar as the Freudian laws of the unconscious have mapped a gravitational field, more intricately whorled than Jupiter's or that of any "simple" physical object (see Volume One, pp. 398–409), ideas and intentions must be mediated always through a distortion or reversal that mirrors the precise strain lines of projection and distortion in the dream. Psychosomatic transformations thus arise from latent metamorphoses of cellular and semantic components streaming through another level in a dream, or across a series of ever more discrete and unconscious levels such that their content may take decades to rise to the level of dream formation (if they should even earn enough currency to get out of the Underworld). Some healing events may in fact get stuck in their own syntaxes in such a way that they reinforce a pathology or transduce only its surface features.

Can dream imagery (outside futuristic idealization) actually catalyze chromosome repair networks into new RNA code sequences or cause an imageless electron-like jump of *"chi"* at the nucleus? Is that in fact dream's evolutionary function? Or do the often ornate and Gothic kaleidoscopes of sleep provide a mere leaching bed, an overflow valve for psychosomatic debris? Is the process beyond negotiation?

A MAN IS WORKING with a dream trainer in waking life (perhaps a Jungian therapist), but for many months this teacher's advice has no impact on the supplicant's dreams. Then suddenly the teacher appears *in* a dream as a guide to an event which neither teacher nor dreamer understands. He is conducting a seminar on swimming in a strangely viscous medium from which people propel themselves into the air; the lesson takes place in an ordinary swimming pool at an old gym. Students from all over the country have travelled to this archetypal pool.

The dreamer is suddenly standing by the ocean trying to track something very complex arranging itself in the waves. The guide-therapist appears here too and makes a banal comment; the dreamer dismisses him. The guide stands looking forlornly at the sea. His presence now directs the dreamer's attention to an even greater complexity unnoticed in the waves. The teacher is gone, but something is beginning to manifest.

The guide is replaced in successive dreams by a master of martial arts, a naive social worker, and an authoritarian baseball manager. He has no identity except as a cumulative disjunction of male and female characters.

Change can only occur by being experienced, and can be experienced only incrementally through a rebus—can be embodied, in a sense, only as some other thing. A cure is a series of metamorphoses, not a hard symbol.

A woman in a dream may not be a person at all, she may be the medicine. She is so alluring at that moment, the dreamer's carnal desire for her is so strong, she transcends her personification and casts a sensual landscape. She may be rendered again among the stings of an acupuncture treatment—the unintegrated female element of the dreamer, intuited also as he thumps lightly on his ear, setting a slight vibration into his jawbone.

The dream guide teaches that all elements of a dream express aspects of the dreamer—the forgotten children in him or her, the tricksters and imbeciles, the disenfranchised physicians, the shadow-beasts, the undines and blue skies of other worlds, as well as the genetic, Yin-Yang fields of her incarnation and the remote cisterns of her uncompleted self. Attention to each vibrating unit of this material compels the dream to deepen, for although dreaming (to occur at all) must allow some of the terrifying unconscious to become conscious (and thus potentially curative), it can never allow unconsciousness itself to become conscious.

A REPULSIVE CAD—bald, misshapen, covered with oil—is scattering children from his house with a shotgun. Before the dream is over, the dreamer must not only embrace him but hold him tight. In another dream (during a bout of diarrhea and a rash for which the dreamer, while awake, has been seeking only herbal aid), a possible holistic doctor has been supplanted by a huckster at a fair handing out slick antibiotic tablets in plastic wrappings astonishingly with the dreamer's name on them. The dreamer asks his therapist-guide for advice within the dream; the teacher recommends ingesting the tablets because one can remedy any side effects later with vitamins. So he swallows these dream objects. Instantly they make him nauseous. He stays ill in the dream, but a dramatic improvement occurs in subsequent waking life. The rash and diarrhea clear up in a day.

In dream iconography these tablets are herbal remedies, homeopathic potencies, expressly by *not* being them; by sublimation they are the thing one would not consider in waking, which makes them the actual medicine inside dreaming. This statement of subliminal contrareity is necessary to break through the lethargy of the system. An act of transsubstantiation is carried out on an unconscious level with depreciated substances of the very allopathic pharmacy one is trying to avoid (conceived of as symbolic poisons), i.e., depreciated aspects of oneself.

Dreams often heal by representing a medicine as exactly what it is not so they then can transform pathology by its distortion into an elixir. In an event dreamed during a flu I was "successfully" prescribed the contents of a can of Red Flag ant poison. The poison when dreamed (when potentized oneiro-homeopathically) radicalized its image, through my repulsion for it, into something uncontacted, medicinal, counter-pharmacological.

Dream "vitamins," as a rule, do not appear even as actual pills; they more likely, for instance, manifest a flood of fertile water over a previously parched and sterile yard. The dirt responds with exotic flowers of all shapes, sizes, and colors. The yard has also moved closer to the sea so that luminescent fish are now mating in it. Trees drop purple and pink maché blossoms into the water. Whether these are symbolic "Bach flower" waters or the dreamer's own auto-medicine, or both, they carry out an actual healing through the dreaming process.

A few nights later the dreamer finds himself in an egg, which he recognizes as an egg only because huge fields of yolk-like matter are separating around him. He has the sense of his entire self shifting in relation to unconscious elements.

In a subsequent dream he uses a technique taught months ago at a seedy pool in a dream YMCA to swim toward the stars. The constellations become Easter eggs in a meadow.

Now the entire cosmic field is shifting; a curative relationship is developing between the rudiments of individuation and the unconscious realms of the self behind the dreamer. This may be as close as he will ever come to experiencing his own embryogenic meridians.

DREAMS PROPOSE A method or a model for a method by which multiple healing systems work together. As one progresses through layers of confusion, non-clarity and disease, one's body/mind accepts different levels of work at different times, different types of therapists and different therapies. Surgery, flower potency, breath, and dream meet and converge beyond modality.

Metaphysical and Karmic Healing

PARAPHYSICAL "SENSES" SUCH as telepathy, voodoo, intuition of distant events, and telekinesis also have medicinal aspects, as we have seen throughout both volumes of this book. After all, we are not completely egoic organisms; we are entities immersed in realms of transpersonal phenomena consciously experiencing only their outer layer.

Much as birds inherit capacities of navigation and spiders the ability to find food immediately after birth, we incarnate a collective unconscious of presymbolic matrices. The Jungian-oriented doctor attempts to put a sick person in touch with such archetypal imagery, which becomes medicine even as seeds from compounds fashioned by alchemists ignite medicinally, first in the act of mixing raw substances and observing (visualizing internally) their fiery and frothy interaction and second by the production of real elemental pharmaceuticals.

Scientologists may or may not believe in an accessible cosmic memory going back billions of years to events in other galaxies, but they attempt to use the pretense of such a memory curatively. Buddhists and Hindu physicians routinely address past lives as a level of karmic disease potentiation. Diseases then literally become guides between incarnations. Generated by events in one lifetime, they can then be healed (their karma absolved) in another. Serious malignancies transcend incarnations; they are epochal opportunities. The Buddhist writer Rick Fields translated his terminal cancer into an opportunity to "heal" others, notably children sharing his plight. He became an exemplar, celebrant, and warrior of the disease process in himself, even writing a small book entitled *Fuck You, Cancer.* Outliving his prognosis by more than two years, he died as a different being, apparently carrying different karma.

It little matters where an ailment seems to be located or *is* located—in ethnic memory, childhood trauma, or past lives. Everything relevant to it arises autonomously from the disease itself or the attempts to heal it. John Upledger tells this story:

In January, 1980, Jean-Pierre Barral was visiting us in Michigan. He examined me "off the body" as he does. He told me that there was an abnormal heat pattern over my upper left abdominal quadrant and over the left inferior costal region. He uses heat or energy patterns to determine how old the person was when the injury or illness occurred. He only needs to know the subject's age. Jean-Pierre moved his hands about for a few minutes. His face developed an expression of disbelief. His voice developed a tone of marked astonishment. He finally said, "John, this is an injury from 140 years ago." This would be the year 1840.

As he spoke I remembered an experience from prior to our move to Michigan in 1975. A friend and I were playing around with hypnoregression. As the subject I had seen myself as a black slave in Charleston, South Carolina. I decided to run away. I ran for a day and hid the first night in an unknown farmer's barn. He found me asleep in the barn the next morning. I came awake suddenly with him standing over me about to plunge a pitchfork into my body. I died of fright before he stabbed me in the upper abdomen and lower left thorax. As I died I flew up above and watched the anger of this farmer plunging the pitchfork into my vacated body. I laughed at him derisively.

In retrospect, I reconsider my behavior at the time of this death. My attitude of derision was deplorable. I see again this angry farmer so controlled and driven by his emotions, prejudices and hatred acting so inhumanely against another human being. I recalled this incident as Jean-Pierre worked with me non-verbally. Suddenly I felt total compassion for this farmer. I hope that some time I can see him and help him as I may be able. He needs to shed himself of this negative emotion. Perhaps we have met again since 1840.

Since Jean-Pierre's evaluation and my resolution of this "experience" I have had no further recurrence of my shingles....

Could it be that we carry trauma from one life to another?[8]

In indigenous tribal healing systems, a pantheon of ancestors and mythological beings is cultivated and summoned through an interchange with channeled forms and replicas of these beings in rituals and vision quests. Healing then becomes a mediation between conscious forces of individuation and unconscious hyperdimensional fields—personal, collective, and cosmic.

"The shaman, himself, is important, primordial," says Calderón, "and without substitution in the field of curing. He uses the San Pedro which affects special points of a person, and gives him a 'sixth sense' in accord with the topic with which he is dealing. Taking San Pedro makes him leap into a special dimension."[9]

A parallel process occurs in Hopi healing ceremonies, African myth-enactments, *ayahuasca* trance conferences with spirit beings, and Australian Aborigine Emu dances—concretely through bright feathers, luminous hallucinogenic landscapes, pigmentation on flesh, chanting to open interior fields of sound, acrid incense, medicinal icons, rhythmic dancing, and secondarily through the collective invocation of mythological "memory."

"The *mesa,*" explains Eduardo, "is nothing more than a control panel by which one is able to calibrate the infinity of accesses into each person."[10] He speaks of the bioelectromagnetic power *(poder bioelectromagnético)* which gives potentiality to his staffs of power in the healing *mesa (potencialidad a la vara)*. The staffs then vibrate precisely according to the account, the reason for the sickness *(la cuenta, a la razón de la enfermedad)*.[11] At an elemental level, the bioelectromagnetic field, the assimilation of massage and herbs, and shamanic mantra resonate together.

Individual Sensory Modalities

Healing by Sound

Sound is fundamental to matter and to life. Some healers believe it is the primary ontological sense, the auditory cerebral placode emerging first among sensory orifices during gestation. Providing a channel for the configurations of cosmic vibration, sound delivers the literal "earmark" of reality; it is the sense by which people ground themselves in this carnal realm. A variety of practitioners over the years have experimented with direct sound as a pathway of medicine—chanting mantras, intoning vibrations, generating vibratory waves in electronic oscillators, or composing music to have a curative effect, for instance, broadcasting melodies to particular *chakras*. Water molecules seem to respond directly to sounds, disorganizing chaotically during heavy-metal and rap performances and forming beautifully symmetrical crystals when played Bach or courted with love ballads.[12]

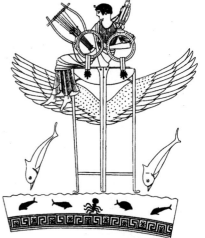

The most refined technique from among these is the one developed by French ear, nose, and throat specialist Alfred Tomatis, who began his career by training singers to increase their vocal range. Later he experimented with projecting electronically filtered music into his clients' inner ears. Different patterns and angles turned out to have therapeutic impact on a broad range of diseases not ordinarily associated with hearing, especially psychopathologies.

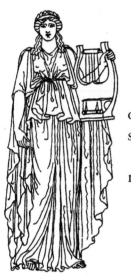

Tomatis took Mozart, Gregorian chant, and, where possible, the voice of the client's mother and electronically filtered out all the low-frequency sounds (below 8,000 hertz). Through special headphones, the client attentively listens to many hours of this filtered music—sixty hours is typical—over three to four months. The idea is to return the client to the sonic atmosphere in the womb, then retrain his or her entire listening function from its formative stages. Gradually, two tiny but important ear muscles are reconditioned to respond to a broader frequency spectrum.[13]

The rationale is that increasing the range of sensation makes the organism healthier and provides more channels for emotional expression.

Sound is also used therapeutically by those caring for the terminally ill:

> In the Chalice of Repose, music is delivered solely through voice and harp, usually nonrhythmic selections (free of pulse or count) with regular alternations between silence and music. The music helps alleviate pain, dissolve fear, liberate the spirit from the body, and enable people to let go.[14]

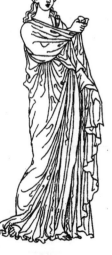

Therese Schroeder-Sheker, a composer who trains people in this method in Missoula, Montana, places the origin of musical healing in the eleventh-century Cluniac monasteries of France. She describes her initial experience, singing Gregorian chant, at the urging of a priest, into the left ear of an irritable, dying man in his eighties:

> He rested in my arms and began to breathe much more regularly, and we, as a team, breathed together. It was as if the way in which sound anointed him now made up for the ways in which he had never been touched or returned touch while living the life of a man. These chants are the power of love. They carry the flaming power of hundreds of years and thousands of chanters who have sung these prayers before.[15]

Music serves as a window, an "'audible glimpse' into the immediate future . . . in the sacred role of mediation between dimensions."[16] In many traditions, we are said to incarnate by increments of tone—sacred chants and drumming by our ancestors delivering the *wakan* into flesh. Panpipes convey a haunting sense of the "beyond," which perhaps becomes biologically resonant at a meta-cellular level, as their notes radiate through molecules. Choirs of voices heal the spirit by summoning remote dimensions into being. Because sound is not conscribed by the linear parameters of sight, alien realms manifest everywhere at once.

Inasmuch as it conducts itself directly to a spirit body, sound is most powerful at the moment of death. During much of life, it may graze over us, tuned and fiddled for worldly pleasures; at the end of life, it regains its esoteric role and rings with the passage between worlds:

> In the darkness something was happening at last. A voice had begun to sing. . . .
>
> Then two wonders happened at the same moment. One was that the voice was suddenly joined by other voices; more voices than you could possibly count. They were in harmony with it, but far higher up the scale: cold, tingling, silvery voices. The second wonder was that the blackness overhead, all at once, was blazing with stars. They didn't come out gently one by one, as they do on a summer evening. One moment there had been nothing but darkness; next moment a thousand, thousand points of light leaped out—single stars, constellations, and planets, brighter and bigger than any in our world.[17]

Healing by Smell

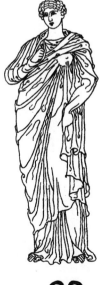

PERHAPS ONE REASON the essences of oil are curative is that scents such as lavender, orange, and rose treat replicas of tissue that once experienced the anonymous reptile healer directly, molecularly. More than sights or touch, and even more than vibrations of sound, smells enter the body as substance. They are the essential component of herbs directly processed through our lungs, heart, and bloodstream. Aroma-essences are hormonal and enzymatic triggers; hence, they may

447

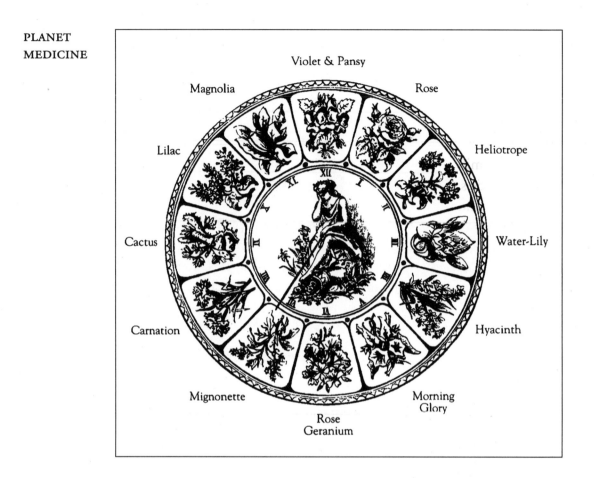

Violet & Pansy

Magnolia

Rose

Lilac

Heliotrope

Cactus

Water-Lily

Carnation

Hyacinth

Mignonette

Morning
Glory

Rose
Geranium

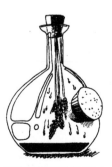

catalyze morphogenetic activity. (See also the discussion of blue oils in Volume One, p. 532.)

The primordial language of smell cannot be abstracted in primate philosophy because it emerges prior to our ocular and three-dimensional reconstruction of the environment. Yet magicians have always known that transformation is available in a poof!

A WIDE RANGE of techniques has been developed to catalyze or cure people through their sense of smell. Leading into proto-reptilian lobes of the brain, the nose activates primitive hormonal chains and instinctual actions of which we are but dimly aware. We can intuit their power by the effects that scents have on our whole being. Aromas are profoundly aphrodisiac and also alert animals with a primal nip of danger. The olfactory canal is the first testing zone of food.

The incense of a fir forest after a rain or a magnolia tree at night in spring is more than just luxuriant or nostalgic. In some inexplicable way their molecules go to the roots of our soul.

Though millions of diffuse scents roam wild in the world at large, the therapeutic specificity of essential oils comes from the concentration of their substance (for instance, 80 pounds of roses to produce one and a half drachms of Rose oil). These essences are triturated and evaporated from leaves such as Lemon Verbena, Fir needle, and Eucalyptus; flowers such as Lavender, Orange blossom, Vanilla, and Ylang Ylang; and fruits, bulbs, rhizomes, roots, and barks such as Almond, Fennel, Onion, Ginger, Cinnamon, and Cedar. They are extracted by distillation and condensation using steam and water or just steam. This craft is at least as old as the solar-powered stills of the Egyptians. Aroma healing is one of the few medicines we know the ancients practiced.

It is no wonder that scents bear medicinal vitality. They are vaporized medicines. On this basis, medical aromatherapy has full institutional standing in France, the nation of its professionalization. Jeanne Rose explains:

> Aromatherapy is a way of treating mental and physical illnesses through inhalation and through the external application of essential oils with pressure-point therapy or simple massage. . . .
>
> The direct inhalation of the odors generally affects the mind psychologically, although inhalation can also have . . . physiological effect via the limbic system in the brain and the blood circulation. For example, rubbing oil of Jasmine on the temples, pressing firmly . . . in a circular motion will definitely ease away a headache. The Jasmine enters into the body both through the skin as well as the nasal mucosa.[18]

Although there is no one-to-one linear chart of aromas to the ailments they cure, among some of the more commonly used treatments

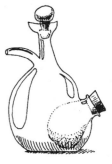

are Turpentine oil for worms and infections of the urinary tract; Tea Tree oil for acne and athlete's foot; Rosemary oil for rheumatism and to speed the healing of wounds; Lavender oil as a sedative, for convulsions, and for burns; Garlic oil for sinusitis, to remove warts, and to strengthen the immune system; Bulgarian Rose oil for herpes; Melissa oil for heart palpitations; Lemon oil for infections of the eyelids and loss of voice; and Peppermint and Eucalyptus oils for bronchitis.[19]

WHEN AROMATHERAPIST John Steele was asked to address a conference of multinational perfumers in early 1990, he knew it was a radical departure of corporate policy for them to even invite him. He shared the podium with marketing experts and executives from Fabergé, Calvin Klein, and Revlon. Whereas the speeches they delivered concerned only the promotion of scents as business, he put forth a theory of layers of consciousness activated by smell. "Most of them hadn't the slightest idea of what I was talking about," he told me, "but

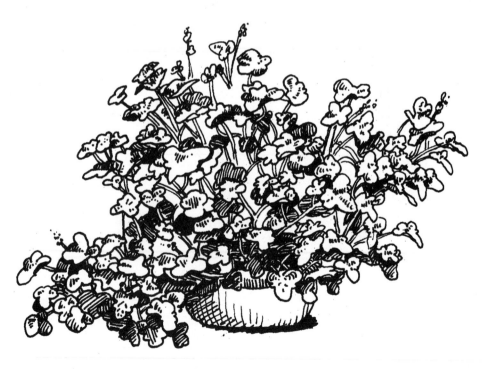

a few were really excited—like this was something they had always suspected but had no idea how to talk about."[20]

"What did they think aromas were if not consciousness?" I asked him.

"The usual things—sexual attractiveness, power, commerciality, the
manufacture of desire. They are totally cynical in that sense. They presume that it's all a seduction and that the goal is to market scents in
such clever disguises that people will be attracted to them but also basically fooled because they are really—well, nothing—you know, wisps
of flavored air, immaterial gas." He pressed his fingertips together and
sprang them apart. "It was as though perfumes couldn't be real, so they
continually repackage them to keep everyone fooled."

"Do they think desire is only artificial and manipulable?"

"I, like you, forget that anyone still thinks that way," he laughed,
"but of course, they do. Notions like 'the earth is alive' or 'the reptilian brain responds to scents' would strike them as the most outrageous
sort of California nonsense."

Healing by Color

If octaves of sound penetrate the body, even subtler vibrations enter it
as light, microdoses which have profound and often unknowable effects
on tissues and energy fields. At least one modern rationale for the healing effects of colors is based on a discovery that 80 percent of the nerves
and receptors of the body are connected directly or indirectly to the
optic nerves. The presumption is that through direct or habitual use,
certain colors then work their way into the viscera and peripheral nerves
and energetically palpate them.

"Gradually, contemporary science has quantified the old folk wisdom that expresses the intimate connection between color, human
health, and subtle anatomy in clichés like seeing red, feeling blue, in
the pink, green with jealousy, black with rage."[21] The implication is
that emotional fluctuations lead to changes in the colors of our own
electromagnetic fields. Likewise, illnesses garb themselves in invisible
colors and are dispersed by complementary waves.

Color is also widely utilized as a therapeutic modality. Post-scientific color medicine began to evolve in the United States during the 1870s. General August Pleasanton, author of *Blue and Sun-Lights,* "reported that blue light, either from the sun or from artificial sources, effectively stimulated the glands, nervous system, and secretory organs of animals and people. In 1877 a prominent physician named Seth Pancoast discovered that sunlight filtered through panes of blue or red glass relaxed or accelerated the human nervous system. In the next year Dr. Edwin Babbitt, in *Principles of Light and Color,* described his 'chromo disk,' a device that projected light through filtered discs onto the body, and his 'chromo lens,' a method of passing solar-potentized water through color filters to produce 'solar color tinctures.'"[22]

In the early years of the twentieth century, various filters and screens (forerunners of Kirlian science) were set up around objects and creatures to make their auras visible photographically. Rainbow patterns shone from within animate fields, reflecting an outer pale blue haze with warmer hues at the interior. In the 1920s M.D. Dinshah Ghadiali, author of *The Spectro-Chromometry Encyclopedia,* applied color similarly, by shining light through differently tinted glass, either directly on his patients or on water that was then drunk by them.

Ghadiali correlated the primary color emission from each element with its known physiological function in the human body, contending that chemical elements were linked with specific color waves and that colors represented chemical potencies of subtler vibrations.... In Ghadiali's model color's radiant energy restored balance at the body's energetic, not physiological, level. In the tonation process, Ghadiali used a set of twelve precisely adjusted color filters enclosed in a projector that shone light directly onto body regions mapped according to chemical element, physiology, and color band.

Harry Riley Spitler, an M.D. and optometrist, hypothesized that colored light projected through the eyes was the key to balance. Spitler, who introduced his new ocular light therapy, called syntonics, in 1927, discovered that alterations in light received through the eyes was the "master key" to the brain's major control centers and, through these centers, to body function, behavior, and physiology. Spitler's syntonics system used thirty-one different color filter combinations, adjusted to each individual's nature, to balance and integrate the nervous system. The College of Syntonic Optometry, which he founded in 1933, is still operating.[23]

MODERN COLOR THERAPY claims a longstanding esoteric lineage, from the Healing Temples of Light and Color at Heliopolis in Egypt, to Buddhist and Hindu curative mandalas, to the mystical color interpretations of Rudolf Steiner and C. W. Leadbetter that take into account scientific discoveries about the nature of photons and radiation and the mechanical principles of the spectrum.[24]

In Tibetan *tangka* paintings, colors are a vehicle of passage between bardos. Meditating on particular brilliances lights the path through cosmic and psychic realms which manifest those hues. Thus, color has not only therapeutic but cosmological implications.

Throughout history and in all parts of the world people have imbued themselves with or meditated on hues. Such rituals are based on a belief in the curative power of colors on specific conditions. Therapeutic colors can be administered in a variety of ways. The spectrum ranges from the greens, reds, and yellows of foods to the colors of sheets and blankets slept in and of clothes worn (for instance, beets, radishes, and red night-shirts to improve blood circulation and relieve paralysis; bananas, curry, and millet, and a yellow hat to increase digestive capacity, relieve constipation, stimulate lymph, reduce the effects of diabetes, and disinfect the throat and eyes).[25] Such a signalling process could be ascribed to the same resonance fields and morphogenetic triggers as in other healing systems.

In formal healing, the yellow-red (solar) end of the scale tends to be stimulating—sympathetic to the rapid circulation of fluids in the body— while the green-blue-indigo (interstellar) edge of the scale radiates neurological and spiritual relaxation. Among traditional applications of

color are: orange hue to stimulate the pulse and to increase the manufacture of milk in the new mother, also to dissolve kidney- and gallstones and heal hernias and appendicitis, and as a burst of
anti-depressant glow; emerald green to soothe nervous disorders, hay
fever, ulcers, influenza, syphilis, malaria, and colds; blue to calm emotions, lower blood pressure (reduce bleeding), treat breathing problems, rheumatism, colic, skin disorders, and burns, and in general to
relax the whole body in its luminous sea of light; indigo for conditions
involving the pituitary gland, also to heal cataracts, migraines, skin
aberrations, and deafness, and in general to sense and sedate the nervous system, particularly the eyes and ears; violet for conditions involving the pineal gland and to increase psychic power, also for psychological
and emotional disturbances, arthritis, and to assist in childbirth; and
magenta for pathologies of the heart and a range of otherwise-untreat-
able psychopathologies.

Colors are also used in combination, for instance, green, yellow,
and violet to treat skin cancer at an early stage.[26]

SOME CURRENT COLOR therapies emphasize the medicinal applications of pure colors on *chakras* and energy fields. Bioenergetic therapist John C. Pierrakos has measured "cloudlike auric envelopes and
their precise chromatic pulsations relative to body metabolism, breathing rates, emotional states, humidity, and air ionization. Pierrakos, like
[Walter] Kilner, postulated that the aura springs from a 'longitudinal
core of energy' in the physical body, possibly connected with the central nervous system, that radiates outward through the skin to activate
the immediate atmosphere and form the triple aura."[27]

According to William Croft, contemporary biologists "have discovered that a weak (quantum) form of coherent light is being used as
a communications medium both within cells and between cells of our
body. In this respect the light appears to be an organizing field which
facilitates communication within whole organisms. Through a technology recently developed, it becomes possible to discover and release

blockages that occur in the light/*chi* communications paths within our bodies. Such blockages can cause imbalance, or dysfunction, or simply keep us from functioning at the full and vibrant potential of our beings. The technology involves shining very pure colors of variable frequency light onto the energy centers of your body. The light produces a resonance phenomenon, not unlike striking a tuning fork next to a harp or piano. The string that resonates with the tuning fork will begin to sound its own note in harmony with the tuning fork."[28]

The Downing Technique, developed by an optometrist in Northern California, uses a machine called the Lumatron to "feed" the body the colors it needs to balance itself. The functional part of the Lumatron is housed in a hood which fits over a person's head. Once within the machine, the healee receives directly illuminated fields of color—red, orange, yellow, blue-green, blue, indigo, or violet—through a lens at different rates of flicker (the particular color or sequence of colors is selected by the therapist during a prior field test). The intensity of a single color is expected to wash gently over the eyes and be transmitted through the optic nerves to the whole body.

The rationale behind this method is that the organism has come to block out certain colors because of stress or traumatic events associated with them, so even someone working all day in full sunlight is selectively assimilating bands of the spectrum. The Lumatron provides stimulation by the lacking hues. It also affords an opportunity for the organism to reprocess events associated with color blockages. These past experiences may take the form of limited vision, blind spots, and startles. Ellen Eatough, a Colored Light therapist, told me that most people see things or experience visual and sensual effects in the Lumatron that aren't physically there. In the center of red or blue, they will perceive a different color or a series of shapes. She uses a form of light hypnotherapy to guide clients to recall and heal the life events underlying these projections.

THE GOAL OF all color therapies is not merely an external impression of a medicine but a sense of its hue arising from within and bathing us in pure light. After direct or indirect treatment, one should have autonomous experiences of that color penetrating the whole being, including sudden visions of the color, scents of it, and even after-tastes of it on the tongue and lips.

Professional color therapists proceed by first consulting with a patient on the various aspects of his or her life and then recommending colors to encourage in the future. This might include hanging paintings with those colors dominant, listening to music associated with those colors, eating foods of those colors, or even bringing the elements of the astrological sign and planet associated with a particular color into one's life.[29] Fai Lloyd describes a favorite breathing exercise of his:

> Holding the visualization of the color, see it as a radiant color breath travelling rapidly upward beneath the outer skin, rising in a spiral about the body and ending above the head in a brilliant swirl of cleansing, transmuting color. At the same time raise the arms above the head in a relaxing gesture. Then exhale, gently feeling the color breath pass out through the pores of the skin carrying all impurities with it.[30]

In this manner one not only invokes a desired red, blue, or green but purges its complement which, physically, *is* its substance (as opposed to the mere illumination with which we are familiar and which gives a color its name).

During one bodywork session with Amini Peller, she suggested that I might be able to "see" *chakras*. As I tried to gauge where I was with my eyes closed, I suddenly noticed a glow of intense orange light. This orangeness was actually present throughout me and could not be diluted by imagining other colors. Scanning up and down my body, I then saw (or felt) the orange glow blending smoothly into a spectrum from red at my genitals and sacrum, upward to intense yellow, green, and finally blue at my throat. These were each dense blankets of color suffusing me.

A few weeks later, after taking a *Chi Gung* workshop from Kumar Frantzis, I dreamed of standing in a kind of planetarium and him conducting our class there. The planets of the Solar System came by above us, and as each one (Mercury, Venus, Mars, Jupiter) passed in procession, with a wave of the hand Frantzis turned its body into a spiralling orb which unravelled toward us in yarns of vibrating color.

Healing by Taste

ALTHOUGH I WILL not explore this modality in depth here, I refer the reader to the discussion of taste in Ayurveda on pp. 315–316 and in Tibetan Medicine on pp. 328–329 (both in Volume One). Additionally it should be noted that in Ayurveda the tongue is considered a microcosm of the entire body; hence its responses to taste and various coatings, discolorations, and sensitivities represents the states of health and disease of internal organs. Ayurvedic doctors give their patients tongue scrapers to clean off the debris at bedtime and upon waking. If the tongue can represent diseases, it can hologrammatically help treat those diseases.

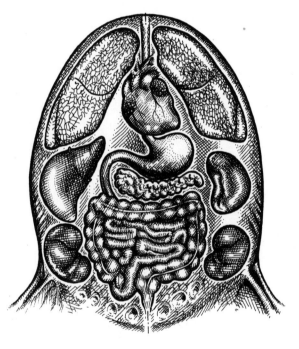

Food

IN THE FIRST (1978) edition of this book I overlooked the role of diet. By ignoring the topic I betrayed my own illusion at the time that disease and health operated on a vital level entirely separate of food and other gross consumption. Right away, a reviewer set me on the right track:

In one respect . . . *Planet Medicine* is lacking. It fails to draw the essential connection between the quality of a people's diet and the quality of their health. The issue of proper medical care cannot be spoken of apart from the quality of a person's food, for the quality of diet reflects also the attitude of a society towards the soil which nourishes it. Writers such as Wendell Berry have argued eloquently the connection between people's relationship to the soil, the food they grow upon it, and the quality of their physical and spiritual lives. To avoid the issue of agriculture and diet is to view preserving public health, ancient or modern, as remedial therapy after an inherent well-being has already been lost. A true planet medicine would place no distinctions between civic health and daily life, and the most healing of all therapies may take place in our own kitchens.[31]

Soon afterwards, Paul Pitchford gave me my first lessons on the importance of diet, and they had such a big impact in changing my consciousness that I encouraged him to write a book so that others might be similarly transformed. It led to seven years of work and the publication (in 1993) of an encyclopedic compendium called *Healing with Whole Foods;* in it Pitchford investigates eating, drinking, and general consuming as a primary aspect of the complexes that heal us or cause diseases over a lifetime. Every food, drink, and mixture in and of itself and in the context of its degree of freshness and pollution, manner of preparation, heat when served, time of day when ingested, etc., has a role in the elemental cycles regulating the energy and health of the organs and meridians.[32]

Pharmaceuticals, vital substances, and osteopathic techniques can all catalyze cures. Eventually, however, one must make an attempt to consume whole foods and unpolluted water and minerals; to stop eating meat, fatty foods and rancid oils, sugar and artificial sweeteners, and pesticided food. Few things are as basic to health as consumption and assimilation, whether one considers food on a physical plane as supplying the actual raw material of life or on an elemental level as potentiated forces necessary to balance the energy in the body. Despite the possibility of biological transmutation of elements, we can hardly count on alchemy for survival—and even transmutation would require the right ingredients.

I violate the relativity of my text to make this one suggestion: if you are sick, change your diet—of impressions as well as of food and drink. At least practice a consciousness of consumption. Challenge unexamined, undifferentiated omnivorousness.

Pitchford points out that much of the medicinal effect of diet takes place on a level where all foods and additives are herbal. In fact, most Oriental healing systems consider foods (grains, vegetables, spices, fruits, meats, etc.) as the equivalents of herbs.

They should be chosen like any other herbs and medicines, individually according to individual constitutions and metabolisms, for their direct effects on the organs. Diet must be seasonally attuned, balanced elementally, and grounded in an intuitive realization of the effects of each food.

O N A MASS CULTURAL LEVEL, Americans end up choosing Colonel Sanders and the chefs at McDonald's as their yogis and dieticians, Coors beer barons and the corporate heads of agribusiness and canned-food conglomerates to prepare the molecular mixes that go into their bodies. As a nation we reify only the mechanical, molecular aspects of food—and then only in terms of the grossest effects of their ingredients, ignoring the trace effects of pesticides and herbicides, preservatives, synthetic flavors, and nutritionless artificial substances by pretending they have no statistically measurable effect on health. Wastes from foods and medicines that are shunted off to the cells must eventually return as at least restrictions, ultimately as diseases.

Grains, fruits, and vegetables are medicines—perhaps dense, slow, dilute medicines, but medicines all the same. Even meats are medicines. They are used selectively to strengthen blood, calm the nervous system, reduce coughs and bleeding, etc. They may induce toxic effects even in small doses, but all foods have some toxic side effects, and the ideal goal should be to consume everything consciously at appropriate times in measured proportions.[33]

Eating and digesting are intricate processes, modes of psychic as well as physical integration. If we numb our systems to the nature of our food, we cut ourselves off from our own true nature, too. Our foods become heavy and deadening, producing wastes at all levels. Eating is not just a matter of gulping down or savoring unknown and unnamed substances in response to hunger—the classic American posture of well-being, even in gourmet circles. Unexamined stuffing of material in one's system is additionally a kind of phenomenological poisoning that may intensify the toxic cellular effects of the food itself. To cut off sensation and awareness of the body and its subtle flavors is to give disease its first foothold, is the beginning of not wanting to live.

It is also medicinal to recognize and acknowledge at some level the suffering of animals that become meats, not only as compassion for fellow sentient beings, but as a decision not to dull ourselves to the reality of our situation. One must assume that Buddha and Jesus were not merely spouting pieties on this issue. Buddha in fact skips over all the subtler and psychological issues of modern existential "Buddhism" and says simply, "Don't eat meat." We don't have to assume that all discussion of the matter stops there, but a reasonable interpretation of his teaching sets compassionate diet prior to philosophy in matters of enlightenment.

MOLECULES FROM FOODS have long-term health effects. Figs moisten the lungs and clean the intestines. Apricots aid in anemia. Bananas with their skin lubricate the intestines and help with constipation, ulcers, and drug addiction. Tomatoes purify the blood. Potatoes strengthen the kidneys and lower blood pressure. Carrots augment the connective tissues and rid the body of parasites. Celery renews joints and arteries and lowers blood pressure. Cabbage heals skin eruptions and warms cold feet. Beets rejuvenate the heart. Radishes clear sinuses. Turnips ameliorate asthma, more effectively when raw. Coconut tonifies the heart. Of course, not all of these foods do this all of the time in all people or at once, and they each have other attributes and side effects. In general, however, as a consistently practiced and lived philosophy, unadulterated whole foods in a balanced cuisine maintain health and discourage pathologies from forming and spreading. The point here is not to catalogue the medicinal foods but to provide a medicinal context for viewing foods and diet in general.

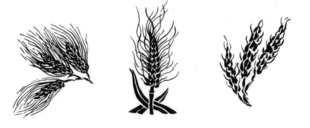

UNQUESTIONABLY SOME PEOPLE override this one, just burn right through the modern cyberworld on a steed of virtual reality, keeping the economy going at the expense of their bodies. But most people are going to get weaker from the modern civilized diet and stronger even just from the conscious attempt to treat food as a matter of practice rather than a neutral body-and-emotion fuel.

One of the most striking symptoms of our civilization is that it is almost impossible (especially in the capitalist countries of the First World and those that imitate them) to find ordinary food. Try driving down the streets of any city or town in North America and look at what the supermarkets and restaurants advertise and offer as normal—synthesized by-products cooked in rancid and chemically mutated oils with overdoses of preservatives, hormones, iodized salts, processed sugars, and artificial flavors and coloring to create the illusion of prosperity and satisfaction.

It is consumption addiction, not nutritional or medicinal eating. It is one more face of the petroleum rush that locates us in our shallow and desolate materialism—a materialism that does not even deign to examine the internalization of the images it floods us with, let alone the substances we ingest through those images.

A constant readiness to eat (to take in food as addiction)—an "I consume" mentality ranging from snacks and coffee breaks to gourmet meals—suffuses existence with dolor and inertia. We become the victims of our hungers, thus never satiate them. It is not just a matter any longer of avoiding gluttony; our collective malady is one of flooding taste cells and tissue with dense superficial "medicines" in order to relieve an existential disease of the soul.

Those in the West certainly mean to protect their consumption empire from the face of Kali, which stares into it from every Third World portal and the homeless lying in doorways (not to mention the eternal famine of unconscious mind and its representation in the night sky).

A person might consider walking *past* those bagel and donut shops and steak barbecues he frequents. Instead of stopping to partake, he simply breathes the aromas and imagines what it is he craves. Microdose replaces compulsive overdose. Suddenly his senses become alert to many different textures and layers of existence. Hunger turns out to be subtler than a desire for food. It is satisfied also by scent, by image, by movement, eventually by fasting. Yogis who famously breathe the air for *prana* and "drink" from the sun through their skin not only prophesy a planet with a healthier ecosphere, they likely taste intrinsic medicinal qualities (sour, bitter, salty, sweet) that Western civilization gets only symptomatically from its roast ribs, fries, and chocolate fudge cake.

If we feed the body predominantly meaty protein and processed meals, we substitute in advance, passively, what the cells must do for themselves in manufacturing and sustaining tissue, and so we rob them of their vitality. Drugs and alcohol are likewise disease agents because they liberate unbalanced forces at the expense of systemic equilibrium. Just because they are hidden and because the body invariably compensates does not mean that the organism is functioning well. As we get older we should move away from what spiritual teacher Da Free John calls the "celebrants" of our twenties—meat, alcohol, sugar, and coffee—to the finer elemental strands on which life is strung.[34] As one eats more consciously, substances are assimilated more fully and consuming approaches prayer. At this level, eating and digesting become internal yoga. Chewing is especially important, first to mix the food with saliva and change it chemically, and second for the experience of that food. We should gradually be able to *feel* which foods harm us and which foods nurture our growth.

Fasts (even short ones) can be surprisingly strong medicines. The effect on the body is obvious: the organs have more time to assimilate and cleanse; digestion goes deeper into the static layers of tissue, reaching older congestion. Da Free John writes: "The stress of fasting favors healthy or growing cells. Defective cells do not function well under stress; they die shortly and are eliminated. Thus the body literally 'eats' its own wastes and diseased or dying cells, and it fully eliminates whatever it cannot consume."[35] Fasting is a form of silence, the beginning of listening. From listening, the mind, tissues, and organs rediscover one another and their intrinsic unity.

When one begins to eat consciously, diet is a different thing. Some people become vegetarians or even vegans (no dairy or other animal products); some people choose organic and/or raw foods. Others avoid processed foods, potentially rancid oils, MSG, food with additives, tap water, refined sugar, industrial sodium chloride, etc. There is no one-to-one relationship between any particular diet or food combination and health. Each individual develops his or her own path through modes of consumption. The act of consciously eating must be its own provenance and guide.*

---

*In the Resource Guide at the end of this volume, I have provided some practical dietary considerations and recommendations, along with ways of implementing them.

Herbs*

PROVEN REGION BY REGION over millennia for their healing precision, herbs are the cream of empirical medicine. Although all foods are medicinal, herbs are specifically "medicinal foods." Foods (most herbs included) start with substance which becomes energy only through its relationship to cells and tissues, but there exceptions: many vitamins and enzymes provide no substance for the organs and tissues to digest. They start close to pure energy. Normal doses of most herbs still have relatively more energy and less substance than other foods.

Herbs are foods that enter the system not so much to provide molecules to digest and incorporate for metabolism but as catalysts for the natural functions of the organs. They are prescribed to reactivate lethargic processes or slow down overactive ones. Insofar as they transfer power, herbs are rarely iatrogenically pathological. Some are given according to homeopathic principles (fever-causing herbs for fever), and others are prescribed by the law of opposites (cooling herbs for fever). Either way, their action is discrete and precise. If one eats iris or black cohosh or quercitron tree bark, they are supplying their organs with raw building blocks that contributed to the genesis of these plants. Of course, the organs of the body will not make plants out of them, but they will use them in ways that would be impossible if the molecules did not originate herbally. The molecules have an intrinsic morphogenetic power.

In place of metabolizable substance, herbs contain fundamental "messages," signatures. We may even discern or taste these. A blend for calming the liver based on peony root has a unique orange-clay flavor; dandelion root is earthy too, but sweeter. The spotted colors and tangled horns of foxglove suggest heart arrhythmia. The sparkle of phosphorus evokes the fragile hypersensitivity of its remedy. Reality is sometimes so basic it is a wonder we lose it in abstractions.

---

*See also Volume One, pp. 530–533.

RECENTLY PAUL PITCHFORD directed me to a traditional pharmacy in Oakland Chinatown. I was charmed to see how raw and unadorned its products were: parts of animals hanging from the ceiling and walls—horns, antlers, fur, cuttlebones; micaceous earth; grasshoppers and cicadas; animal galls; dried earthworms and smaller worms; huge chunks of fungus, rind, and bark; roots of all sizes and topologies; whole fish; and other unidentifiable items that looked disconcertingly like the exports of cannibals. (One might wish we had access downtown to Australian Aborigine and African pharmacies, too.)

When I asked for my prescription of abalone shell the clerk couldn't find it, and I had to wait for her to fetch the proprietor. He consulted his chart to the many drawers that lined the wall behind the counter. This series of exchanges between me and them was carried out uncertainly and in painstaking English with the help of other customers. Any fear I had that the language barrier might lead to my getting the wrong "herb" was quickly dispelled when he opened a seemingly random drawer and pulled out a handful of distinctive whole iridescently glistening shells. He slid them into a sack, weighed them quickly in midair on a delicate scale, then said, "Fifty cents."

I wasn't ready for such a literal response, so I tried to explain that I needed to make a tea. He agreeably unwrapped them and dumped them in a metal mortar; then he beat and crushed them with a pestle until they were chips and powder. Every tenth stroke he hit against the side of the mortar, setting it ringing. This demonstration of the transposition of raw shells into "medicine" was quite dramatic. Any mere trope was demolished. When I poured hot water over the midden I knew what I was drinking. I even imagined the mineral shimmer asking interesting questions of my cells as they encountered it—questions they likely had not heard for many years.

FLOWERS ARE AMONG the most prominent herbal physicians: blossoms of elk clover for bronchitis, dandelion and yarrow for purifying blood, saffron to stimulate liver *chi*. Herbal berries include rose hips for soothing nerves, quisqualis and may apples for tumors; among medicinal seeds are poppy, wild carrot, pumpkin, and oat straw (the latter providing minerals for bones and connective tissue). Fenugreek, flax, and fennel combine with comfrey root and dandelion root to make an effective intestinal mixture for absorbing liquids and eliminating wastes. The leaves of horsetails are prescribed for teeth and prostate, raspberry for checking menstrual flow, and parsley to dry mucus; the leaves of mugwort are medicinally burned into the meridian points in Chinese burning-ash acupuncture (moxibustion). Apple bark is used to lower blood pressure, cherry bark as an astringent, bayberry bark for ailments of the gall bladder.[36]

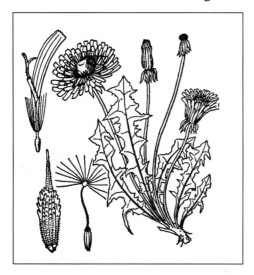

Echinacea and goldenseal cleanse the blood and remove infections. Lobelia oil reduces congestion. It is combined with drops of citrus seed extract to form a powerful "antibiotic." A combination of wormseed and wintergreen oils is used both to kill parasites and to raise congestion (as from bronchia). An "acute sinus" blend of ragweed, yerba mansa root, and cayenne pepper fruit helps clear nasal and pharyngeal passages of lingering effects of flu and industrial pollution. A related Ayurvedic potion containing brahmi leaf, calamus root, and skullcap in a base of sesame, olive, and eucalyptus oils is squeezed directly into the supine nostrils.

Garlic is a mythical cure-all, providing heat for circulation, lifting stagnation, and inhibiting viruses. A clove of garlic wrapped in cotton and soaked in olive oil may be placed gently in the ear sometimes to treat infections. The garlic gradually seeps into the nasal and oral cavities.

No plant is a more honored physician than ginseng. Apparently wild ginseng root is such a deeply rejuvenating medicine that the Asian variety was stalked to extinction, and all we have left are the semi-domesticated varieties. Stephen Fulder describes ginseng as a true stimulant, a medicine that restores energy and harmony and confers long life and *yang* without draining the system as pills and coffee do. He quotes from a Russian writer's description of finding one of the last wild roots in 1934:

> I sat with the Chinese and we were all staring, when to my great amazement I noticed that the root had a human form: here was a separation between the feet, there were hands, and there, a neck, and on it the head and even a little plait. The fibres of the hands and feet were like long fingers.
>
> I was ... overwhelmed by these seven people wrapped in contemplation of the root of life ... I could hardly bear their faith. The lives ... of millions of people seemed to me to be in relation to the enduring faith like the waves are to the sea. The waves began rushing towards me, the living, as to a beach, begging me to grasp the power of the root. Not with my flesh, because that will soon go, but with the wisdom of the stars and the constellations and maybe something beyond that.[37]

Can one doubt the living figurine of a planet shaman in this sinewy, subterranean elf?

In non-Western cultures, the herbal materia medica includes such varied ingredients as olive oil; wheat germ oil; walnut husk tincture; bamboo sap as an expectorant; honey to neutralize toxins; crystal; bear gall*; fungi of all varieties; kelp, kombu, and other sea vegetables for diseases of the nervous system; haliotis and oyster shells; pearls for headache and insomnia; animal excrement; rhinoceros horn* and toad secretions to cool and detoxify the blood; the scorpion as a nerve

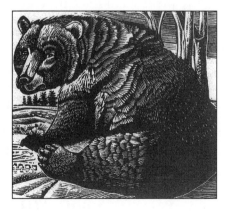

---

*Endangered species are no longer considered acceptable to hunt and kill for medicinal uses.

tonic; and the fossilized bones of dinosaurs as tranquilizers and anti-spasmodics. In China a variety of substances is used to cure fevers with different qualities: the whole earthworm, the exuviae of the cicada, the rhizome of the cnidium, and the tortoise shell.[38] The Chinese also calcine and powder human hair as an astringent and dry human placenta for impotence, infertility, and for ailments that do not improve with other treatments.

Cinnabar, sulphur, fluorite, and many other minerals can be made into medicines. Ayurvedic physicians form very pure and fine wires of metals like gold, silver, copper, and tin, and after dousing them in plant juices, convert them into a powder which is then mixed with botanicals. Supposedly metal can be ingested in this fashion without aggravation. Herbal iron enters the blood faster than in an allopath's intravenous injections and without gastric side effects.[39]

True sea salt is a great herb with "clarifying, alkalizing, purifying, and centering qualities."[40] It cools the body; counteracts toxins; aids the kidneys in moistening; helps move the bowels; reduces hardness in glands, muscles, and lymph nodes; and, in diet, balances beans, peas, grains, and other acidic foods. However, salt is reliably medicinal only in a now rare form of gray seasalt which contains the complete complement of trace minerals. French bathing salt is one of the few guises in which medicinal seasalt can presently be legally imported.[41] Otherwise, herbal salt cannot be sold in the United States for internal consumption. First to be marketed as a condiment, it must be "purified" so that it is toxic. Then it contributes to high blood pressure, kidney damage, reduced absorption, cancer of the stomach, and weakened bones, nerves, muscles, and heart. This is the salt that pervades the Western food industry in place of whole salt with minerals.

Enzymes and Minerals

ENZYMATIC PROTEINS AND natural minerals may be ingested in specially prepared dietary supplements (like edible herbs). Enzymes are critical macromolecules for all bodily functions, as each cell houses over 100,000 enzymatic particles to aid it in carrying out its life alchemy. Enzymes function as nutrients and catalysts of metabolic processes; for instance, they transform other proteins into amino acids and extract minerals from food in order to convert acidic and other toxic wastes for elimination.

Natural enzymes in food are mostly nullified by cooking them over 110 degrees Fahrenheit—the fate of much of what civilized men and women imbibe; yet, without these components alive and active, it is difficult for the upper part of the stomach to liquefy the bolus of food that continually enters it through the digestive tract. As expected, a large number of enzymatic products are now sold in health-food stores, by mail order, and even in standard drugstores and supermarkets. These are generally in pill form, to be taken before each meal (see Resource Guide). Enzymes can also come from consumption of raw foods— fruit and vegetable salads; sauerkrauts (Korean kim chee, etc.); "meats," breads, and vegetable crackers made from sprouted grains (often the burger plus the bun); cold vegetable soups from juicers; almond and other nut milks; seaweed salads; nut-based pâtés; plants eaten directly from fields, streams, woods, and gardens; and even raw fish and shell-fish (sushi), the latter, though, at risk of some unwelcome hitchhikers (parasites). These so-called "living meals" may be found at a number of newly popular restaurants throughout the West.

Minerals are necessary to create the distinctive internal cellular environment and to catalyze the work of enzymes. To manufacture the biochemical products necessary for their many bodily functions, cells enlist an astonishing variety of molecules, often in very minimal trace amounts but always in subtle balance with one another. The lack of any single mineral will distort the entire life system, putting a strain on some organ or tissue; in fact, a shortage of one trace mineral may make other nutrients functionless or inefficient.

Vitamins, proteins, enzymes, carbohydrates, fats, sugars, and oils all require key minerals to act biologically and are pretty much quiescent in their absence. Those biologists who believe that subcellular transmutation of elements is a key to life's miracle consider every trace mineral a *sine qua non* of healthy biology.

Minerals are also critical for cells in maintaining osmotic equilibrium—a balance between internal and external cellular pressures—throughout their internal milieu.

Human bodies have quite limited capacity to combine metallic with nonmetallic ions in the assemblage of molecules; they chelate only a small portion of the inorganic minerals they need directly from nature. In fact, all animals require plants to put minerals into a form that they can assimilate; this leaves modern humans in a uniquely vulnerable position because of the degree to which the mineral content of their soils, fruits, grains, and vegetables has been abrogated by petrochemicals, synthetic fertilizers, heavy processing, and cosmetic adulteration. Organic foods grown in mineral-rich soil may well supply some of the lacking ions. For a more thorough approach, trace minerals are commercially available in various brands of nontoxic colloidal forms—as treated water circulated or steamed (for less gamy taste) through Jurassic clay deposits. Utah provides enormous beds of these prehistoric vegetable-based residues that contain essentially all the biologically required elements. Trace-mineral products prepared from Deseret clays have been analyzed chemically to show a startling array (72 to 75 colloidal configurations) of just about every natural mixture of protons and electrons synthesized from original stellar dust, including iridium, gadolinium, dysprosium, zinc, rubidium, thallium, yttrium, gold, erbium, zirconium, and minute amounts of uranium, manganese, and europium. (See Resource Guide.)

One whole system, Body Electronics, combines doses of trace minerals and enzymes with palpation to generate a quasi-crystalline phase on multiple levels of body/mind (see Volume One, pp. 534–535) and then to hologrammatically purge it. First, tissues are flushed and rejuvenated through ingestion of large doses of papaya, malt diastase, cellulase, and other enzymes; trace-mineral waters are drunk concurrently in amounts varying from a few tablespoons to a few cups a day, depending on the speed and depth of healing sought. Toxins are then gradually exuded along with rigid patterns of thought and emotion by a method of sustained acupressure known as "pointholding."

Drugs

I HAVE PLACED medicinal herbs with food at the fourth level; these begin a treatment, but the patient must complete the cure by responding systemically. Both food and herbs can appear anywhere on the chart depending on how they are used. However, drugs are antibiotic or anesthetizing "herbs" that are meant to "replace" the organs in carrying out a process in relation to a particular pathology. Their after-effects are intrinsic to their nature: the body/mind can respond to them only as outsiders, initially as brilliant physicians from out of town with swift and incredible effects, but secondarily as thieves who have left the organs with only relative powers to carry out their own functions.

There are many strong herbs that resemble drugs, in fact are the forerunners of specific modern drugs, but they do not work as indiscriminately. Careful diagnosis by pulse, color of tongue, palpation, etc., is crucial to their use, as are precise preparation, dosage, frequency, and assimilation.

Refined pharmacy changes the characteristics of its "herbs" into more immediately activating substances that are less subtle and internal, hence more toxic. The classic medicinal smell of the hospital is really the "chemo" odor of the industrial laboratory. It is also the liquor of embalming fluid, the new bitter malignancy-killing taxol brew.

A NTIBIOTICS KILL GERMS, but they do so at the expense of the immune system and the overall vitality of body/mind. Directly toxic medicines may sometimes be necessary (even as guns may be necessary confronting a direct adversary). In a community context, though, they lessen the ability of our species to fend off germs arising even naturally in the environment. They numb the biological responsiveness of the planet as a whole (or perhaps they transpose it to the realm of microscopic bugs).

While the tundras and rain forests breed mostly healthy life forms, antibiotics (and pesticides) breed more and more virulent germs (and "pests"). Our mindless attack upon an imagined world of germs and parasites has left us weaker than our supposed enemies, for we not they are the ultimate victims of relentless mutations. They in fact are beneficiaries for they take the new information and mutate. There is a growing belief that the host of newer immunity-related diseases is at least partially the side effect of antibiotic residues in people's systems. Cattle feedlots and hospitals in particular, with their indiscriminate use of antibiotics, have become rich breeding grounds for exotic viruses and bacteria.

Commercial pharmaceuticals are both gross and abstract—gross in their chemistry but abstract in their relation to the body-mind's actual dynamics of survival. These highly synthesized medicines are often more semantic than substantial. They originate in and then generate clichés and presumptions that apply so-called objective biochemical research and prescribing. A gap, however, exists between the semantics of drugs and the reality of mind-body after their ingestion.

It is not as though drugs and diseases speak the same language. Plus, neither of them have anything to do with the propaganda of pharmaceutical marketing. One ingests someone else's fantasy, a cumulative guess as to what a standard condition and its range of potentiation are. People do not realize that the drug "action" they experience is often a combination of autogenic process, placebo effect, and cultural conditioning. They accept the marketing at face value. After all, it is written in the language of desire.

This is vintage seventh-level medicine, and it works extraordinarily well in heading off or postponing major crises. When enthusiasts hear that a medicine is effective they often rush to the "word" with the same

obsessiveness and unconsciousness with which they have accumulated

disease. Too collapsed or lethargic to respond to treatment, their systems ultimately become weaker.

At a party I observed a traditional Chinese doctor informally take
the case of a middle-class American woman who had never consulted
such a practitioner (and wouldn't have considered it outside the fortuity of the social event). She had major digestive problems, and the
doctor was trying to be of service. He wrote down her complete diet.
Many times he asked her not to leave anything out. Then he prescribed
an herb.

Several days later he made a special trip to her house to find out
the results. After listening to her carefully, he said, "Are you sure you
didn't eat anything else?"

She thoughtfully went back over her actions and meals of the last
few days. "No," she replied with certainty.

"Think. Is there anything else at all?"

"Well, I took Gelusil. But you don't mean that?"

"Of course, I mean that. How much?"

It turned out to be a full package a day!

"This is the most important part of your diet."

"But it's just Gelusil. It's not even a drug."

"It is a drug. It's supplying you with calcium which you should be
getting from elsewhere."

Talk of cultural categories masquerading as medicines! In this society the packaging is so soporific and disarming we often have no idea
what we are consuming or whether it is even real.

V ACCINATIONS (especially the routine childhood DPT shots) may
be even more hazardous than antibiotics. Who knows how the
body reacts at the deepest level to being fed deadly disease products to
induce an immune response? Although no links to serious ailments
have been proven, a number of researchers believe that isopathy may
have far more significant consequences than simply to immunize against
specific diseases. It may transpose aspects of pathology into overall sys-

temic homeostasis and thereby set in motion intractable and exotic neurological disorders, including the compulsion to commit crimes. One would be advised to consult the references available on this topic and carefully weigh the pros and cons before taking any "shot."

Sedatives, anti-depressants, anti-anxiety drugs, psychotropics, and the like are stopgap measures that numb one's organism to pain, hence to the real crisis. They are police measures in a security- and property-conscious state.

The other "drugs"—crack, heroin, ice, etc.—are hardly the toys of a kick-happy society. They are last-resort medicines for people who cannot handle the input of a materialized, external-value, bottom-line-only culture in which family and community are already nostalgias. Environmentally we may have some margin left, but psychically and in our inner life we have reached *Blade Runner* and *Mona Lisa Overdrive*. Recreational drugs are medicines of despair, not fun. "Just say, 'No!'" is the most ironical of jokes when everyone who takes these medicines addictively has already said a far deeper "No!" than Nancy Reagan or any George Bush could fathom.

Notes

1. Paul Pitchford, from a lecture at the Pacific College of Naturopathic Medicine, San Rafael, California, 1982.

2. Bruce Kumar Frantzis, personal communication, 1994.

3. Nyanaponika Thera, *The Heart of Buddhist Meditation* (New York: Samuel Weiser, Inc., 1969), p. 71.

4. Father Berard Haile, recorder and translator; in Leland C. Wyman (ed.), *Beautyway: A Navaho Ceremonial* (New York: Bollingen Foundation, Pantheon Books, 1957), pp. 141–142.

5. Chögyal Namkhai Norbu and Adriano Clemente, *The Supreme Source* (The Kunjed Gyalpo): *The Fundamental Tantra of Dzogchen Semde,* translated from Italian by Andrew Lukianowicz (Ithaca, New York: Snow Lion Publications, 1999), p. 86.

6. Michio Kushi, *The Book of Dō-In: Exercise for Physical and Spiritual Development* (Tokyo: Japan Publications, 1979).

7. Jacques de Langre, *Dō-In 2: The Ancient Art of Rejuvenation Through Self-Massage* (Magalia, California: Happiness Press, 1978).

8. John E. Upledger, *SomatoEmotional Release: Deciphering the Language of Life* (Berkeley, California: North Atlantic Books, 2002), pp. 175–176.

9. Eduardo Calderón, Richard Cowan, Douglas Sharon, and F. Kaye Sharon, *Eduardo el Curandero: The Words of a Peruvian Healer* (Richmond, California: North Atlantic Books, 1982), p. 42.

10. Ibid., p. 45.

11. Ibid., p. 42.

12. John Douillard, "Ayurveda and Reaching Mainstream America," talk at Ayurveda International Symposium, California Association of Ayurvedic Medicine, Berkeley, California, May 4, 2002.

13. Richard Leviton, "Healing Vibrations," *Yoga Journal* (January/February 1994), p. 63.

14. Ibid., p. 124.

15. Ibid., p. 125.

16. Ibid., p. 124.

17. C. S. Lewis, *The Magician's Nephew* (New York: Collier Books, 1970), pp. 98–99 (originally published in 1951).

18. Jeanne Rose, *The Aromatherapy Book: Applications & Inhalations* (Berkeley, California: North Atlantic Books, 1992), p. xiv.

19. Ibid.

20. John Steele, personal communication, 1991.

21. Richard Leviton, "The Healing Energies of Color," *Yoga Journal* (January/February 1992), p. 48.

22. Ibid., p. 47.

23. Ibid., pp. 47–48.

24. Ibid., p. 47.

25. Nevill Drury, *The Healing Power: A Handbook of Alternative Medicines and Natural Health* (London: Frederick Muller Ltd., 1981), p. 53.

26. Ibid., p. 53.

27. Leviton, "The Healing Energies of Color," p. 47.

28. William Croft, C. S. T., "Light Energy Practices (Yoga/Qigong/Aikido) and *Working with Light*—a Synergy," flyer, 1993.

29. Leviton, "The Healing Energies of Color."

30. Quoted in Drury, *The Healing Power,* p. 53.

31. Otto Max, review of *Planet Medicine, East West Journal* (August 1981), p. 80.

32. Paul Pitchford, *Healing with Whole Foods: Oriental Traditions and Modern Nutrition* (Berkeley, California: North Atlantic Books, 1992).

33. Ibid.

34. Bubba Free John (Da Free John), *The Eating Gorilla Comes in Peace: The Transcendental Principle of Life Applied to Diet and the Regenerative Discipline of True Health* (Middletown, California: The Dawn Horse Press, 1979), p. 178

35. Ibid.

36. Pitchford, *Healing with Whole Foods,* plus a variety of other sources.

37. Stephen Fulder, *The Root of Being: Ginseng and the Pharmacology of Harmony* (London: Hutchison Publishing Group, 1980), p. 86.

38. Rechung Rinpoche, *Tibetan Medicine* (Berkeley, California: University of California Press, 1973); Hong-Yen Hsu, *How to Heal Yourself with Chinese Herbs* (Los Angeles: Oriental Healing Arts Institute, 1980), and a variety of other sources.

39. A. Lade and R. Svoboda, *Tao & Dharma—A Comparison of Ayurveda and Chinese Medicine,* unpublished manuscript at the time of publication.

40. Pitchford, *Healing with Whole Foods,* pp. 159.

41. Ibid., pp. 156–164.

CHAPTER NINE

Beyond Ideology

Levels of Healing

THE INFORMATION IN this book—or in any book of medicinal etiology or self-help—exists disguised on a number of levels in relation to any reader, the author as well. The modalities I have described operate as not only competing brands and businesses but often-rival paradigms of disease cause and effect and cure. They locate pathological processes (hence, diagnoses and treatments) in different layers of mind and body and at different levels of manifestation of matter and energy. One theory tells us that medicine must be vital and energy-oriented, as disease is; another, that insofar as incarnation is physical, only herbs and bodywork (or drugs and surgery) operate on the carnal plane. The global pharmacy now offers us a choice of potions, distillations, essences, saturations, syntheses, potentizations, images, and archetypes of the same basic substances. Of a given plant, does one ingest the seeds, soak the petals in water, succuss the pulp into an ultra non-physical dose, combine in complex formulas with artificial substances, or meditate on its signature? Should the bones be manipulated, the viscera palpated, or the meridians activated to affect the organs? How does a person choose?

Virtually every holistic practitioner has some blind spot, is closed to some other method. An acupuncturist may attribute poor eyesight to *chi* stagnation with age and deem the Bates Method antiquated auto-suggestion. Yet a Bates practitioner may improve her visual accommodation without ever *directly* affecting the meridians through her eyes. A Rolfer may dismiss the notion of potentized microdoses as effective somatic agents. Many a Feldenkrais practitioner has denigrated Breema or Reiki as "hippie" bodywork. A Reiki healer or Polarity therapist may propound that diseases are solely impediments of spirit and *all* physical methods are merely rituals to awaken cosmic energy. A high proportion of homeopaths and diet-oriented practitioners ignore both psychological issues and tissue cysts. Yet an equally high proportion of body-workers overlook diet and herbs. Most homeopaths wouldn't ask their patients to breathe more deeply or begin massaging intestines. These are not part of their modality. It would be just as inappropriate for a Reichian to prescribe a microdose. As long as we stay totally in either system, the other domain does not even exist.

Can a homeopathic remedy remove layers of "Reichian" armor from the ocular muscles and belly? The simplest answer to this question is no—at least as an operating premise most of the time. Somaticized trauma is structured deeply and rigidly in the mind/body and can usually be dissolved only by a process of palpation, breathing, exercise, and internal imagination akin to the pathways by which it was imbedded. However, a homeopathic dose might well alleviate a digestive ailment associated with belly armor and thereby participate in its bioenergetic dissipation. A potency might also release the miasmatic and dermatological aspect of a "mask" and so energize the dissolution of facial armor. Some osteopaths now work with homeopaths or acupuncturists to mobilize such an effect. A visceral manipulator may say, "I think I got all of that block, but there's a small stuck part around the dura. Have a high-potency homeopathic remedy prescribed and see if that will do it."

Each system elicits its own categories of reality and devises processes relevant to these, but it can also collaborate with other systems. Treatments cannot be substituted literally; yet the therapeutic grammar behind each of them can override separate ideologies. Cases of complementary or reciprocal healing, even embracing conventional allopathic treatments, are in fact quite common now. One modality (usually surgery or pharmacy) deals with the immediate crisis; the other addresses overall health at a deeper level of cure. Chemotherapy and acupuncture/diet have become a relatively familiar complementary pair, with the latter used to counter the former's toxic effects.

Conversely, there may be another system of medicine claiming that the real disease lies deeper or that the cure of symptoms by a rival modality is pure placebo or merely displaces the pathologizing force. Allopathy commonly plays that role.

When the renowned Greek homeopath George Vithoulkas spoke a few years ago in San Francisco, I overheard a cluster of Reichians outside the auditorium chortling over how deeply armored he was—this present paragon of a homeopathic physician. From a different part of the room a local homeopath pointed to the circle of Reichians and told his colleagues: "There you see the pure sycotic miasm* on the hoof."

Such a lack of empathy and appreciation is a failure of holism, for on some deeper level these dichotomies must converge. There is only one incarnation, one body template, one consciousness, one life energy, one physical universe. True systems all heal, even if they enter at different points and work through different levels. How can we be sure that the active elements of homeopathy, acupuncture, chiropractic, or even allopathy are not mainly psychokinesis guided by a therapeutic mythology?

As one observer notes, the key to healing lies in something other than the utilitarian logic or linear function of a particular modality:

---

*"Sycosis" (literally "figlike pathology") is the homeopathic name for gonorrhea; a miasm, homeopathically, is a deep-seated, often-inherited disease complex.

Every method of treating illness works. High-tech laboratory-tested therapies of Western medicine work—so do the ancient techniques of Eastern medicine. Laser surgery and chemotherapy, crystals, ginseng root and echinacea, low-fat diets and vitamin megadoses, as well as the whole armamentarium of New Age medicine—such as aromatherapy, music therapy, Therapeutic Touch, Reiki, macrobiotics—they all work. Every possible decoction of forest and garden, and yes, a rag, a bone, and a hank of hair, have been used to heal and have healed. In the history of the world, there has never been a medicine or treatment that did not heal someone.

How is this possible? What is really going on here?

To compound the puzzle, why doesn't a given treatment work on everyone who has the same disease? And, if a treatment is effective in Switzerland, why doesn't it work in Swaziland? And, if a treatment worked in 1800, why didn't the identical treatment work in the year 1900?[1]

This is because the actual domain of health and disease lies at a deeper level than the transient symbols and artifacts used to address it. Medical symbols and artifacts, while engaging meanings more or less literally at the body/mind surface, set in motion much deeper fields and phase states that are always in process and come to no firm resolution either way, until they do, in death and conception.

There is a level at which no one ever has a real idea of what medicine or event cures an illness. A sick person may try dozens of different modalities without results and then find that the ailment dramatically improves, perhaps because of the treatment proximate to the improvement, perhaps because of the collective effect of the treatments, or perhaps because the complex of factors underlying the illness changed over time or changed in catalysis with the treatments.

Each organism is a miracle of development; thus, it should be no surprise that homunculi from signaling errors attach themselves to growth networks and become part of everyday life. These are true miasms, and their ultimate genealogy goes too deep to be rooted out by most medicines. Living itself is hard to explain—why we stay healthy so much of the time for so many years. Disease is far more obvious; yet some invisible tissue synergy keeps it at bay.

Systems of alternative cancer therapy generally set as their absolute requirement a specific drug (apricot pits, shark cartilage): a dietary change (macrobiotic, vegetarian, raw foods, vitamin B, iodine); a lifestyle modification; the elimination of a particular microorganism, toxin, radiation, or proto-cellular substratum; the replacement of mercury dental work; a bioenergetic or primal-scream therapy; an injection of embryonic trophoblast; a potentization or serum of the tumor itself to stimulate the lacking immune response; or some other concrete modality. Each system claims uniquely to have discovered the sought-after cure, and each presents itself as a victim of orthodox medical prejudice against unsanctioned methods. Likely, some cancer patients will be successfully treated by each of these methods, leading its supporters to presume universality. Yet I doubt that any of these methods is, by itself, the answer, though each may represent a possible vector to the core, a clue to where an answer lies.

Cancer may also be a complicated set of interacting causes, catalyzing physical, embryogenic, viral, emotional, and psychospiritual layers. It may not be a unique disease. It may not have a singular cure.

Misplaced concreteness is as much a hazard of alternative systems as it is of mainstream ones. It may finally be the case that an authentic cure for any condition is the one that confronts and extricates a patient along her unique line of resistance—diet for some, herbs for others, bodywork for others, prayer for others, etc.

The human organism is a fragmented entity and must be addressed level by level, persona by persona (some levels and personae will not even appear in a lifetime). Surgery and drugs may effectively penetrate one level; Gestalt therapy, another; Bach flower remedies, another; chiropractic, another; and so on. Some levels may be touched only by magic, love, or a song.

Yet because these levels are interpenetrating fields, medicines and meanings introduced into one will be transmitted to all. Such is the potential and legitimate promise of holism. A medicine may be directly curative only on the level at which it is introduced. What it translates to other levels may or may not be immediately functional; it depends on the integration and receptivity of the organism and the timing and synchronicity of the cure.

A successful herbal treatment—or pill or operation—does not eliminate core disease; it merely shifts it to another, ideally less debilitating level. It changes the body-mind configuration. A homeopathic remedy sometimes requires concurrent psychological work for its completion; otherwise the condition it was treating may lapse into dormancy, re-energize there, and return either in its previous guise or as some other ailment. Oftentimes psychosomatic and even serious malignant conditions gestate because an existential rip occurs in the social, biological, and/or psychological continuum of an organism. The body creates deviant cellular material in response to a discomfort—morphogenetic/emotional patterns that were initially innocent, i.e., without pathological implications. Once the new material becomes fixed in tissue, it develops its own weird integrity and enhances itself for no other reason than that it occupies an unconscious organismic zone; it steals space from mobility and natural function, developing its own metabolism and identity and eventually ossifying by institutionalizing itself in the body-mind's configuration and developing its own iconography and even a crude ego structure. At this point it has almost as much claim on the organism's energy as the creature's own healthy patterns. And because the "disease" has rooted itself in subliminal territory, it makes itself "normal" by attaching to kinesthetic awareness in a way that it doesn't seem parasitic or strange.

Ailments originating as secondary compensations for other problems—perhaps a minor physical defect or idle personal crisis—take on lives of their own and claim a facet of tissue structure and proprioception. Even if the surface distortion is ultimately dissolved and its anatomical obstruction alleviated therapeutically, an underlying field

482

may eventually reimpose it, probably in a slightly different form representing a new trajectory and energy balance. When a chronic ailment's material aspect has been substantially removed, the holistic factor imposing it may seek to reestablish the familiar longstanding and compensatory pattern. The ailment mysteriously returns, or a variation of it develops with a different rhythm or in a new locale.

It is possible too, as we have seen at various points throughout this text, that an effective treatment, even a vitalistic one, may have secondary pathological consequences if it introduces energy into an organism that cannot contain and integrate it. Perhaps this is why Edward Whitmont preferred not to use homeopathy separate of psychoanalysis. He was concerned about setting in motion forces that the personality would then either cathect neurotically or suppress.[2]

CURES ARE NOT always dispensed in proximate time and space. There is a mistaken tendency to expect a doctor of any persuasion to diagnose a condition and offer its remedy in the form of a pill, regimen, physical adjustment, prayer, or some more esoteric currency; the petitioner assumes that he or she "gets" it then.

This is often the case. Yet on another level medicines may contact such deep-seated conditions that some of their effects will not be felt for years, or even decades (this is axiomatically true for autogenic "medicines" like dreams, life experiences, and insights that change orientation to one's own character and to the world). Thus, any medicine is simultaneously short-term and long-term, exoteric and esoteric, activating and internalizing. While a dose of comfrey or a papaya enzyme mix instantly energizes an intestinal condition, a concurrent use of barley grass or microflora may begin flushing the liver of deeper-seated toxins. The person may experience some degree of immediate relief from the comfrey (more ease digesting, less frequent constipation), but also a painful intensification of other symptoms (chronic pain, emotional distress, burning tears, diarrhea) that attend longer-term cleansing.

Alternative medicines generally (if unintentionally) encourage the demedicalization of healing. Their practitioners suspect that certain regimens or remedies tend to lead to cures within a broad holistic context, so they prescribe them with confidence. By contrast, conventional allopathic medicines try to capture the precise locus of cure within medical liturgy. This is how they get sanctioned and licensed. Either way, though, the match between putative cure and actual cure is often pure speculation, either makeshift aesthetic theory or scientific totemism.

Although the mystery and complexity of curative cause and effect are not just attributes of alternative modalities, the custom in allopathy is for the patient to attribute cure in an absolute and linear fashion to the category proposed by the doctor. Very often this is more religious catechism than scientific verity. It can also be dangerous insofar as it implants false beliefs in the patient regarding future health and curability. Only naive or vain doctors need to demonstrate with "surety" a cure's trajectory.

Many allopathic treatments may well incorporate placebo effects, powerful projections from a physician as shaman-priest, or mysterious systemic resonances that either abet or operate *instead of* the ostensible therapeutic vector. In the last decade of the twentieth century a new allopathic treatment was developed for Parkinson's Disease, a deteriorative pathology of the brain leading to involuntary shaking of the limbs, discoordination of muscles, and slurred speech. The remarkably successful remedy involved implanting tiny electrodes in the Parkinson's area of the brain, a perilous surgical feat by itself. Many of the lost neurological functions returned to the patients instantaneously as long as the charge-generating machine was functioning. Why? No one is certain. The treatment was discovered by doctors experimentally probing the brain during Parkinson's research. When electricity was applied to explore this region, the symptoms coincidentally seemed to improve, so doctors decided to formalize the side-effect by concentrating and aiming it. The result was a dramatic and functional cure. The cause of its success apparently lies in some unknown resonant relationship among the brain tissue and its neural pathways.

Other than the fact that electrical brain implants are an extremely hi-tech solution outside the range of any alternative clinic, they are similar in innate effect to many resonant osteopathic palpations. They represent the kind of remedy that could result from a merger of osteopathic, homeopathic, and other alternative modalities with advanced allopathic technologies. A whole new spectrum of otherwise inaccessible paradigms and remedies might unfold.

INFORMATION SYSTEMS OPERATING at the level of soma, cell, DNA, and perhaps even in uncertainty phases in molecules and atoms determine the fate of an organism. It is foolhardy to think that anyone can see or track such discrete, deep-seated, and fast-moving originations through the camouflage of seemingly more explicit physical events. Like allopathy, many alternative medicines identify healing with a protocol of treatment, but they often also "augment" it in their minds with some impalpable or ineffable factor such as *chi* energy, homeostasis, an activation of the life force, an affirmation, or the magical effect of holism itself. As we saw in the chapters on faith healing and linguistic codes, symbolic cures may penetrate the disease core, even without modality or linear cause-and-effect. When we most seem to know the path of a cure is often when we least know it.

A naturopath may conclude a session by handing a client with a digestive disorder a page of prescriptions—herbs, dietary changes, modes of exercise, a homeopathic constitutional, a biweekly bathing ritual, and points on the body on which to do self-acupressure. The sincere patient may well undertake all of these things but forget about pressing two Intestine points at the creases of his elbows. Ten years later another healer from a different tradition may emphasize *only* those points—and this time the person remembers, and the result is the true cure. That does not mean healing was not taking place all along or that the points were the "right" medicine: the body/mind's vibration merely changed frequency and amplitude, which it does anyway throughout life.

A different person with a similar diagnosis might never remember to press those two points but then unknowingly (and efficaciously) incorporate their meridians in a sequence of *Chi Gung* exercises, intoning "kaaa!" or "ssss" within a cycle of "animal form" motions, breath-awareness, and light massage of her heart meridian.

Perhaps a person visits both a homeopath and a psychotherapist and gets gradual relief of chronic indigestion and flatulence. Years later the same person may replace twice-a-week red meat in her diet with biweekly chicken, then drop meat altogether and develop a dish combining brown rice, miso, seaweed, and carrots. Along the way she may undergo periods of susceptibility to colds, irregular menstrual cycles, and a range of unfamiliar emotions, but then, with the more vegetarian diet, she experiences new feelings of lightness, freedom from colds, and general well-being. Each phase doesn't simply emerge like a new image popped into a slide projector. Homeopathic and psychological cures probably begin a process of change on the vital and emotional planes that leads to a shift in attitude, that leads to a change in awareness and food taste. Then the entire metabolism responds to a new identity. Psychological work rouses something *pre-psychic* in an organism. Quite likely, dietary attention alone (initially) could not spark a character change and might not have the same healthful and profound physical effect. On the other hand, another person might follow diet to psychotherapy. Someone else might never alter their diet and experience a similar change from a series of craniosacral and visceral treatments.

A rebirther emphasizes her in-breath for accumulating *prana;* then she joins a Zen meditation group and learns to accentuate her out-breath for dissipation. Both are real; each has discrete results relative to the other it would not have alone.

It is a subtle, even evasive point at which the true healer works both toward curing the disease and giving the patient the lesson *from* the disease, i.e., leading her to walk the labyrinth of the disease rather than

simply to airlift out. Native healers, as we have seen, cultivated this well.

We have lost and are forced to regain that component in our own medical complexes because, as we have turned mechanical and doctrinaire, we have come to treat diseases only as external destructive agencies.

Recently an acquaintance with a severe lung malady sought both explanation and (of course) relief by visiting a succession of renowned allopaths with different specialties. She heard diagnoses ranging from exotic respiratory parasites to lupus, but none of the treatments for these brought any change in her painful symptoms and mood of despair. Then with no cure in sight and her pain so searing she was at the point of suicide, she scheduled an appointment with a homeopath as a last resort, got diagnosed according to different parameters (as having the disorder currently euphemized as Chronic Fatigue Syndrome), was given potentiated microdoses, and experienced an immediate marked improvement. Her pain and despair became less deeply rooted. But she was still quite weak until a form of Korean finger acupuncture relieved a whole other cluster of symptoms. Later, a different doctor offered a series of *dō-in* exercises and dietary transitions (eliminating all forms of sugar and meats). This ameliorated some remaining symptoms. She was a different person by then. The disease had come to seem the trademark of a more passive, less mature self. A subsequent stage might involve Jungian therapy to transform the layer of self that accepted the disease initially on an archetypal level. Or she might just live her new life until the next challenge. In her own mind the original pathology had been reconceived as a harbinger of growth, a death-like blow dislodging an even more profound systemic morbidity.

Admittedly, I have presented a long pilgrimage with an optimistic outcome. But I am trying to propose what is possible when things *work,* not to recount the all-too-well-known ravages of progressive pathology. This succession of treatments—or even anything resembling it—would also likely not improve another person diagnosed with the "same" Chronic Fatigue Syndrome but having a different constitution, individuation process, or etiology of disease.

During the mid 1990s someone close to me was stricken for two years with a seemingly undiagnosable and untreatable ailment. In retrospect, he was probably sick for at least another year and a half before that, but it took that long before he recognized something intractable settling in him.

The year-and-a-half etiology began with a case of pneumonia and continued with increasingly severe ankle pains and muscular stiffness. After he dropped out of graduate school and came home, he was seen by a series of physicians, starting with a family doctor for an exam and eventually including, over the two years, two podiatrists, an endocrinologist, a rheumatologist, a "sports medicine" surgeon, two separate doctors at a pain clinic, and a foot surgeon. He underwent extensive lab tests plus a variety of X-rays, bone scans, and MRIs. Although doctors speculated on a number of conditions throughout this odyssey, its conclusion was an inability of all of these people to find anything wrong with him. It should be noted that at different points in the examination process, three of the doctors and radiologists did think they detected deterioration in the ligaments around his ankles (one even said, "it is as though he jumped out of a six-story building and landed on his feet")—a diagnosis that was routinely refuted by the next physician to whom he was referred. Additionally, none of their symptomatic treatments (orthotics, anti-inflammatories) seemed to alleviate his pain.

During the same period of time he was treated by two homeopaths, a chiropractor, a Rolfer, a Feldenkrais practitioner, a Lomi therapist, and two doctors of Traditional Chinese Medicine. Except for the homeopaths, each of these practitioners had a significant demonstrable positive effect on him. His posture and metabolism improved, his breathing deepened, and he got stronger and generally healthier. Yet none of them could alter the basic condition—pain in both ankles making it impossible to walk more than a short distance. In fact, the Rolfer, while stating clearly that the condition was outside the range of his practice, expressed doubt as to whether the pain actually originated in the ankles since he could not affect it either positively or negatively at the ostensible source.

Near the end of the second year the patient took to getting around in a wheelchair most of the time. The last doctor he saw was a prominent foot surgeon who wondered if the disease was in his mind and then suggested casts on both feet for six months as a last resort. He had no particular rationale for making that suggestion, merely that he could find no cause for the pain. He boasted dryly that he was well qualified to diagnose absence of pathology because he had written the textbook on surgery of the particular ligaments involved. "The buck stops here. You've either got *me,*" he said, "or you've got someone who's been trained using my textbook." Undoubtedly this was true. Yet at the end of the quest stood a surgeon with a waiting room full of patients concluding, "Pain of unknown origin. Deer hold up their wounded limbs. Maybe immobilizing both feet will help."

At the beginning of approximately the third year the patient was seen informally by John Upledger at the end of a workshop. Within forty-five seconds of beginning his palpation, Upledger felt "it." "Holy shit," he exclaimed. "It's a wonder you even get up in the morning." After the hedging and bafflement of the other doctors, to Upledger the pathology was immediately obvious and unambiguous. It was located not at the ankles but in the meninges of the spine. The pain at the ankles as well as other symptoms were probably, Upledger thought, areas of prior weakness. They expressed chronic structural and developmental problems that had begun to be successfully treated by the Rolfer and chiropractor but could not be improved any further without getting at the core illness. The failure of the spine to transmit free cranial motion had congestive and restrictive ramifications throughout the body, more severe in some areas than others but clearly both pathologizing and symptomatic. "I haven't a clue why the greatest pain ended up in the ankles," Upledger said. "But if we succeed at the core, it is likely that the periphery will follow."

He began his regimen two days later. This consisted of himself and an assistant mutually stretching out the restricted tissue, restoring its elasticity from the top of the spine and the sacrum, respectively. Of course, enacting this was not as quick and direct as pulling off a rubber glove. The process had to be accomplished by minute degrees from different angles along vectors suggested by the tissue itself over half a year, with intervening periods for rest and integration.

Upledger's cure was completed by two bodyworkers (one a visceral manipulator, the other a chiropractor). Within a month the patient was out of the wheelchair. After six months the condition had improved to the point where he was functioning at around 75 percent of his former strength and mobility and beginning to deal with other physical and emotional issues.

Although no precise cause was ever given for the disease, Upledger thought it possible that a series of unusual vaccinations (followed by a fever) three and a half years earlier (just before the pneumonia) had provoked the acute condition, a meningitis-like reaction. The patient had received these vaccinations so as to be qualified to handle raw sewage safely while building alternative waste-treatment plants. It was possible too that a toxin from the sludge had gotten into his system. The disease itself (whatever it was), Upledger emphasized, had long since passed; that was why so many doctors reported the patient was healthy. The after-effects of the disease were his ongoing stiffness and pain from constricted tissue and fluid flow.

The power of simple educated touch—of being able to set hands on a body and feel its visceral and neuromuscular restrictions—is becoming a lost art in the face of ever more complex microchemical and cybernetic techniques of diagnosis (often missing the forest for the trees). The former attends to the inner physician; the latter consigns the patient to statistical purgatory.

Most doctors now do not know how to or even want to "feel" the disease, and they are not outcome-oriented. That is, it is not of great concern to them to find a precise and complete remedy; they are satisfied to alleviate symptomology (even if it involves lifelong medication) and to forestall blatant tissue damage. They want to identify a

category of pathology, propose an acceptable, defensible treatment, and not get sued. And this, according to one dropout M.D., is in truth the fate of all conditions—not just chronic or intractable ones— brought to doctors in today's clinical environment. "We are in the dark ages of medicine," he said, "but nobody realizes it." Note that immobilization recommended by "the buck stops here" guy was contraindicated and would probably have made the condition worse by further restricting the natural rhythms of the skeleton (doctors have prescribed cutting ankle tendons for the effects of cerebral palsy as well as a host of other, similar quasi-functional, simplistic solutions for numerous complex problems). While the surgeon did not himself have a surgical resolution, Upledger, in a sense, recommended a kind of surgery, a deep gradual holistic surgery with subtle course corrections and adjustments along the way. Each step of the treatment was followed by a week or so of ordinary life; then the "surgery" continued. This was surgery at the innate rhythm of life.

The best allopathic surgeons probably wield their blades with similar responsiveness to tissue and care.

Regardless of the actual cause of this condition, one is led to ask, "What would have happened if the person had not been lucky enough to see a John Upledger and had continued his search among allopathic physicians?" After all, this is the plight of most people in the Western world (and many in the developing countries as well). It is the plight of thousands of Gulf War veterans "complaining of persistent headaches, rashes, nausea, chronic fatigue and body aches. Military doctors at first said their symptoms had nothing to do with the war. One man was told that his rash was age spots, his low red blood cell count a dietary deficiency, and his hacking cough a function of pollution. Others were told they were suffering from stress."[3]

As long as the goal of medicine is to validate prior categories and serve a variety of civil, political, and economic agendas, it can never return to even the depth of diagnostic and therapeutic clarity that existed a hundred years ago or to some extent among the ancient Hippocratics. We may have a dazzling new technology that allows our doctors to do things their forebears could not imagine, but only when that technology is applied with real empathy and insight can it be a true ally of cure. Otherwise, it is a blind and dangerous robot, shredding tissue and reducing life functions to molecules and cells that are their mere transient commodities.

Holistic Caricatures*

MANY PEOPLE INVOLVED in holistic health look to it for answers it cannot provide. They assume something has become wrong in them or was always wrong and that a radical treatment will correct it. Then they become the representative of their idealized correction instead of who they were. And they remain sick.

There are health and therapy junkies who go from treatment to treatment, looking for the one that has the insight to recognize them or the power to intercede in their behalf. Their overly earnest quest for a cure becomes another symptom, and the longer the search goes on, the less chance there is that they will regain their own systemic integrity. Flaunting their holism, they can become solipsistic and righteous. They begin acting like the parody of a medicine, which is really like a disease.

Many of the current male and female initiation rites (notably the empowered males drumming and dancing to confront the symbols of

---

*This section was originally written in 1978 for the first edition of this book and updated in 1994. Though it is clearly obsolete now, I have left much of it in because the issue it describes (New Age inflation) is still a dilemma for many people. Divine posing is a mainstay of human folly and will probably always be with us. Shakespeare presented inflated clowns and fools for comic relief amid *The Tempest* and *A Midsummer Night's Dream,* while D. H. Lawrence in *The Plumed Serpent* foreshadowed the darker side of self-proclaimed enlightenment. The snake-oil salesman, a familiar burlesque trope of the American Western, is alive and well in new guises throughout gullible alternative-medicine circles.

their weak but tyrannical fathers—and their counterparts, the newly shamanized females of the once and future matriarchy) are *ideas* masquerading as acts. Playing at being shamans and warriors shows how we overendow image and product, how we are incorrigible spiritual materialists.

It is healthier finally to get instruction from a master of *chi*. By engaging with a tradition going back generations one at least is not naively trying to reinvent all of mythology and all of ontological ritual. The old masters require hard internal work and keep things real.

One bioenergetic therapist tells of leading a group in a simple breathing exercise on the floor when a man unexpectedly crawled onto an adjacent young woman who had recently given birth and tried to suckle her. When she pushed him off, he shouted "Bitch!" as if *she* had violated the spirit of the exercise. Then he added, to the group, as if in explanation, "I'm expressing myself."

The therapist told me, "I found myself wondering, 'What are we teaching these people? What kind of a world are we telling them this is?'"[4]

The most abiding holistic illusion is that there is no planet, no history, no context, no undeserved pain or injustice, only empowerment workshops and enlightenment intensives, shamans and spirits in the shaman or spirit business, inner psychic powers, forgotten victimizations, and lost lives. If this planet is wasted, another higher dimensional domain (it is presumed) will replace it.

Among the New Age masses it becomes an unabated (and unabatable) appetite for spiritual experiences and goods that will somehow confirm their own flimsy existence. One does not have to universalize the implicit pessimistic (and decidedly un-New Age) message of political refugees from Asia, Africa, the Middle East, and Central America or our own homeless mendicants to realize that they are telling the truth when they report: "There is a world out there, and it's got teeth." On 9-11-2001 it came right into the largest North American city. The karmic situation in which we find ourselves cannot be replaced by an imaginary

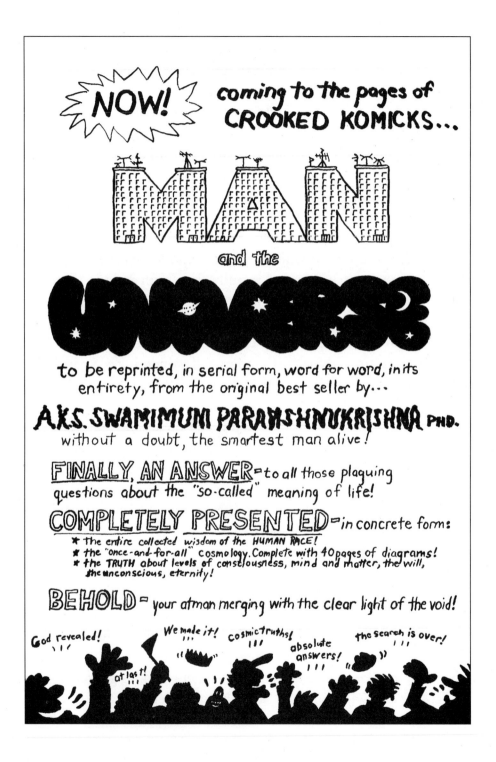

clinic or asylum. There is not only no one to blame but nothing that blame can expiate.

The same therapist concluded at the end of another fable: "Having a sixty-year-old man run around in diapers crying may have therapeutic value, but as a statement on the human condition, it's fucked."[5]

It is not a matter of lying on the floor pounding and breathing more fully or escaping on a science-fiction journey through Reiki rays or herbs and needles of the Yellow Emperor. Each episode comes to an end, and the same issues in the world-state prevail. Despite these bizarre artificial villages in which we live, we are still wild animals in tribes howling at a totem moon. From the beginning of the Ice Age till now, nothing has been solved, nothing has truly changed, nothing at all. People live and die and, as Montreal Leonard Cohen sang, *"The poor stay poor and the rich get rich ... Everybody knows...."* So holism is hardly a ticket to the big carnival or ultimate Whole Life Expo.

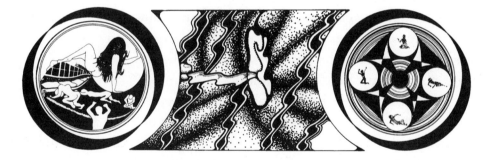

IN THE LATE 1970s a plague of naive, "enlightened" M.D.s and psychologists adapted versions of acupuncture, chiropractic, homeopathy, and macrobiotics into their general standard practices. Some attended holistic meetings as authorities and gave papers on "wellness," biofeedback, shadow pain, biodynamic nutrition, and cosmic healing energy. They preached a mixture of religion, lifestyle, health, exercise, seduction, and charisma. Yet they had no more training in these fields than an average educated person would have in surgery from scanning a few textbooks.

The 1977 edition of *Planet Medicine* presented a caricature of such a doctor that by now reads as a caricature of itself: suntan, leather pants, astrological or Tibetan medallion hanging in his chest hair, a beaming holistic smile; jogs, does *aikido;* acts as though ancient wisdom has come through all of history to anoint him. If challenged, he will quickly cite his training in physiology and the "hard" sciences. Another version is the cosmically receptive and annointed shaman-lady with her Ph.D. My pretenders may still exist but they are hardly as blatant. Instead we have new holistic posers.

For instance, one chiropractor claims to have been "kidnapped by a tribe of sixty-two aboriginal [Australian] natives and forced to go on a walkabout. For four months, she walked barefoot through the desert. She was subjected to various privations and indignities. She was required to listen to muddy spiritual chitchat from people who chose to speak in capital letters. Finally the purpose of her journey is revealed. The earth is in such terrible shape that the aborigines have chosen to have no more children. There is war and killing and pollution, and the aborigines are fed up. Before they die out, they have chosen one person, one 'mutant' to carry their warning back to civilization. They have chosen a chiropractor from Lee's Summit, Missouri. . . ."[6]

This is the sort of cosmic prophecy that presently muddles and corrupts spiritual healing—self-glorifying myths on one side and, on the other, ascended homeopaths claiming to represent the Knights Templar and the Order of the Solar Temple while leading fifty-three people in suicide, murder, or both. Throughout Eastern Europe and the Westernized Orient, exorbitant guru regimes, messianic quasi-political therapies, reverse cargo cults, Reiki and *chi* machines, and other mind-over-matter apparatuses abound. A "Whole Earth" plague of messianic cults and apocalypticists pile up personal fortunes and arsenals from decommissioned and still shell-shocked Cold War troops.

Journalist Jon Carroll refers to the supposed mutant-message walkabout as "another example of white people using brown people as man-

tel ornaments or game tokens. It's cultural imperialism masquerading as harmless New Age spiritualism. Its racism is no more lovely for being unwitting." In fact, the author was paid $1.7 million for the rights to her self-published account and, though promising that a portion of the proceeds would go to the Doonooch Self-Healing Centre run by Aborigines in Mowra, New South Wales, had sent not a penny as of September 8, 1994.

Carroll concludes:

> The real message of the aboriginal peoples is: Give us back our land. It's a nasty, greedy, materialistic message; it's one that requires us to do something other than think good thoughts. So much better to make aborigines passive children of God, praying for the misguided white people while committing cultural suicide....
>   *Mutant Message Down Under* is fiction; it's also a disgrace.[7]

Something new *has* been emerging, from within our individual and collective souls—but it is different from the entire holistic health and New Age movement. It is both more and less—potentially more but presently less. There are in fact two movements—the true political medicinal revolution and the one in flight from it which borrows its symbols and tries to masquerade as the same thing. The true one comes from within our historic process and *is* our historical realization. The other seeks to enlist every passing fad, in hopes of postponing any real change. So close together are these two that for a moment now (in 1978, still in 2002) they seem to merge.

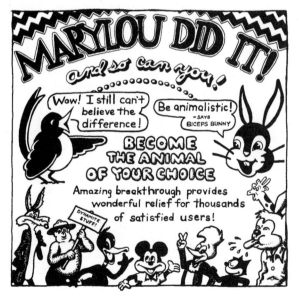

Despite obfuscating fads, there is, finally, a gut sense of wellness whose "symptoms" are a lucidity and the freedom to act, an ability to move without internal resistance. We may never be totally cured, but we can have intimations of what it would be like to be healthy in a healthy world, and we can set ourselves on that path by the guideposts that are intuitively most true. If this book has a practical purpose it is to sharpen people's senses of how to recognize those guideposts and how to keep their options open when either medical or holistic rhetoric clouds the issue.

The trouble with our revolutionary insights and belief in the holistic cure is that these are too good to be true. They have nothing to do with the lives most people lead. Pursuing exogenous images of enlightenment and energy, men and women lose the sense of what it is to experience *themselves.* They attach themselves religiously to their craniosacral unwindings, muscle-testing regimens, vitamin and enzyme elixirs, radionic and affirmation waves, or quantum jolts of homeopathic doses; they see environmental illness, psychic and bacterial parasites, and industrial allergies lurking everywhere, wear masks while walking in the streets, and guard their diets zealously; they become workshop junkies, worshipping Byron Katie or Stanislav Grof and taking the same classes over and over again in search of connection, romance, health, and enlightenment. Doing nothing and entertaining their own shadow would be more efficacious than even the most energizing therapy.

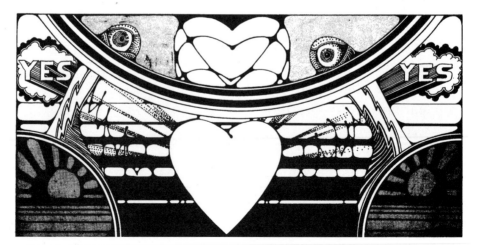

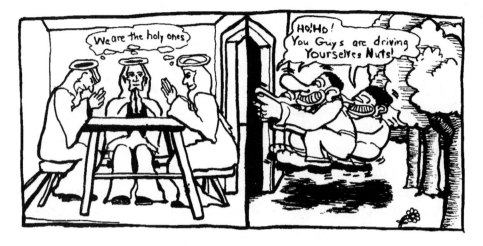

Carl Jung diagnosed the holistic disease as long ago as 1929:

One cannot be too cautious in these matters, for what with the imitative urge and a positively morbid avidity to possess themselves of outlandish feathers and deck themselves out in this exotic plumage, far too many people are misled into snatching at such "magical" ideas and applying them externally, like an ointment. People will do anything, no matter how absurd, in order to avoid facing their own souls. They will practice Indian yoga and all its exercises, observe strict regimen of diet, learn theosophy by heart, or mechanically repeat mystic texts from the literature of the whole world—all because they cannot get on with themselves and have not the slightest faith that anything useful could ever come out of *their* souls. Thus the soul has been gradually turned into a Nazareth from which nothing good can come. Therefore let us fetch it from the four corners of the earth—the more far-fetched and bizarre it is the better! . . . Were it so, then God had made a sorry job of creation, and it were high time for us to go over to Marcion the gnostic and depose the incompetent demiurge. . . . But man is worth the pains he takes with himself, and he has something in his own soul that can grow.[8]

The Problem of Authoritarian Evangelism

THE YEAR I wrote the first version of this book, I reported on Ruth Carter Stapleton's visit to the Berkeley Holistic Health Center to perform Christian healing ceremonies on the week's calendar with a Celestial Rainbow Healing Evening and a *t'ai chi* class. This was a hopeful glimpse, at the time, of the emerging "planet medicine." In the same month her brother Jimmy Carter, President of the United States, appealed to the Black African continent in America's behalf as against the state atheism of the Soviet Union. These loosely paired events evoked a mythic allusion to a legendary time. One could imagine a global-political fusion of spiritualism, voodoo, and evangelism—United Churches of Africa and the Mississippi in alliance with the Rosicrucian Temples of Bohemia and California. That moment has since passed, some of its potential realized in a new unaffiliated global energy medicine and a breakdown of authoritarian Communism, some of it degraded into religious fascism, anarchy, mob rule, and ethnic cleansing.

Occult medicine, faith healing, and the invocation of spontaneous cures unfortunately tend to spawn their own corrupt gurus and authoritarian institutions. The mysterious and often hierarchical nature of healing requires unquestioning faith and invariably a charismatic leader not under the social constraints present in traditional tribal situations. The healer is literally one who makes contact with spirits, gods, death, or unknown forces. He is the hope of all who view him and put their fate in his magic; thus, he (or she) can control the lives of clients and disciples, or even whole communities. All charismatic healers are susceptible to fraud and betrayal—sometimes intentionally perpetrated, more often the result of their own unconscious ego inflation. It turns out to be difficult even for the most enlightened and carefully trained masters to care for their compliant disciples. "Healing" has thus become the tool of hierarchical, nonhumanist, and nonprogressive movements throughout history.

At the moment the physician loses interest in and compassion for his patients, they serve merely as objects to aggrandize him and increase his power. This process, as noted earlier in this volume, is not limited to the politics of esoteric cures. Conventional allopathic doctors, non-Western spiritual gurus, and charismatic revolutionary leaders equally run the risk of ego inflation. All cures are to some degree esoteric and power-transferring. All healers exchange treatments for power: their implicit obligation is to return that power to the patient.

Many healers and gurus want the lives of their devotees as gratitude for their spectacular deeds of prayer and energy mediation. The transition from healing to maiming—from respect to contempt—is subtle and often imperceptible. It is a small step from mass evangelical healing to mob lynchings, cult enslavement and brainwashing, oppression of women and infidels, genocides, etc. What cannot be saved is cursed or wounded (out of frustration or as ransom against future healings); what cannot be healed is fed to demons who inhabit the zone between grace and malignancy (*they* must be fed, too). In fact, the organized militias and spontaneous gang violence that distinguished the twentieth century (and continue, past 9-11-01, into the twenty-first) draw on the same ecstatic and intrinsic energies that served occult physicians.

The danger of diseases of the spirit is that once they have numbed individuals, their victims turn the pathology blindly against an exterior "evil." The parapsychological becomes the paramilitary; the voodoo priest is suddenly part of the junta. Zombies kill the innocent, or order the innocent to kill each other; hence a whole people can be sacrificed for the health and affluence of another people, as though *they* were the disease.

The lineage of medicine must always bear the caution of these abuses; it provides the healer with an array of magics, so it must also provide him with their ritual antidotes. Spirit forces that heal are not merely pliable allies in the service of good: they are also agents of disease and madness that occupy the border-zone between epiphany and apocalypse. The collective numinosity of a Navaho sand-painting ceremony is under strict sanction and ruled by lineage and ritual. All its mythological references, symbols, and internal legends conspire to keep disjunctive forces at bay. The fact that no one may remember their exact relationships and applications is an advantage because everyone is subject to their unconscious meanings and egalitarian order and no one can appropriate snakes or vultures or lightning for personal use.

On the other hand, healing in the theater of apocalyptic religion is devastingly and fundamentalistically specific; it awakens the mute masses and calls out what is deep and silent (and unwilling to be cured) in them. It is medicinal shamanism on a mass scale at the same time that it is diabolic sorcery and voodoo—different faces of the same mystery. The dark forces—precisely along the same tracks and with a different attention and relationship to *chakras*—shadow those of light.

The collective spirit of a populace in economic and social turmoil is under no sanction and potentially ruled by psychopathology and pandemonium. The faith healer, in different guises, becomes the McCarthyite politician, the hooded inquisitor, the prophet demanding collective suicide unto a golden world. Adolf Hitler practiced his street politics and theater in the time-honored tradition of charismatic healing. He converted collective kundalini "tingling" into gas chambers and machines of death. Since his downfall, humans have institutionalized such medicine, creating more ingenious and antiseptic machineries in the name of ethnic therapy.

Chairman Mao Zedong was considered the beneficent modern father of the Chinese people; even in the West, he was a shining Left Wing hero. Yet, it appears that he horrifically abused his power. For decades, while he was revered as a Marxist philosopher king, egalitarian general, and founder of a new epoch of agrarian reform and class justice, he was actually replicating the most debauched feudal emperors of China. Alienated from his comrades and isolated from most human contact, he held nightly orgies with proscripted concubines, in part to gain longevity according to the Taoist theory of taking on *chi* during intercourse. His personal physician for more than twenty years, Dr. Li Zhisui, describes how Mao ordered women brought to him from peasant homes and from official acting and dancing troupes.[9] This same Mao, the author of brilliant texts on the plight of the poor and hungry, rose to power as a savior of the disenfranchised masses.

While partying and indulging himself with consorts, he was presiding emotionlessly over the slaughter of millions, unleashing saturnalian waves of Red Guards murdering, disembowelling, and cannibalizing those unfortunate enough to be fingered as class enemies. When Dr. Li told Mao he was spreading genital herpes to his sexual partners, the Chairman seemed puzzled at his concern. "If it's not hurting me," he said, "then it doesn't matter." In the same spirit, he refused to take a bath. "I bathe myself in the bodies of my women," Mao boasted. He meant that he was bathing in their *chi* for the good of the nation. "The Chairman is such an interesting person," one liaison told Dr. Li. "But he cannot tell the difference between one's love of him as the leader and one's love of him as a man."[10]

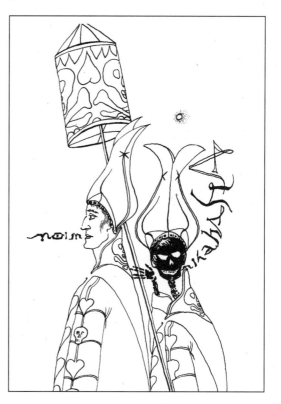

The charismatic physician must transcend duality in himself or herself before practicing on others. He must be able to tell the difference between himself as a healer and himself as a man. He must not bathe in the bodies—or spirits—of his subjects. In that context, egalitarian political influences on healing are crucial. This is in fact the major accomplishment (despite widespread individual abuses) of institutional allopathy.

Blaming the Sick Person

ONE OF THE flaws of holistic and affirmation-based ontology is that often the victim of disease is blamed for something that is functionally out of his or her control. Nowadays cancer is spoken of in some circles as retribution, as a disease of repressed anger, or another archetype, the cells themselves ostensibly picking up the nihilism of the person, punishing emotional inauthenticity or a lapse in faith with disease. Conservative preachers likewise blame the gay "lifestyle" for the AIDS infection.

Whereas karmically disease is destiny and is not arbitrary or meaningless in terms of the life of the organism, most of this happens in such a deeply unconscious dimension that no one but the most enlightened avatar or advanced yogi could control his absolute health and destiny, and these can only for a period of time before they too submit to natural law and decay. Those born into African epidemics are surely not responsible for their diseases. At most, one interacts creatively with their environment, situation of ancestry and birth, and present historical conditions in a balance of health and sickness.

Edward Whitmont points out that,

> [W]hile relatively valid as one particular view of the illness dynamic, the exclusive [dependence upon the ego] as the sole focus tends to place too much emphasis upon the ego's deliberateness, power and freedom. Our historical patriarchal and heroic religions, myths and cultural viewpoint have tended either to burden us with full responsibility and guilt for becoming ill, or conversely, in the nineteenth-century positivistic-mechanistic backlash version, to present us as hapless victims of random "accidental" events or malfunctions.[11]

Illness, like injury and murder, originates from below without regard for belief systems either way. The worst curmudgeon, even an assassin or hit-man, may thrive, while a compassionate "Florence Nightingale" or "Mother Teresa" may struggle with lifelong disease. Sickness is not MODALITIES itself a judgment.

Whitmont spells out the true psychosomatic thermodynamics of health and disease:

> There should be no need to emphasize that, even in the case of secondary gains, it is not necessarily the conscious ego personality that "wants" to be ill. Neither, as a rule, is one able to produce illness by conscious volition, nor is one necessarily aware of the underlying dynamic that leads to illness.
>
> Illness is the "invasion" of a dynamic that arises out of the Self field and leads to a dramatic conflict which encodes itself psychosomatically. The form impulses that motivate our life's dynamic in terms of need for love and emotional closeness, power and assertion, and meaning and self-expression (the domains of Freud, Adler, and Jung respectively) imprint themselves in the codes of our vital, behavioral, emotional, and mental fields without necessarily reaching conscious awareness. (Even thoughts can be unconscious; we may, for instance, feel and act on the basis of convictions which we take for granted as "obvious" facts.) ... We may suffer stomach cramps without being conscious of the fact that we are afraid of something, or rheumatic stiffness without realizing our existential stiffness. The formal patterns simply "become" innervation, ways of moving, of behavior, emotion, or thoughts, depending upon the code form of their incarnation. Our wills, thoughts, and emotions, hence, are not necessarily the originating causes of our psychosomatic ailments. Rather, like their bodily counterparts, they are forms of enactment of archetypal impulses.[12]

Because no one gets to control the molecules, cells, neurons, or emotional drives that make us up, no one should pretend to be responsible. Grandiosity only increases negative innervation. Whitmont emphasizes the importance of observing this mystery and not drifting into sterile holistic ideology:

> To challenge the sufferer with questions like "Why did you want to get ill?" or "What are you doing wrong to make yourself sick?" has become a not infrequent implication by "New Age" practitioners. Such challenges are cruel and burden the ego with a responsibility

for unconscious incursions which are not in its power to stop or prevent. By adding guilt to the already existing suffering, they may, in fact, increase ego defensiveness and thereby delay the receptivity to helpful insights into the possible meaning of the suffering. . . .

We must beware, therefore, of apportioning guilt, shame, and blame to ourselves or others for not "individuating adequately" or not being able to heal ourselves, whether psychologically, by "right living," or through "sufficient faith." The very assumption that we can always do the "right" thing amounts to hubris of assuming that god-like powers can be available to us always and just for the asking. For anyone at any time, even for the "strongest" or "most conscious" and responsible person, the invading claim of the new can be too much. Therefore, while in principle at least, every illness can be healed through the "appropriate sacrifice," not every ill person may always be curable. While we are alive, illness as a potential or actualized fact is our constant companion.[13]

Of course, one should try to put mind over matter, heart and spirit over pathology, because sometimes molecules respond to a ballad and a prayer. Every disease has a shadow through which it is curable, but not necessarily in this lifetime.

The Addiction to Therapy

THE PROFOUND EFFECT of ideological myths in uncentering people was seen in the late twentieth-century fad whereby many individuals replaced their own memories and sense of self with induced memories, often under hypnosis or from some more "holistic" trance. People became so unsure of who they were that they no longer know if they have been abused sexually by their fathers, kidnapped and probed by aliens, or (for that matter) reigned as kings and queens in Atlantis and served with Alexander the Great. Their own existences seemed incomplete, so they asked someone else to tell them who they were, to lead them inside themselves, invariably to a "memory" imprint they then adopted as their guiding star.

Just interview anyone who has been "anointed" with rape, alien abduction, or execution during the Cathar massacre. They serve these images as faithfully as if they were recent experiences. They give up the immediacy and priority of the self as lived.

Yet reality is everywhere, now as well as then, here as well as after death. It is never a matter of where one has been. It is where one is now, which is always "bardo." If memory were that crucial to being, we would never forget.

In the most recent fad of "recovering repressed memory of sexual abuse," so-called victims are selected by overly eager therapists as anyone who suspects or comes to believe that such abuse must have taken place or even anyone who "feels different from other people."[14] Sexual promiscuity and lack of interest in sex are taken equally as confirmatory symptoms. Patients are encouraged to stifle all doubts about whether such abuse ever took place.

> The recovery movement, it must be plainly understood, is not primarily addressed to people who always knew about their sexual victimization. Its main intended audience is women who aren't at all sure that they were molested, and its purpose is to convince them of that fact and embolden them to act upon it.[15]

"Acting" has taken the form of women accusing their fathers of rape, Satanism, necrophilia, and murder of other children with consequent lawsuits and criminal trials. The so-called process of healing is "not about surmounting one's tragic girlhood but about keeping the psychic wounds open, refusing forgiveness or reconciliation, and joining the permanently embittered corps of 'survivors.'"[16]

This has evolved into an unexamined ritual in which therapists come to prefer the recovery of molestation fantasies to the difficulties of present life. Of course, there *are* real victims, but this ceremony has little to do with them, except insofar as it requires their very real testimony for its own survival.

As a rule of thumb, any physician (alternative or allopathic, psychoanalytic or physical in orientation) should question himself as soon as every patient (or most patients) start showing up with the same condition—or can be talked into the same memory. Memory and kinesthesia are so subtle that they can be inculcated externally as if from within.

Contemporary psychotherapy too often provides a person with a new story or pseudo-memory to replace a so-called wounded or fragmented one. That fiction can be based upon the Freudian notion of an "original trauma," or it can be highly visioned, as many neo-Jungian and shamanic versions are, with gods and goddess functions, Amazons and heroes, reenactments of ancient myths, and socially constructed images of masculinity and femininity. (Jung himself would be appalled by the present worship of the archetypes.)

The goal of therapy is always adaptation to a therapeutic story. And by whose authority is one tale truer than another? The lives of Christ and other great teachers have been scandalously abused by various denominations of preachers as well as by Church hierarchies themselves for centuries, i.e., have been used to steal people's own mysterious lives and replace them with blind allegiance to a literalized account that can be managed and exploited. Even the most benignly expansive healers and gurus run the risk of habituating their disciples to the utopian cure and themselves to their own authoritarian system.[17]

The person seeking clarity in the marketplace of therapy is reduced finally to choosing among models of co-dependency, primal violation, archetypal quest, and low self-esteem. But what about the actual and immediate life he or she is also leading? Does it just become a shadow of therapeutic reality and imagined or real victimization? Can it be made one's own without first shattering therapeutic authority and its act of clan initiation?

It would seem that our soul-doctors have blundered into just the confusion of psychological and spiritual authority our Constitution sought to guard against by separating Church and State. Tithing to a therapist for personal growth and vision is perhaps only superficially removed from tithing to a priesthood. And who is to say that the psychiatric profession is not the priesthood reinvented?

On the other hand, this is not a hardhat anti-therapy position. I don't accept the "pre-psychotherapeutic" trashing of therapy. If one has little sense of an internal life or of the cause-and-effect cycles of their emotions, then they can be healed in remarkable ways by working with someone who is emotionally resonant and skillful at transference. As long as both parties are clear about the limitations of the exercise and neither has heroic goals, then the therapeutic dialogue recovers not only the patient's true memory but, more crucially, his or her emotional authenticity.

One casts his or her voice into the void and takes the answer that returns, no matter who is speaking or if the void is inhabited or not. Oftentimes traditional divinatory methods (like Navaho myth-chanting and sand painting) or oracular therapies (like reading the *I Ching* or medical dowsing and astrology) can have profound and creative impacts by supplying totally novel images in circumstances where an imposition of the rigid archetypes of Westernized shamanism would represent only a continued assault of an authoritarian consciousness. And this is because the unconscious answer is always liberating, always a process-oriented response to the mysteries of psyche ... as long as one doesn't literalize or become superstitious about its meanings.

The casting of astrological charts, for instance, has the possibility of revealing cycles which are beyond consciousness and unconsciousness (and are routinely ascribed to stars and planets for lack of any other metaphor). That is, they are consciousness-mediated cycles outside of ordinary objective viewpoints. "Uranus and Venus in opposition" or "three planets in the twelfth house" are potentially radicalizing challenges. They become programmatic myths only if the astrologer or diviner (or even the planets themselves) are elevated to the level of authorities.

I would recommend Polarity Therapy, *Chi Gung*, craniosacral work, and, in some instances, Gestalt and other vision quests as substitute "psychoanalyses"—in other words, therapies that energize one to make a new life rather than tell a new version of an old story. In the end life itself is what the gods of Egypt (or any nome) put on the scales; they make no dispensation for sanity or insanity, no extraneous distinction between myth and reality. They say simply: "Live!"

Wanting to Get Well

MEDICINE HAS NO MEANING. That is, medicine cannot supply the missing meaning or direction to a life. After the healing, deep-sea divers return to the sea; musicians return to their music; philosophers go back to language and reality. As Werner Erhard, L. Ron Hubbard, and other "human potential" business people have proven, money-makers continue to make money—more money. Those who looked out for number one continue to look out for *Numero Uno,* etc. A medicine can be proposed around any process and play into a variety of possible meanings. The same skeletal adjustment can lead to quiescence in one person and aggression in another.

In the emphasis on hidden process and the unconscious mind, we have forgotten consciousness, where our lives and selves (as we know them) occur. It is mostly in the awake mind that systems of medicine form and the doctors do their diagnoses. It is in terms of the ego that will is aroused and a decision to get better is initiated. The intentional discipline required by the most powerful societies of ritual magic and healing reminds us that the conscious mind is a critical player in this affair.

The modern student of *t'ai chi ch'uan* holds himself up with a habitually stiff torso; what is trying to sink is the *chi,* which is supposed to sink; but against a history of tissue and mind tension, the pain is unbearable—for the disciples of Ida Rolf and Matthias Alexander, too. Gravity is a dread opponent.

These exercises must be repeated thousands of times, tens of thousands of times, day after day, for years, and finally for a lifetime. The teacher (doctor) cannot do *t'ai chi* for him any more than he can eat or sleep for him. All he can do is demonstrate and correct, demonstrate and correct. At some early point, any student runs into insurmountable difficulties; it is so painful to move through the positions in the prescribed manner that he adjusts to take strain off his weaker areas. The teacher corrects this, and ultimately the student is asked to correct it himself, to learn to observe when one part of his body tightens to allow another part to carry out a difficult movement. The corrections are profoundly painful, but the goal is to move with integration and cohesion, according to life principle, despite the pain.

There is always a relationship between conscious will and the emergence of internal intelligence. In order to grow and heal, one must suffer, either in redirecting attention under hardship or in having life itself shift painfully after being healed passively. Systems that involve direct suffering allow a person to participate consciously in changes rather than become a straw in their wind. Such bringing to consciousness is one of the things life *is*. In his spiritual school in France, Gurdjieff hung educational aphorisms on the walls of the Study House, including:

> The worse the conditions of life, the more productive the work—always provided you remember the work.[18]

> Only conscious suffering has any sense.[19]

I am reminded also of the culminative moment of Jean Cocteau's *Orphée,* where Death and her helper Heurtebise struggle to force Time backward in order to undo their damage. Heurtebise screams that it is impossible. An invisible wind ripples his hair; his every muscle strains. But they lean back against the flow of events and force the film to unravel to its beginning. All the while Death continues to shout at him—Death as the woman, the actress he loves, urging him to use his will, reminding him, "Without our wills, we are cripples." Even "Death" is.

Medicine men and women have long known that the organism must want to get well in order to get well; it must want to live in order to live. We have seen through this book that such wanting comes from the core of one's being and has little to do with surficial greed for life. It does not mean that all diseases are finally curable if the patient wants to live. It means that the medicine itself is not the final court; the individual is. The medicine sets into action the healing force and reminds the body of its implicit desire to be well (the same desire that originally led it to *be* at all). This must be a single message and not a mixed message; it must be a specific unignorable shot, a homeopathic simillimum. The body famously knows how to resist mixed messages.

A sting or irritation is more compassionate than a salve because it is more definite and communicative. It is brief, swift, and precise, like a microdose or chiropractic adjustment. The acupuncturist uses a fine needle. The bioenergetic therapist seizes the pinpoint edge of the patient's compulsion and fear and exacerbates it.

Nurturing is curative too. After all, an organism can be irritated into exhaustion or terror unless there is something in the irritation to which it can respond positively. It is important to say, "There you go! You're doing great!" at key moments. This confirms that, even though "breaking through" hurts and sometimes terrifies too, it is the right—not the wrong—direction. Encouragement from the healer is pure, instantaneous energy.

Any shift in bodily attention is communicated back to the will, to express itself in the life of the person. It may not even be recognized as coming from the doctor or medicine.

Discussions about whether a person wants to get well are doomed to go around in circles, for wanting and not wanting can be indistinguishable ploys of the self. Not wanting to get well is itself part of the disease, but it also can be the irritant catalyzing the cure.

Arguments in our culture about what is legal death and when we can stop trying to save someone who does not want to live or is brain-dead and on life support are telling indications of our dilemma. When we don't know why we are alive and have bodies, nor how to inhabit them happily, we put the issue to every desperate test. At the same time, we stand stupefied before legalistic and problematic definitions of things we must ultimately know from the inside if we are to know them at all.

It is as though people try only partially to be healed, only partially to be alive. The dichotomy becomes: now I do this/now I am me. When they are being cured of something, they withhold their more sophisticated part, making the experience as if a cure of someone else to whom they are allotted privileged access.

During a seminar in Vermont in 1977, the poet and homeopath Theodore Enslin was being questioned along these lines when someone raised the issue of the relative nonhierarchy of importance of symptoms in homeopathy, implying that the wish to get well *must* be a more significant symptom than calluses on an elbow. Enslin objected:

> If you're really trying to get into homeopathic thinking, you have to erase those artificial boundaries—that thought is different from a hangnail. It's not. It's a manifestation of you. I've always loved that story about the guy who went to [Charles Godlove] Raue, who was one of the Philadelphia school, a really very eminent homeopath. And he was an old man. He had many many things wrong with him. He had gout. He had prostatitis. And he had loose teeth. And he had all these things. So Raue gave him a pill. He said, "Well, now, is this for my gout? Or is it for my loose teeth?" and so on. And Raue finally said, "Your name is Miller, isn't it?"
>
> "If you were really going to be a good homeopathic patient, there wouldn't have to be any more discussion. You simply realize *it's all one thing.* You cannot consider one ailment or another. You have a burn on your arm which doesn't heal. The aim of usual medicine is to clear that one spot. Cure it. Fight it. Homeopathically, we don't think that way; we think about the whole organism. Because there is that one disease manifestation, there is an indication that the entire organism is diseased and you've got to treat it that way."
>
> "But still," the questioner persisted, "isn't not really wanting to get better such a basic and serious symptom that one won't even seek out a doctor in the first place? How do you overcome that?"
>
> "Well, that is a personal decision," Enslin replied. "There are cer-

tain medicines that can bring you to the place where you *do* want to. But sometimes not. Some so-called failures of treatment can simply be traced to a personal resistance."

"But then isn't a personal resistance just another symptom?"

"Yes it is. Yes it is. Of course we're always looking for the miracle that will cure us of everything. I don't think that homeopathy or very much of anything else will ever do that for us. And when people weren't talking about psychosomatic disease, Hahnemann himself was the first one, by saying, yes, the mental symptoms are equally important. But they are sometimes hard to deal with. You get to the point of [James Tyler] Kent and the mental symptoms are more important than anything else. I think he got to the place where perhaps he *over*emphasized them. He did because there was absolutely no support for them anywhere. I mean there *is* a balance. The thing that we really need to do, the thing that more than anything else can get over that kind of resistance, is simply the admission that there is no difference between any kind of symptom and any other. The old division of mind and body—with all our philosophizing about it—means we still think we are superior to the animals, we still think that somehow our thinking brain is going to bail us out."

He paused for a moment and then continued:

"You asked in our earlier talk: 'Would you say we are, as a race, diseased?' I would say, 'Yes we certainly are.' Because we place an emphasis on something which has nothing to do with what makes us move. We think that—we *think!*—that is the problem."

The questioner still proceeded: "Whose chances of cure are greater: the person who wants to get better but doesn't take a homeopathic medicine or the person who doesn't want to get better but has the right medicine prescribed for him?"

"Well, the chances of cure without a homeopathic medicine are far greater than without a feeling that one wants to be cured. I mean there are many instances of the whole placebo thing. A person is convinced that this *will* do it, and he *really* wants to be cured: therefore he *is* cured! That, in a sense, is a homeopathic high potency. It is a strong enough wish in the person to outrage the system to the point where it will cure itself, which is the principle behind all of this."

"But where does the resistance to being well come from in the first place? How do we get to the bottom of it?"

"There is a direction to your repeated question. You're hammering at this one particular thing. But you see, in doing that, you're actually doing what we all do when we depend upon our thinking processes. It's a very difficult thing, because somehow we're going to have to do it in reverse if we're ever going to get to the place where all of these things are in balance. But there are places where probably this is the wrong direction to take—if you really want to know. If you really want to know, don't want to know! I mean, enlightenment never comes if someone wants to be enlightened."[20]

This is a shared paradox in the history of medicine and philosophy. The wish to be cured *does* locate in the will, but it is not the conscious self-expressed will we understand in language; it is the real inner will of the body. The conscious will must, at some point, work counter to literal intention, to itself, in order to incorporate the "meaning" of the deeper will. For "healing to be possible, we must desire this healing and yet have no attachment to it," writes Body Electronics practitioner Douglas Morrison. "We must be willing to put our full effort into the process and yet have no attachment to the outcome of that effort."[21] The way a person expresses to himself that he wants to get well may in fact be the very way to stay sick. One thing is clear: the ambition itself is not the desire; the ambition is usually the disease. So the person must suddenly discover how *not* to want to be well (which is certainly not the same as wanting not to be well).

Enslin continued:

"I think the only real problem and the only real resistance to this whole way of thinking is this refusal to admit that there are no divisions. You can sit and talk philosophically about it, and it's very popular to do that. You can talk about a holistic universe and so forth and so on, but we don't *think* that way. If we started to do that, probably there would be far less disease. And homeopathy or any other specialty would fade away. You wouldn't need this particular way of looking at things because everything was looked at in the same way."

"What would our lives be like if we did think in that way?"

"I have no idea. It would seem to me, from every indication that I've had personally, simply looking at animals, trees, or anything else, that it would be far easier to do things that we really want to do, or say we want to do. We have simply forgotten. We think. We think we are the masters. We forget that we aren't any more important than a raccoon. We think of *our* lives, the preciousness of *our* life. Even a man like Schweitzer: he is a humanitarian, but he is not a totalitarian—the reverence for life; there is always the feeling, 'human life—this is more important.' If we could just drop this, maybe we wouldn't have to go through this backward trip through the labyrinth to get to where we could really function."

"Well, we can say we're going to do that. We can theorize it—"

"Don't theorize it. Do it! Of course it's impossible: therefore do it!"[22]

Notes

1. Lolette Kelly, "Faith and the Placebo Effect," in *Ions: Noetic Sciences Review,* March-May 2002, #59, Petaluma, California, p. 5.

2. Edward C. Whitmont, personal communication, New York, 1975.

3. Anna Quindlen, "Gulf War's Killing Legacy," *San Francisco Chronicle* (October 10, 1994), from *The New York Times* wire service.

4. Ian Grand, personal communication, Berkeley, California, 1979.

5. Ibid.

6. Jon Carroll, "The Odd Saga of Marlo Morgan," *San Francisco Chronicle* (September 7, 1994), p. E8.

7. Carroll, "The Odd Saga of Marlo Morgan," *San Francisco Chronicle* (September 8, 1994), p. E10.

8. Carl Jung, *Psychology and Alchemy,* translated from the German by R.F.C. Hull (London: Routledge and Kegan Paul, 1953), pp. 95–98.

9. Tai Hung-chao (trans.), *The Private Life of Chairman Mao: The Memories of Mao's Personal Physician, Dr. Li Zhisui* (New York: Random House, 1994).

10. Ibid.

11. Edward C. Whitmont, *The Alchemy of Healing: Psyche and Soma* (Berkeley, California: North Atlantic Books, 1993), p. 15.

12. Ibid., p. 129.

13. Ibid., pp. 130, 168.

14. Frederick Crews, "The Revenge of the Repressed, Part II," *The New York Review of Books,* Vol. XLI, Number 20 (December 1, 1994), p. 50.

15. Ibid., p. 49.

16. Ibid.

17. See Charles Poncé, *The Archetype of the Unconscious and the Transfiguration of Therapy: Reflections on Jungian Psychology* (Berkeley, California: North Atlantic Books, 1990), for a full discussion of this issue.

18. G. I. Gurdjieff, *Views From the Real World: Early Talks* (New York: Dutton, 1975), p. 273.

19. Ibid., p. 274.

20. Theodore Enslin, at a seminar at Goddard College, Plainfield, Vermont, recorded in May, 1977.

21. Douglas Morrison, *How We Heal: Nutritional, Emotional, and Spiritual Fundamentals* (Berkeley, California: North Atlantic Books, 2001), p. 38.

22. Theodore Enslin, at a seminar at Goddard College, Plainfield, Vermont, recorded in May, 1977.

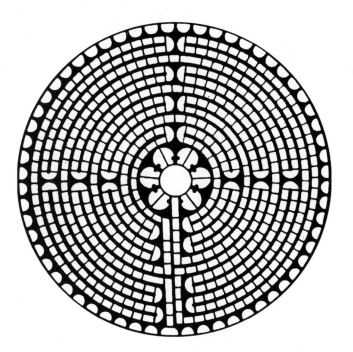

*Beyond
Ideology*

CHAPTER TEN

The Politics and Spirituality of Medicine

Ecological Update

PLANETARY DISEASE now threatens the continuation of our species and all other species on this world. We cannot exist indefinitely in an escalating carbon-dioxide climate with a fraying ozone layer, spreading deserts, radioactive lakes, and an increasingly devitalized biosphere—even assuming legendary *Chi Gung* and *feng shui* masters and future homeopathic potencies applied to oceans and rivers. After all, faith healers and shamans cannot turn Mars or Venus into habitable planets on a physical plane. Even leaving aside matters of intra- and interspecies slaughter, even conceding nuclear winter and atomic waste as politically addressable issues, there remains a foolhardy and mindless squandering of farmland, rain forest, oceans and atmosphere; an offhand poisoning of the layers of life; and an arrogant extinction of species (and with them, their unique ecospheres, genes, medicines, and spirits). Some have observed that the planet itself now has AIDS, its immune system weakened to a degree even Gaia cannot reconstitute it without hard yoga from its inhabitants.

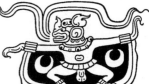

If this is the case, as sooner or later it will be, then the big medicinal task of the coming decades is to understand that issues of individual health and planetary health are inextricably linked in increasingly shorter and simpler loops. It is probably not too late for people to heal themselves and then begin healing the environment (or vice versa for those of more social-activist bent), but both are necessary. Just like the body, the world is incarnate; it responds to realities and physical laws, to molecules of carbon and oxygen, photons radiating from the sun, and whatever vital and psychic energies obtain. The ecological crisis has no agenda; in fact, it is no more a crisis than chlorophyll or fog are. Thus, it cannot ultimately be solved in an arena of legislation and discourse. With drug addiction, Bloods and Crips, child pornography, corporate profiteering, and school shootings on the mere surface of American life, there are hardly "50 simple ways."

THE PRESENT DEMOGRAPHY of homelessness is more than a growing cadre of people who have either the courage or desperation to bottom out on the streets. We are all blown by the same careless wind. This planet is stirred up like a hornet's nest, and none of us any longer know our true ancestral homes. The streets are at least real. They keep no illusions of meaningless repetitive labor for tawdry wages or fake possession of fortress-spaces that must then be paid for again and again with toy money. They offer only the reduction of time and breath and landscape to what it is, what only it is—that we are here in a mystery and "bound away" to a mystery, even as the "wide Missouri" was to an earlier ragtag people.

The sense of forced migration, which has famously displaced the native peoples of North and South America and much of Asia, Africa, and Oceania, we now understand is displacing everyone, if not geographically, then economically—or both—sometimes with poverty, sometimes with heavy artillery. The wind is strong enough they are blown to sea in paper boats and driven shoeless across snowy mountain passes. Those who remain in the lands of their ancestors suffer global-mafia intrusion, guerrillas and terrorists, and multinational displacement of the meaning (and crops) of their lives. The basic road gang is Indonesian loggers in the employ of the Chinese People's Army, taking apart tribal Laos and Belize equally. Or it is Arabs, Chechens, and Pakistanis in the employ of Saudi and Egyptian corporate terrorists raping and devastating Afghanistan and Somalia. Even algae and microbes have been set adrift in poisoned waters and air.

Those Indians and Aborigines who continue to conduct old-tongue ceremonies on the landscapes of the Dreamtime are one by one being enticed and corrupted by the global New Age packaging of their epochal ways. The dominant culture is desperate to be loved by everyone, even those who carry the last embers of another reality. It is in the interest of the cocaine/virtual-reality megastructure to seduce every lama, shaman, artisan, and Divine Feminine, if not with power, material goods, and sex, then with dreams of flying the cargo-cult airplanes and saving the soul of Mother Earth. The money that is paid in greater and greater decimals to blackmail even Cassandra to stop crying out to us to see who we are means less and less as we are more and more spun each year in the cyclone World Market. No wonder some choose to stop living this hollow cinema and sit begging on the streets. The shadow of our decimation must be cast somewhere. Cassandra must occupy her given throne.

A sense of being afloat in oneself infects the dwellers of urban ghettos and lavish suburbs, as endemic to lords in their British castles suffering their own sexual decadence as it is to Mexican Indians displaced by agricultural and timber barons and the radioactive propaganda of a bankrupt state apparatus. No wonder the "aliens" in all their guises, from the denizens of unearthly biology to the most intimate members of our own families, come to abduct and abuse. Yeats' rough beast does indeed slouch closer and closer toward Bethlehem to be . . . . Is the word . . . "born"?

Medicine and Society

M EDICINE IS A CONFLUENCE of practical techniques, remedy provings, scientific experiments, acts of transference, and mutative symbols. It is a *cul de sac* but also an infinitude, for there is nothing in the cosmos that is not an aspect of a disease, that is not potentially a medicine too.

The first volume of this book began with the proposition that the new healing paradigm was more a mythological than a medical statement. I would restate that bias now in different words: healing modalities arise from ecological, psychospiritual, and cultural imperatives and address diseases of the social and karmic body. This process can be represented at two esoteric levels:

First, diseases originate as totemic categories; categories of cure match them in kind. Despite much seeming evidence to the contrary, there are no purely natural diseases. Parasites and toxins may approach lightning and snow in their guilelessness, but even germs and poisons must make their way through various differential layers of code, clan, immunity, cell identity, protective *chi,* body-mind resonance, etc. Their passages through these and any other manifestations are always funnelled into quasi-congruent taxonomies and delegated to cultural classifications. Likewise, there are no medicines not mediated at some level by social constructs and belief systems. The shaman, reggae singer, and voodoo master are phases of the surgeon and the war chief.

Second, the large-scale environmental and cultural diseases of the Earth give rise to new pathologies and modalities of cure. The relationship between disease, cure, and society may be even more basic than that: the present plague of pathology (cultural, physical, psychological, and spiritual) is precisely its own first stage of cure. If we want to know what is wrong with us, we must look to our wars, crimes, diseases, and injustices (especially those that cross lines of clan, class, and species). If we want to discover what the treatment should be, we may observe its homeopathic proving in the disease manifestations themselves. Look to our planetary plague and you will see, albeit draped in executioner's robes, the first ugly stages of our arousal to self-cure. Functional remediation may be a hundred or more years away, but it has already begun, as much in Palestinians blowing up their bodies in Israeli cabarets and African guerrillas cutting off civilian limbs as in new modes of palpation and herbal compounds. The body of the disease *is* the body of the cure.

Alternative medicines represent actual traditions, legacies, and innovations of cure in respect to specific states of disease and dysfunction, but they also comprise a metaphor for an improvisational and radical response to the universal disease crisis. Collectively they are more than a metaphor; they are the second tier of treatment of planetary disease, after the diseases themselves. They arise from a species-wide immune reaction to profound loss of body, self, and heart. At the level of subtext, their modalities invariably address what is awry with the Earth as well as what is ailing in any one client.

"Planet medicine" is this: social, political, ecological, and economic change must occur simultaneously in the body/mind of man and woman; in the forests of symbols that make up global culture; and in the physical forests, seas, and atmosphere of the planet. We must change our beliefs and behavior regarding just about everything: cause and effect, life and death, human society and animal-kind, disease and cure, liberty and the pursuit of happiness. We can posture all we want toward social and corporate change through direct action, plus upheavals of governments, laws, and constabularies to enforce them. However, opposition to these changes (even by their ostensible advocates) will always express itself by exponentially greater force through and against the bodies of actual men and women. Companies will bully their way around regulations and deposit toxins where they want; scientists will engineer and set loose whatever life-forms they care to. Terrorist legions will behave likewise, arming children and burning farms, flying airplanes into buildings regardless of moral or ecological import. There are too many of them, and they have access to much more direct and Machiavellian techniques for carrying out their will. We can scream "Scoundrel!" and "Thief!" all we want, but we are paper tigers. Laws and ethics are flimsy superstructures compared to the brute power of the body. The Thirty Years War in seventeenth-century Germany, with its Halloween cast of armies sweeping over populaces, is a better indication of what we are up against than the antiseptic, cybernetic meltdown of the Gulf War. Cocaine is a perfect modern weapon (disease), operating as it does simultaneously on the body/minds of men and women and the economies of nations, building its own gargantuan bank accounts, raising its own armies from unlimited equity. It is a virtual-reality weapon; there is no way to stop it by conventional means. Germ warfare and military computer viruses are not far behind.

As one East German skinhead put it, "Radical ain't bringing your aluminum cans to the recycling center. 'Radical' is holding a gun to the butcher's head and saying, 'Give me that steak!'" We have ignored this voice so long now, it is speaking as directly as it must—with Uzis, car bombs, street gangs, bioterrorism, and oil wells on fire. Leonard Cohen again: *Everybody knows the war is over./Everybody knows the good guys lost. . . ."*

Yet we are not paper tigers, although we must pretend to be because, frankly, if we showed our teeth we would simply become one of them—Tutsi and Hutu, Palestinian and Israeli, Muslim and Hindu, Serb and Albanian interchangeable. If we are going to join the battle, we must learn how to be the alchemical Lion, not just another predator in regal guise. We must release the philosopher's stone, the elixir from our subtle bodies into rivers, jungles, and winds. We must find the source of energy circulation, of *chi,* in a state powerful enough to transform this stubborn, trenchant manifestation with its armors of ideology. That is why palpation (happy touch) is ultimately the equal of cocaine. It is the body, hence the antidote. Guns and prisons are not.

Despite the growing fad of nihilism and despair in our present state, hope lies in a reciprocality of diseases and their cures. All of these pestilences, environmental disasters, and bombings are medicines—medicines in their raw and unrefined state, alchemical Lions unborn. The "planet medicine" paradigm, which I will discuss at length in the Epilogue, is an early clue to a new direction. Whether it is too little too late we will not know for a long time, probably long past when we have

concluded the opposite.

I would offer that the promise of radical medicines is that by addressing the body directly, they are assimilated in tissues and cells and translated into new mind-sets. They change the meaning of life and death, revise our ethics, and give us new goals and responsibilities as life forms on a planet. More than ecological imperatives or grass-roots action, they get inside people and make them different. A radical medical paradigm is a social paradigm coded in medical language because social and economic disruption is now so widespread and trenchant it is unamenable to other reifications. The cure does not vote, lower the interest rate, or spread global markets. Ultimately, social change must become medicine if it is to be anything more than talk.

I do not mean to argue against ecological and political activism. These are aspects of a therapeutic process and inevitably mutate into medicines too. I mean to suggest that in our present constellation of ideologies, "planet medicine" is the one that bears the most urgent message, for, like disease, it proposes to invade the body/mind and to carry out the work of destiny (or karma) in the living fabric of the Earth. Alternative medicines are a means of opening our core and putting us back in touch with our spirits.

Until a second or third tier of cure is infused directly into the body of the species, medicinal language, i.e., the language of this book, is directed as much at the corporate devastation of the world and of meaning as at clinical alternatives for medical orthodoxies. "Planet medicine" means an injunction to "planet healing," but only in the largest sense.

The Present Status of Medicine and Disease

WATCH THE PLAYERS on the field in a sporting event. Despite all else that is happening (the millions of dollars, the equipment, the attention of masses of people), they too are involved in a struggle to rectify some condition, the same condition that makes their exercise possible. When they are done, it will end—not only the game and

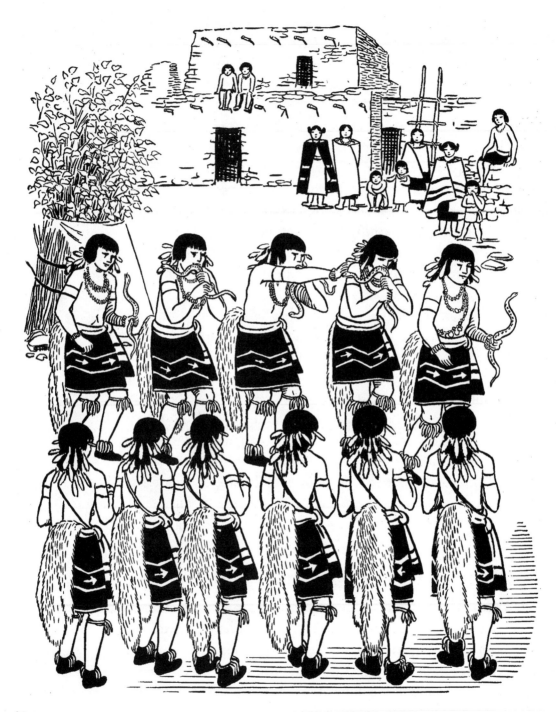

their lives, but the leagues, the records, and any of the rules. They are
not doing it only for themselves, and what they are drawing out and
shaping will not become visible for millennia. (Warfare puts its participants up against opponents far more lethal than they have developed the power to handle—today far more lethal than they could
develop the neutralizing medicine for in a thousand lifetimes.)

No one is innocent, no one is immune, no one is safe, and no one
gets off with a plea of insanity. We must climb to the level of the giant
and meet his gaze with ours.

Our elite establishment would prefer to face petty crises of markets and dangers of terrorists and military adventurism than to address
global poverty and inequity at the roots of our existence. The reality
that is served with the morning newspaper and chatters twenty-four
hours a day on radio and television runs a meaningless gamut from
Democrat to Republican, greed to humanitarianism, nihilism to ecstasy,
but it is all a clever mirage in place of real activity. We reached the point
(election year 2000) when there was no true campaign; the candidates
tried as hard as possible *not* to say who they are or what the consequences of electing them might be. Actors playing politicians, they
aimed only to perfect faux sincerity by which they presented their characters (e.g. George W. Bush as the champion of the poor much like
O. J. Simpson as the misunderstood innocent). They may even have
convinced themselves that the role they were acting was who they really
were.

Only the future will tell us what the real issues of 2000 were; I imagine them to be: the increasing disparity of wealth and resource use
between the wealthy and poor in the world at large, the altering of climate as a by-product of heedless technologization, the destruction of
the biosphere, the relatively short epochal life-span of cheap oil, the
national and international growth of fundamentalist ideologies, and
the spread of gun culture, atomic technology, and virtual and biochemical weaponries among regional and transnational disenfranchised
groups and suicide bombers.

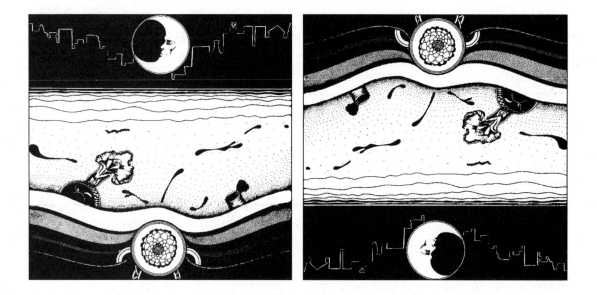

Given the seriousness of these situations and their impending global crisis, ceaseless discussion about trillions of dollars in surplus wealth and how best to use or squander it (as if America were in some special utopian time-warp, untouched by even global warming) not only sounds bizarre but presents to the world (outside our delusionary time-warp) a naive and dangerous act of hubris. Candidates who speak as though this is a time of unprecedented prosperity rather than an unprecedented hell realm for life and spirit on Earth are either shameless deceivers or benighted xenophobes. Either way, they are panderers and beneath the supposed dignity of the offices to which they aspire.

How we behave and how we treat the other entities on this world affect relative disease and health. Until all living things are healthy, no living thing can be healthy. But that incontrovertible rule is going to take a long time to get our unflinching admiration.

A civilization of drugged junk-food addicts working at psycho-spiritually vacuous jobs will not respond to the crisis in time—no matter how many aluminum cans they recycle, contributions they make to Greenpeace, recovery groups they join. When the patient has AIDS

MODALITIES

you don't simply berate the manufacturers of fluorocarbons. You speak to the hollow at the heart of the modern world.

Ailments run banshee from the village doctor into the hills, return armed as revolutionaries. If they were deeply sick, their illness has been transformed by a new possession; but it is not cured, for history merely deals a succession of diseases. They sit behind corporate desks, granting lives and deaths more mundanely than any sovereign or surgeon. Their symptoms and medicines abound on every street—autos, currency, billboards, cigarettes, microwaves, reflections in glass, unknown substances that speed through air and liquid and become part of every impression and breath.

Poisonous urban sprawls and military machines mark the range of interior devitalization. Like the capacity to kill heartlessly, these are marks of powers suppressed and distorted, not powers achieved—true shamanic powers naked somewhere else in the universe. Gangs of juveniles preying on the old and homeless are site-specific eruptions of profound collective diseases. They vibrate, then shriek with the rhythms of raw life. They *want to live.* Within the planet's homeostasis they are statements of relative health, for as long as there is a vital force left, we will not see the disease, we will see only our desperate stands against its ravages—rockets aimed at hospitals, protestors tossed out of planes, mass executions in stadiums, and anonymous anthrax and other vitriol. We will become the disease in a desperate attempt to find the cure. Diasporas stretch from Apache lands, Maori villages, Palestine, Sudan, Tibet, et al.; the exile of jungles, tree spirits, fish, amphibians, reptiles, birds, and mammals fills the akashic records. The scourge of the 1994 *interawahme* in Rwanda is the karmic equivalent of the nuclearization of Tibet and the despoliation and depopulation of its forests and monasteries. This is what punk-ritualized decadence, car-jackings, ritual torture-murders, suicide attackers, and the global "epidemic of guns" must also reflect: our natural resistance, our desire to be here; to liberate the deadly Frog and Spider doctors, the most extreme and dangerous

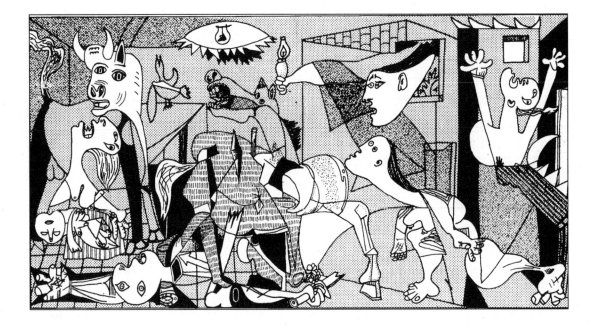

shamanic forms (so close is the malady now to the heart). When the poisons start to eke out, know that the mother serum has also already been prepared.

To become the disease is, esoterically, to strike at the disease. This remedy may well not cure the single junkie or reclaim gang members and the dead victims of their attacks, but its vibration will slowly fan out to the society at large. The process may take generations, but it is inevitable if our planet is to survive.

To spiritual warrior Andrew Harvey, the Indian teacher Mother Meera gave a vision:

"'*Now I will show you the twentieth century.*

"'Gaze with all your courage into its darkness.'

"I saw writhing bodies, burned, flayed, spattered with blood, I saw bombs flowering, the faces of mad dictators as they cut open the eyes of living children, torturers masturbating over the women they had just electrocuted. I saw all these nightmares arising out of the darkness and returning to it.

"Then, just as I thought I would faint because I could not bear the sight and smell of so much horror, I realized, with a clarity and certainty beyond my power to express, that this terrible, unparalleled filth and depravity, this unspeakable desolation spread out over every continent and enacted in every culture, was feeding the New Light.

" *'The spiral of light rises out of the darkness.'*

"She had come because the cries of the tortured and mutilated had called her; She was here because a million tears and screams had pulled her to her torn and battered creation. The horror that humankind had revealed to itself had driven it to call for a new hope, a new world. The depth of that cry was answered, I saw, by a force, a passion, a height of Divine Light that sprang directly out of the heart of the horror, that flamed out, invincible, from its center."[1]

He asks her:

" 'Has the evil of this century happened to make humanity aware of the madness of living without God?'

" 'Yes.'

" 'So humans can turn to God now and take the leap into another Being that God is preparing for them?'

" 'Yes. This leap is certain. It will happen. It is happening now.' "[2]

That God, imbedded in us and wreathed around our cells, our densest and finest fibers, is also a shaman, a yogi, the Christos.

A PARADOX LIES AT the core of this book. On the one hand, we are sick as a species, and getting sicker. On the other, we are beginning to realize that we can heal ourselves, even with the mind alone—perhaps not by a patter of simple thoughts but by a process akin to intention, mentation, and meditation. We are realizing it historically for the first time as a combination of empirical science and internal practice. This synthesis is not even half-born, so we have no idea if it is even real, let alone how far we can go with it. At this point we are still trying to get machines to do all the work without realizing that machines are merely other projections of our mentation.

Right now, while clearly all is lost and the world is submerged in millennial miasm, we are drenched with a universal medicine, and upon the slightest impulse in the right direction we are capable of curing ourselves of just about anything. At each moment we see both sides of the polarity. We are children of the universe and the night. An incalculable darkness is there at the best moments, rejoicing in our freedom and song, warning us in our epiphany. For being one of us, it requires integration too.

Healing is painful because so much remains unconscious or has been forgotten in us. We are working against time to save what is left and transform what is active—as crews are assembling apartment buildings and power lines in transient cities. We worry now about whether there are resources in the sense of minerals and fossil fuels and fish in the sea for another century of this, let alone an eternity. But even as the disease is not visible, the true energy is not within our present frame, either. We do not know where this world is headed, materially or psychically. So we pretend, with our Federal Reserves, free trade, insurance pyramids, and automated clinics, to conserve mere time and restore quantifiable matter.

THERE IS SOMETHING ELSE at hand—equally dangerous and unfathomable—an intruder in the house. The creative energies assigned to *chakras,* auras, meridians, and thought-waves throughout history have their negative counterparts in curses, vampires, malevolent aliens, and "evil eyes." The modern therapist and his comrade surgeon cannot begin to diagnose a plague that so-called primitive shamans were thousands of times closer to than we. It is a joke to think we can cure such a disease. We cannot even tell when our own headaches begin. At the moment the first symptoms (of anything) are perceptible the condition is already irreversible. To "banish" our troubles with palliatives is to waste our time and delude ourselves. Imagine—those who cited "a clear and present danger" thought that by arming ourselves with nuclear missiles (or canisters of germs) we could become safer! Not when the elemental forces of voodoo still rule this world.

"It may be one of the most tragic paradoxes of history," writes parapsychologist Jule Eisenbud, "that throughout the tortuous course of what is somewhat charitably referred to as 'the ascent of man,' the repudiation of such an aim (the 'destruction of the enemy,' to use the utterly emotionless military abstraction) in the ordinary transactions of everyday life has led to a never-ending assault on an omnipresent and protean enemy-by-proxy on a scale that would have been unimaginable to the primitive."[3]

No wonder the Tlingit shaman's chanting sounds positively demonic, even to his followers around him. We are all engaged in witchcraft. "One creates devils when one acts badly," says Eduardo Calderón. "... We should not confuse ourselves that . . . the evil shadows frighten us, kill us. One frightens oneself; it is not the shadow that frightens one."[4]

All healing and pathological processes are finally latent. Meanwhile other forces that do not share our consciousness—or at least are not integrated—dart and weave throughout us. Given the violence we carry out routinely toward one another and with "mere" external tools, and given our undiscovered psychokinetic power, our death wishes and curses may be collectively more pathogenic than all the bacteria and viruses and malignancies on the Earth combined. Our responsibility for this ongoing murder spree, from the large to the small, in wars, plane crashes, and heart attacks, may be the primal guilt that Freud displaced onto a mythological Oedipal event because he would not acknowledge the full and present impact of mind on matter. Our whole technological civilization might then be one vast denial of the diathesis of our voodoo and true powers. (See Volume One, pp. 183–185.)

The whole of Western technology was once an attempt to make life safer and easier by progressive externalization of the gross properties of matter and refinement of the products of that externalization to channel and control cosmic energy. Such an attempt had to be made, and we are now the millage of its experiment and the captains of its gears. Passing through this monstrous metallic-petroleum externalization is crucial to all, from the Yellow Emperor proposing harmony in a shattered world to the Eskimo shaman cursing the cold he cannot cure while the children die around him. He prayed through a glass darkly in an olden time for a sanctuary, a sanctuary of machine-like entities in which we and he now sorrowfully dwell. Better it might still be to face the cold, the night, the wild beasts, the spirits; in fact the present milieu is our only answer to the deep and dark voodoo of nature. It is this relief we requested collectively and perhaps psychokinetically, and it is this disease we must now heal.

Doctors like yogis must begin to treat the nuclear weapons and environmental pollution within all of us, the internalized war from which the external armaments come. It does not mean abandoning science; it does not portend a return to the abuses of traditional magic. It might be no more or less than an enlargement of science to include all its faces, inward and out. The mindfulness and bare attention of the Buddhist monk, the visions of the Peruvian shaman, and the directed intention

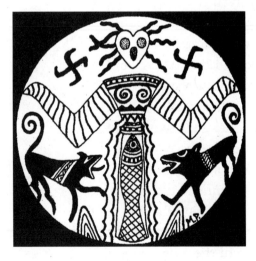

of the craniosacral therapist are relevant to the medical effort necessary to gather the tremendous, unruly energy now on the loose, to return it to its causes which alone can detoxify it.

In our ideal medicine of the future, doctors will treat how the nation is ruled as well as its rulers, and how goods are transferred as well as the buyers and sellers, but they will not be called doctors; likewise, there will also be no politicians or police by the present meaning. "Polis" will stand as a synthesis of justice, production, and healing. What doctors practice will not be called medicine. Senators and corporate directors will be philosopher-scientists.

Some may insist that such a "polis" has already been, in Atlantis or

Old China, and we have destroyed it, and continue to obliterate its bare motes today; but this must not be true, or we would not be in such disharmony; we would not have inherited millennia of war. Or maybe it is true, and we have lost all memory in a cataclysm. In any case, we have only the present Earth to work from. So we begin again.

Lomi founder and aikidoist Richard Heckler was hired by the U.S. Army (1985) to teach meditation, spiritual discipline, and Oriental martial arts to the Special Forces because these skills might lead to higher performance levels. Despite his misgivings about his new students, Heckler found that, compared to therapy junkies in the counterculture, the Green Berets were quite willing to make the sacrifices necessary to become planet healers. They were frustrated shamans—seeking vision quests but offered only the technology of war. They were willing to jump out of airplanes and perfect submarine sabotage as their skills of initiation. After Heckler's training, they had intimations that a Green Beret was first a samurai and a samurai was once a medicine man. This is the kind of medicine soldier needed by the planet, one who cannot be co-opted by its separate warring nationalities.[5]

In 1859 Charles Dickens wrote of the irreclaimable cycle whereby oppressor and oppressed succeed each other generationally in positions of power and abuse. He was describing the peasants of eighteenth-century France who, having seized power from the monarchy, turned against their own populace with the guillotine. Almost a century and a half later, he could have been portraying the Red Guards of Mao's China or any number of post-colonial African military regimes:

> Along the Paris streets, the death-carts rumble, hollow and harsh. Six tumbrils carry the day's wine to La Guillotine. All the devouring and insatiate monsters imagined since imagination could record itself, are fused in the one realization, Guillotine.... Crush humanity out of shape once more, under similar hammers, and it will twist itself into the same tortured forms. Sow the same seed of rapacious license and oppression, and it will surely yield the same fruit according to its kind.

Six tumbrils roll along the streets. Change these back again to what they were, thou powerful enchanter, Time, and they shall be seen to be the carriages of absolute monarchs, the equipages of feudal nobles, the toilettes of flaring Jezebels, the churches that are not my Father's house but dens of thieves, the huts of millions of starving peasants. . . .

Changeless and hopeless, the tumbrils roll along.[6]

The radical Left and the sciences have both failed us, as has the People's Revolution. Once those were our cutting edge, paths to new worlds. But they became arrogant and inflexible; they did not change our lives, and then they denied that anything could change our lives.

If the new samurai-doctors achieve their destiny, they will practice more than medicine. They will bear the seeds of new values that might

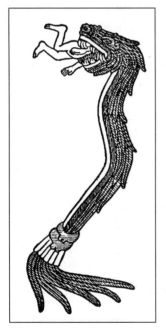

not be the same hierarchies in new clothing, nor merely other tyrants bankrolling the overthrow of the present regime. This will be the first People's Army—meaning, protectors of habitats and sentient beings.

EVEN THOUGH THERE is every reason to be pessimistic in the midst of so much pathology, there is equal reason to be optimistic because we are alive in an unbroken flow of breath and insight. Though we are behaving like hungry ghosts in the global marketplace, we have many other sides to us, unexperienced and untested. As we struggle against this decay of culture and contamination of nature, we are individuating and externalizing. The very process of life that brings us into being and sets our uniqueness and agency against the vastness of nature is medicinal. We have phenomenal untapped powers (if we cultivate and earn them), and some of the changes we might effect could heal not only ourselves but the world (and the invisible planes that attend it).

All of us are already wandering in life as the teachings tell us we

will between lives. Home must now be found inside us, in our hearts, from where the embers of compassion might be rekindled, from where alone our feeling of isolation might end. This does not mean the sentimental heart, the fantasy of "home sweet home." It means the actual bloody heart, the esoteric body represented—in fact manifested in—the physical body, in its manifold fields and sheaths of energy and layers of nerves and flesh. Here we might begin to be the kind of creatures who can live for five minutes in a place without depleting it with cynicism or greed (masking terror).

When we can look out again into the vast field of stars (we now know contain homelands of billions upon billions of creatures beyond imagination), when we can acknowledge our nativity without diminishment but with a sense of the universal affinity and eternal domain of spirit, then we will find, even now in the midst of degradation and polluted city slags, an intimation of coming home.

Harvey laments to Mother Meera:

" 'But the power and force of evil are terrifying.'

" 'Stop being afraid.' She has raised her voice slightly. 'Root yourself in the Light.' She pointed to the plants in the windowsill. 'Live on the Light like those plants live in their earth. Make the Light your earth, your food, your strength, and nothing can destroy you.' "[7]

Art

ONCE WE DROP the idea of medicine and think instead of wanting to live, it becomes clear again how everything is a medicine.

People remark offhandedly: "That woman is my medicine." "My work is my medicine." "Dancing is a medicine." "Rock and roll is a medicine."

Interviewed on TV, the rock singer Bruce Springsteen recalled: "When I was a kid, rock and roll was the only thing that always came through. It was the only thing that never let me down. Now I can't let those kids out there down. I let them down and I let myself down."

It is the same for the Cherokee chanter. He grew up hearing the voices, the rumbling tune. They were his medicine. They delivered him into life. Now he is *their* voice.

Not a medicine? Watch how the audience responds rhythmically, expressing a collective pulse and resonant feeling. Not a doctor? See how the wave emanates from him and how he leads them through the exegesis, the riff.

Song and glyph are natural folk medicines. They need not be literate; in fact, they rarely are. Rap, hip-hop, and break-dancing liberated inner-city kids. Their hearts may not stay open, but at least they knew themselves profoundly for a moment in time. Young graffiti artists cultivate highly personal traditions and styles. They are medicine men too. *Saturday Night Fever* was both the medicine and the disease for which it was the cure. Nothing but disco then could carry these dancers into a sense of their desires, unshaped personalities, and potential for absolute freedom. In the dance, they were alive. Without it, they were inert, trapped. Rock 'n' roll and the twist arise from the very fact of human life in the biosphere. They express the direction and the yearning of that life, the immense satisfaction at its biological and spiritual core. That is why they are so effective in melting and transforming the difficulties people bring to them. The language of poetry is valuable exactly because it is the language of the self. A dance, if done authentically, is the dance of the self.

When people live for something, that thing becomes engaged with their psychic and physical process. The will to live may not be expressed as that directly, but it is expressed through life as an art form. When disease is encountered, it is at least partially transmuted through desire. If we can learn to convert the seeds in their raw primary form, we can enact a cure prior to a disease. The more complex and true to the heart a dance or painting or religious ceremony, the more access it gives the maker to the depths of his or her own being.

The artist, whether she knows it or not, works side by side with her health. The development of a style and work, initially in youth,

becomes part of her maintenance system. It unfolds on a level prior to division, hence prior to remediation. The inspirational moments in an artist's work, as well as the plunges into the depths, are entanglements with the roots and petals of life itself.

Sometimes these adventures stir up material that the artist cannot deal with; after all, many have lost their health in their work, too—Vincent Van Gogh and William Faulkner are modern examples.

Moby Dick was Melville's cure, given how sick he was writing it and the calm that came upon his life afterward. *Pierre,* his next novel, reads as the sweating off of a profound ague in its last vestiges. Laura Dean's choreography of spirals, performed in 1978 in New York, shares features with the colors and positional codes of a Navaho sand painting ritual; they are both psychosomatic objectifications. Why shouldn't they contain incipient healing possibility? Cecil Taylor's and Blind Lemon's musics were old African medicines, a lineage Pharaoh Saunders "named" by his *Healing Song.* Art and politics are as old as medicine, as the bison on the cave walls at Lascaux and the X-ray turtles and serpents on rocks in the Australian desert—why not as primary? Why not as overseers and handmaidens of our initiation?

Stan Brakhage, an experimental film maker, spoke of his early works as medicines for his asthma because of the way in which the splicing and montage taught him to breathe in visual rhythms and put his lungs and heart into a visualized landscape.[8] Poets like Charles Olson and Diane di Prima long considered the breathing in poetic syntax a declaration of how to get right, how to be well. They—and the whole school of Beat and radical artists—were self-declared geomancers and shamans. Dr. William Carlos Williams wrote:

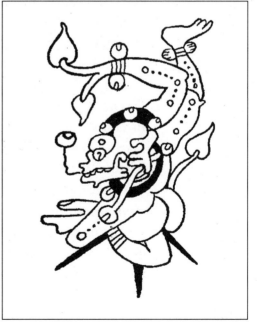

My heart rouses
            thinking to bring you news
                        of something
that concerns you
            and concerns many men. Look at
                        what passes for the new.
You will not find it there but in
            despised poems.
                        It is difficult
to get the news from poems
            yet men die miserably every day
                        for lack
of what is found there.[9]

It is, literally, "my *heart* rouses," not the mind and not the voice, which later give it shape.

Existence is primal and pagan, and Coleridge's "negative capability" is probably still a more accurate gauge of our potential for growth and change (and cure) than even the most healthy regimen of Whole Earth Medicine. That is why we have to be careful not to be too "good" and why we should remember how "bad" the natives were when they put on costumes and practiced for real. The Osage Rite of Vigil (with its vapor baths, Sun Turtles, sacred moccasins, war clubs, and House of Mystery)—and the Navaho Beautyway Ceremony (with its Mountain Gods, Magic Tobacco, Big Snake with No End, and Monster-Slayers)—remain the micro-encoded infrastructures for a true "planet medicine" yet to be born.

We see anew that medicine is real not because it alone heals or because it can finger the agent or the cure, but because it alone contains the metaphor for change. Despite their failings, the new medicines fill us with joy and hope and give us something to do during the long hours. When the clouds descend to ground zero and we cannot find a surface or a direction, these sacred practices provide the skin with which to inhabit and shape the fog. All other materials and events fall back into the relativism of the world and mystery of not knowing who we are and how we got here.

Notes

1. Andrew Harvey, *Hidden Journey: A Spiritual Awakening* (New York: Henry Holt & Company, Inc., 1991), p. 191.

2. Ibid., p. 186.

3. Jule Eisenbud, *Paranormal Foreknowledge: Problems and Perplexities* (New York: Human Sciences Press, 1982), p. 229.

4. Eduardo Calderón et al., *Eduardo el Curandero: The Words of a Peruvian Healer* (Berkeley, California: North Atlantic Books, 1982), p. 38.

5. Richard Strozzi Heckler, *In Search of the Warrior Spirit: Teaching Awareness Disciplines to the Green Berets* (Berkeley, California: North Atlantic Books, 1989).

6. Charles Dickens, *A Tale of Two Cities* (New York: Charles Scribner's Sons, 1898), pp. 431–432.

7. Harvey, *Hidden Journey,* p. 186.

8. Stan Brakhage, personal communication, Rollinsville, Colorado, 1964.

9. William Carlos Williams, "Asphodel, That Greeny Flower," from *Pictures from Brueghel and Other Poems* (New York: New Directions, 1962).

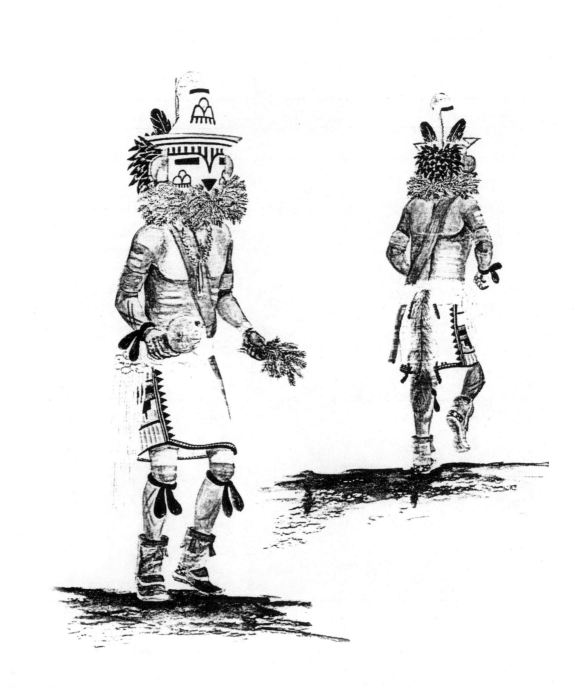

Planet Medicine

Training

WHEN I ENTERED Randy Cherner's somatics seminar in the fall of 1990, I was the least experienced "practitioner" in a group of approximately thirty, and one of only three who were not professionally engaged in some form of somatic or psychotherapeutic practice. Most of the other enrollees had seen clients for periods ranging from five to twenty-five years. I was also farther than anyone else toward the intellectual side of an "intellectual to sensory-motor aptitude" scale, so I lagged behind the group and I tended to pick up different things from others.

I was expecting to learn a range of techniques and methods. However, the main "technique" I encountered was the complex nature of "palpation" itself, which is less a set of physiological skills than an intuitive exploration of direct touch and sensation, a way to activate tissue, and an expression of energy in structure. The skills themselves arise from nondiscursive levels of touch rather than vice versa. Coming to trust one's touch and learning to think and move in terms of it involves a monumental shift, especially for one who started out viewing his hands and fingers as mere tools for possible acts of dexterity. All the fields of somatics require this degree of sensitivity. I soon found out that no repertoire of skills could compensate for an invasive and overly mechanical touch; yet a subjective awareness of how to touch and how not to impose rigid patterns could overcome almost any lack of technique. In one sense, the single effect of my three years of study was to bring me to a starting point where my training in somatics could begin.

The most frustrating aspect of intuitive "expression through touch" was learning to sustain and replicate success and to recognize when a particular piece of work was completed and so to make smooth transitions to the next. Conversely, the most exhilarating aspect was achieving therapeutic results before having mastered a full choreography of techniques.

I experienced these same dichotomies in the work of classmates. Some were more mechanically proficient than others with often negligible or even countertherapeutic results; others always got good results and, more importantly, led their training partner into new ground. From this experience I am convinced that receptivity of connection is the heart of healing, and the techniques, while critical to any sophisticated and discriminating practice, mean nothing without subtle awareness.

Two years into the training, Cherner asked us to write down the things we either had learned or were wanting to learn during the remainder of the course. I include my own list here as a kind of gloss, after the fact, not so much on bodywork *per se* but the text of this book and the impediments readers might run into in exploring the paths I disclose.

    ꞛ I can't ever do any better work on someone else than I can on myself. If I treat myself impatiently and mechanically on a daily basis, I can't suddenly switch and magically treat someone else with care. If I demand unrealistic performance from myself, I will demand it from another. Even if I try consciously to make the switch to being an impeccable practitioner, my attitude toward myself will translate into an impatience or distractedness in my touch.

    ꞛ When I am unconscious, spaced out, or generally grumpy, the answer—meaning the dissolution of that state—is in-toward, not abstracting myself further and thinking to be aloof from it, which merely tightens its grip. The mistake is to think that melting is an act of inattention. Melting can be an act of the sheerest emotional authenticity and attention.

જ Always do less. And then do less than that. Attention is critical here. It is only possible to do less if I am aware of what I am doing. Few techniques are more dangerous than an urgency that "nothing is happening," thus trying to rush things ahead by doing more. The habit is to think, "This sure isn't working. Do I have any more tricks?" Or, in the worst scenario, one escalates from technique to technique, always up the invasive scale.

If nothing is happening, do less. If nothing is still happening, then do less than that.

Wait for something—anything—to begin on its own.

જ Right at the cusp of profundity I try to make things more profound—and that's where I lose it. I have to trust to let profundity develop by itself and emerge, not to overwhelm it by "amping" in impatience for a big experience. Amping diminishes. It turns an authentic experience emerging in its own time into melodrama or theater. Adding emotion does not enlarge or deepen experience. Quite the contrary.

જ Stand by what I do. It is already done anyway and, if it is "wrong," it cannot be negated. Don't be ready to give up a technique the moment someone questions me or I look around the room and see everyone is doing a different rendition. The game is not "Simon Sez." Don't judge my work only against someone else's proficiency.

જ There IS time.

જ I don't have to know what a technique is in order to be able to do it. Manocher Movlai has his students repeat: "I don't know what I am. I don't know what this is."

જ When Ron Sieh was teaching me *hsing-i,* he said rather unexpectedly one day, "I'm trying to teach you to be as good as you can, but you obviously have some other agenda."

~ I can't underestimate the number of ways in which I am addicted to giving up. Anxiety to change technique or the compulsion to flee comes uncannily at the moment when something is about to happen. It is always a matter of waiting *a little bit longer,* as long as I don't count the seconds while waiting.

~ I occupy more space than I think I do.

~ My tendency is to assume that affectations and unconscious gestures, little "faults" in myself I apparently can't correct, are residual matters to the overall task of training. In fact, filling unlived spaces, however incidental each unlived space seems, is the path in. Often the more minor the habit, the more central it is as a means of access to one's center. The over-effort at improvement, imposed by having external goals, is simply a reaffirmation of not being able to fill in my own gaps. The same is true for the person one is working on.

~ It is not important to be "correct," at least not at the expense of the above. Being correct—being liturgical—is often just another excuse for not doing it. Anyone can be right theoretically. But not everyone can do the right thing, especially when there are no "theoretics" to back it.

~ The most damaging impediment we put in our own way is looking at a task and presuming it can't be done, thus flailing away in sorry imitation of it, demonstrating mostly our conviction of personal incapacity. Any technique, or new skill, is learned in pieces, piece by piece ... piece by piece. Any task undertaken, no matter how monumental, is accomplished a step at a time. The cliché is correct.

If you stare at the wall and plan to get there some other way than by taking a step at a time, you have found the one sure way never to get there. Many people spend their lives not taking the first step because they have convinced themselves they could never reach the wall, be it healing touch, relationship, writing, real compassion for sentient beings, etc. They'd just as soon not undergo the tragedy of taking years worth of steps and falling short anyway. Or they fear exposure and embarrassment along the way.

People don't love because they assure themselves in advance that their love isn't enough, that another person won't love them, or that they will never love enough to make a difference. The essence of somatics work is teaching oneself and others *how* to take "first steps."

∾ In a difficult technique, instead of trying to do everything right, how about first doing *one thing right.*

D URING A WEEKEND intensive the second year, our class as a whole spent a day participating in the Prison Integrated Health Program at the Federal Correctional Institute at Dublin, California. One of our group (Kathy Park) was co-director of the program.

After going through the Medieval routine of prison entry, we met a self-selected group of about thirty women in a rec room set aside for the joint training. We from the class were white with one Asian; the inmates were mostly African American and Hispanic.

The structure of the workday was an extended version of our training. Cherner led the entire group through a "lesson," which was a series of "Awareness" exercises based on Feldenkrais work, designed to teach us to explore new modes of feeling and movement as well as to understand the basis of techniques he was about to teach. We lay on the floor in a mixed group and carried out his instructions for about forty-five minutes, differentiating movements of our arms from our torsos and neck, our legs from our pelvis. Afterwards, using "client" models from the prison group, Cherner demonstrated how the same techniques functioned as neuromuscular and visceral healing modalities. Then we shared lunch at the prison cafeteria.

The bulk of the afternoon was set aside for each of us to treat an inmate.

Giving a session in that environment meant going into the teeth of every ambiguity and inequity present. It was difficult for me not to experience a profound disquiet relating through touch in a prison, and additionally with a woman who was cut off from any other intimate contact with a man. The already fine line between, on the one hand,

Card sent to author by women in Federal Correctional Institute at Dublin, California, after day of lessons and treatments there.

the therapeutic and kinesthetic aspects of touch and, on the other, its sensual components was further narrowed by the poignancy of incarceration. After an awkward beginning and three false starts, I fell back on our teaching, which was to work in response to situations exactly as they arose, to blend appropriate techniques into each other, and to foresee what kinds of touch might be experienced as disturbing or invasive. It meant "being present" in a situation I would normally space out from; in fact, it trained "being present" because any lapse in attention left one excruciatingly exposed.

The goal of somatics in general is healing which arises experientially, incorporates movement awareness and mutuality, and works to

MODALITIES

enhance well-being through feeling, visceral adjustment, and kinesthetic reorientation. The mere introduction of such a form into a prison—no doubt without the full understanding of its implications by the authorities—augurs a society (not this one, 2002) in which there might actually be a way of guiding inmates (including so-called violent offenders) into new modes of being (Palmer and Park have also taught these practices in similar circumstances in men's prisons with dramatic results among even some of the more hardened inmate populations).

Stealing and killing arise from somatic substrata too; their "attitudes" take root in the same layers of flesh in which love and healing are nurtured, and they are cultivated and hardened likewise as habits and modes of practice. Being able to pull out a gun and shoot someone requires layers of deep neural support. It is not, despite seeming evidence to the contrary, a simple, mindless act. Once embodied it cannot easily be renounced or abandoned.

Without a somatic vocabulary in our culture, we rarely consider or teach how one energetic state leads to another; we fail to provide people with the means to rescue themselves from habits of violence and crime until it is too late. We expect them to carry out their own miracle in a vacuum (e.g., in prison). Some people can (and do) catalyze their emotions and change on a dime (unfortunately, this sometimes means toward destructive as well as creative acts). Others need to be supported and educated somatically in order to act from a new place. Yet rehabilitation rarely considers the somatic component.

At Dublin there is a secondary benefit to the Health Program, for at the same time that it provides healing for those desperately needing it, it trains these women in a potentially remunerative occupation which they were unlikely to discover on their own (especially given their cultural milieus) and for which they are, in some cases, particularly talented from the same energetic charge and charisma that may have led them to jail. So while they are encountering their shadows, they are training skills they can bring back to their communities when they leave. They might be able to earn a living from these, and they might educate others in them. The techniques themselves might provide answers for despair and addiction in the slums. The prison sojourn can be an invitation to a vision quest.

T OWARD THE END of our visit to Dublin, Cherner held a question-and-answer session. It quickly became a raucous exchange of jokes, with riffs and teasing by the women, directed alternately at one another and us (as they ran back and forth across the room to deliver apparently accustomed taunts and jibes). Bawdy sexual humor dominated, and no one was spared. The bodywork had so charged the room with energy, the potentially distancing innuendos of the occasion were tossed indecorously on stage and blasted away with laughter. Personal styles of those present and enmities among the inmates were caricatured and cleared.

The event closed near five o'clock with a singing circle. Popular folk songs were followed by the ballad "Harbor Me." Different parts of the circle were assigned sequential choruses at changing pitches: *"Har-bor me. Oh, won't you harbor me. Har-bor me."*

This was another world, *another country* (James Baldwin), another time.

But that was not the grand finale. After the conclusion of "Harbor Me," different women led us in the national anthems of their homelands: Chile, Colombia, Mexico, and Puerto Rico (three of them had been arrested as members of a Free Puerto Rico guerrilla group, and an untold number were South American nationals taken into custody because of husbands or boyfriends in the drug business). Most of us by then were in tears.

True medicine *is* finally a matter of communal solidarity and planetary survival. And though we should be able to achieve that without extreme rituals in extreme places, we have little choice in the matter. Our huge (and ever growing) prison population is itself testimony to our loss of the ability to touch one another. We need new rituals and tools that have the capacity to heal not only individuals but communities and perhaps one day nations.

There is no present groundswell to develop these, but then, in this hyper-commoditized, bottom-line world, there is no present groundswell for anything that addresses our actual crisis. The most fanatical religious zealots, in league with various corporations, oligarchies, and gangs, fight against true self-realization the hardest.

Rewriting the American Health Plan

THE CLINTON HEALTH PLAN was not a health plan. It was a money plan. Nowhere did it say anything about health except as a legal commodity. What the Clinton plan did was redistribute costs and profits arising from a system of treating human bodies as medical and statistical products. It proposed legislatively to adjust relative balances within a regulated marketplace of HMOs, insurance companies, lawyers, and businesses. As one cocaine addict on the street remarked about the heralded arrest of a Colombian cartel kingpin, "It don't mean nothin'. It's just a corporate thing, a change in middle management."

Thus, all the debate about the Health Plan and its relative distributions of expense was so much verbiage about who got the bucks and who paid the bills. There wasn't any change proposed in health care. Although the role of the insurance companies in pulling their greedy share of unearned profits out of the potential pool of health-care resources was directly challenged (especially in single-payer versions), the legislation in *every* version presupposed the continuing commoditization of health care.

To try to assuage pain, dislodge pathology, and cure disease is an act of service and compassion. To medicalize lives is an act of power and control. To require everyone to submit to the clinic and the hospital is to imprison individuals in artificial systems of meaning that take away the autonomy and novelty of their existences and steal their bodies and minds for capital agendas. It is enforced donation of live organs.

Planet Medicine

The blatant commoditization of the body-mind and health care and the empowerment of medical conscription have vaulted far beyond any nineteenth-century fantasy of, say, Mary Shelley or William Blake. The medical constabulary has disenfranchised individuals in an unprecedentedly systematic and profound manner. It has disenfranchised them on a cultural basis and, just to make sure, it has disempowered them on a skeletal-visceral basis. Real health and cure have become pawns.

No national plan has yet questioned that commoditization, and none gives the inkling that there is anything wrong with viewing disease and medicine solely in market terms.

Needless to say, the Clinton Health Plan did not even begin to address the underlying assumptions of the reigning medical paradigm or the explosion of iatrogenic disease. It only peripherally dealt with the shoddy level of diagnosis and treatment guaranteed by putting accountants, lawyers, actuaries, and other bureaucrats in charge of health. Allopathy has enough problems with the complexity of disease categories even before those categories are further simplified and manipulated to serve HMO and insurance margins of profit. Trained primarily in technological methods of diagnosis and treatment, doctors know an extraordinary amount about some things and virtually nothing about others, but they pretend both categories are the same and under control. Why pay a fortune for medical school now unless you want to become a bureaucratic technician? To this, add legal liability and you have a mess.

Clinton did recognize and then took a direct stand on the relationship between the availability of guns and the high cost of health care. This was a step in the right direction. But there were a lot of other blatant social factors that needed calling out. In fact, it may be impossible to improve health care without first confronting the pathologizing effects of the public education system, the food and meat industries, and the advertising-media cartel.

To give a monopoly to one company is a classic way to set costs skyrocketing. Yet even Republicans are mesmerized by the allopathic paradigm and (except for Orrin Hatch backing the Utah herb and supplement industries) have been willing to strip away that most sacred tenet of capitalism: free markets and open competition.

Competition brings prices down and encourages commerce. Lack of competition ensures prices will rise, while siphoning resources to shareholders. No one tells auto manufacturers they have to design one kind of engine or use only one alloy. No one limits Apple and IBM to only one kind of disk operating system. But politicians of all ilk are so buffaloed by the medical lobby and indoctrinated by the chimera of a proven model of disease diagnosis, etiology, and cure that they are willing to give the AMA the sole and exclusive right to manufacture a health-care product.

Why? To protect the public from quacks? To prove to themselves that they belong to an advanced civilization on the cutting edge of even greater future technologies? From the mythology that the ultimate medicine of the future will be carried in silicon chips or transmitted by a handheld computer like the one wielded by Dr. Leonard McCoy in *Star Trek*? To avoid looking like anti-scientific fools? To reassure everyone that pathology is under control and that the current economic hierarchy is the best of all possible worlds? To maintain the doctor as a bulwark of social authority? To serve the gods of materialism and quantification? To suppress a revolution in values that could spread to government and the military? To avoid the consequences of an admission that generations of service to a single template were benighted? To elevate the AMA and allopathy to the status of a modern priesthood or cabal?

This much is certain: the governmental protection of one kind of medicine has led to wildly inflated prices for services and goods. The monopoly of allopathic health care not only devours an increasing share of the GNP but threatens to suck up *all the surplus wealth in the society.* And this is the real problem, not how the bills are paid.

As CREATURES WHO have lived in artificial villages so long, we are afraid of going back onto the open road, of having to define our own meaning again. We want to be protected from our depths by rules, brand names, sanctions, trade guilds, and the weapons of litigation. We want to play by our own rules rather than the rules of nature, so we have medicalized our incarnation even as we have suburbanized the wilderness. But we are not doing too well thus far living the lives deeded us by the "hospital," the protected lives (and deaths) of medical statistics.

What would constitute a radical change in health care in this country—and on the planet as a whole—would be a recognition of different actual modes of healing, a legitimization of each of them relative to one another, and a strategy for making them all available in appropriate circumstances. Allopathic medical treatment could certainly be one of these, but sharing a venue with cranial osteopathy, *Chi Gung,* shamanism, psychotherapy, Body Electronics, homeopathy, Feldenkrais, etc., it would be less expensive, less rapacious, less exclusive, and more acutely self-critical. Simply from the diagnostic and therapeutic repertoire expanding—the medical monopoly ending—the cost of health care would plummet. People's lives would be less commodities to be arbitraged, homogenized, and experimented upon and more mysteries to be lived. We would become responsible for ourselves, using diet, herbs, exercise, yoga, while developing rudimentary skills of energy flow and self-palpation. We would begin to experience the visceral synergies and complex resonance patterns that make us up and less often seek simple mechanical and chemical solutions for ailments. Doctors would no longer get to tell us who and what we are or pretend to write marginalia excusing us from fate or sacrificing us to imaginary futures. We would have to become real. We would have to recognize our actual place in the universe.

Better to call it now and change the system before we tinker grandiosely with the method of payment.

Once health care is fundamentally redefined, then it might be just to offer "Universal Coverage" and to attempt to balance the cost of that coverage among the segments of society that could best afford it.

To pretend to do this without first reformulating the entire meaning of health care is to saddle our country—in fact, our whole civilization—with a Medicare system rooted in culturally prescribed disease categories, a ridiculous, unmaintainable algorithm in which actual health and well-being have no meaning except an actuarially defined longevity and an illusion of protection from certain arbitrarily isolated categories of diseases (and in which the legal right to such pseudo-health replaces any responsibility for real health).

THE GAP BETWEEN a widely nondenominational range of alternative medicines and the highly sophisticated specialties on which the medical establishment pins its hopes is demonstrated by routine everyday occurrences in clinics, hospitals, and doctors' offices throughout the Western world. For example, many of the typical procedures of cosmetic surgeons would not be permitted if doctors were forced to take responsibility for the overall and long-term health of their patients and were required to check the effects of their work six months afterwards, a year later, two years later, etc. Insulting tissue that is carrying out its natural function in order to achieve a mirage of youth not only denotes a dangerous attachment to a temporary and superficial cultural guise but, beneath its fair surface, distorts and obstructs fluid structures with prosthetics and scar tissue. Surgical effects spread from skin, musculature, and skeleton deep into viscera where they spawn pathologies that are then assigned by other doctors to other, often random causes. A provincially nonholistic approach almost guarantees disturbing the subtle homeostases of an organism while disguising its own iatrogenic tracks.

A method as unlikely as botox, which involves injecting botulism into nerves to make people look younger (i.e., by essentially blowing up the neural junctions that form wrinkles), in effect robs their faces of neuromuscular control and emotional expression (compromising even their capacity to smile) while introducing a substance which, if ingested, could be fatal. If syphillis spores can survive in a semi-dormant state for fifty years in eye orbits before invading a brain, and chicken pox can return after decades as shingles, certainly one would think twice about inviting botulism innocently into their tissues.

Osteopathic science demonstrates the complex, functional links among the spinal column, neck, limbs, jaw, teeth, palate, and other bones. Dentists with craniosacral training are able to minimize damage to the skeletal and visceral organs of their patients not only by treating teeth with recognition of the larger circuitry but by later releasing any structural lesions caused by drilling, crowns, braces, etc. Yet in 1990 the Colorado Medical Association sued W. M. Raemer, D.D.S., for adjusting the sacra of his patients on the basis that spinal treatment was a violation of his dentistry license. By demonstrating beyond a doubt the relationship between the sacrum and the jawbone, Dr. Raemer won in court.[1]

If Alzheimer's is caused in part, as some believe, by the destruction of neurons from cerebral stagnation of heavy metals like lead and aluminum, then craniosacral palpation might well help irrigate those deposits. As people age, their full exchange of cerebrospinal fluid slows from four to two cycles a day. Techniques stimulating this flow and flushing the brain and spinal cord would seem at least worth a try; yet manipulation has long been consigned to the scrap heap of allopathic medicine while neurologists have such a clamp on the business of Alzheimer's that there has been no systematic attempt (to date) to apply any alternative methods to treatment of it.

Other difficult-to-cure diseases might also yield to osteopathic palpations or homeopathic microdoses. It is possible that multiple sclerosis has a psychosomatic etiology shielding it from standard pharmaceutical intrusion. Many acknowledged psychological conditions such as depression, autism, and dyslexia have improved markedly with palpation (for instance, balancing of the temporal bones in the case of dyslexia). In a holistic medical system, physical and other empirical approaches could be combined with psychological and neuropharmacological vectors to find a curative medium appropriate to each condition.

MODALITIES   A woman who, after a serious automobile accident, developed the condition generally called reflexive sympathetic dystrophy was referred to the Upledger Institute Clinic only after she had already been treated unsuccessfully at Duke University, Mayo Clinic, and a number of other advanced medical facilities. She was in so much pain that she could not even be touched. She was also allergic to Demerol, so it could not be used as a pain-killer. Reasoning that her nerves were firing in overdrive, John Upledger attached a copper wire to her toe and led it to a water pipe at the other end. (From within the box of orthodox medicine, the ultimate treatment for this condition is more or less to sever the entire sympathetic nervous system.) Remarkably, when the wire was connected, the pain was alleviated enough for her to be palpated. Repeated palpation gradually restored her health. However, until she was well enough to function without it, she kept a spool of copper at home to allow her to do housework and move about without pain. Imagine the confusion when the lawyers for the insurance company came to depose Dr. Upledger. After all, this woman had been to the highest centers of Western medicine and seen their most learned physicians—the best minds of our generation. "No seriously—you did what?" They had to hear it three times and they still didn't believe it.

When the path of thinking is dictated in advance, science is replaced by belief systems and indoctrination, and investigating nature and healing the sick take a back seat.

WE THINK WE CAN control time and space by quantifying them. We don't understand what temporality and spatiality are beyond grids of streets and avenues and orbits of clocks. By defining health and well-being likewise, we think to prioritize the ego's control of meaning and to reify each individual by the templates of prior individuals. In truth, we are abandoning people in a quicksand of genes, drugs, and cultlike science and losing the unified whole known as health. Men and women hardly know any longer whether they really want their lives prolonged and their diseases abated, but they grab for a medicalized solution because it makes them at least as real as their cars and laptops.

There is no meaningful theoretical limit set on how long bottomless resources can be poured into nonfunctional and even iatrogenic responses to the allopaths' favored disease modalities. In theory, the entire resources of the Earth could be put at the service of prolonging one person's life—and even that would not ultimately be enough. One might as well pave over the topsoil, use the oceans as garbage dumps, raise all the planet's food in greenhouses and fishponds, and jail the youth of the expanding underclasses. Each of these is more expensive than we can afford, and they are ploys to evade the reality of our plight and to pretend that the universe is a place of business not of destiny.

We will lose. And we will lose big.

A New System of Health Care

IT IS PERHAPS absurd for anyone to recommend a practical alternative to the present medicine monopoly with the thought of it being adopted and working, but it would be irresponsible to come this far without taking at least a shot in that direction. I don't expect my suggestions to be taken seriously at a level of policy, but they provide a critique of the bill of goods we are being sold. In fact, I challenge those who disagree to demonstrate why my fantasy is any less practical and economically feasible than the jumble of bureaucracy being offered by the AMA or various Clinton-Bush administrations.

What I propose is a six-part medical system. For clarity of illustration (alone) I will place each sphere within this system in a different region of North America. This region shall be its research center, its university, and its chamber of elders. Satellite clinics and practitioners will also be spread throughout the other regions. Needless to say, all systems belong in every region.

In New York and the greater Northeast I will place the high-civilization allopathic schools of surgery and pharmacy—in other words, the majority of what passes now for modern medicine, including most
forms of psychoanalysis, nutrition, immunology, allergology, genetic

medicine, and laboratory research. These are the most scientifically advanced therapeutics and the ones requiring the most refined technologies. In the future, pharmaceutical companies can continue to do advanced research, ideally discovering new vaccines, antibiotics, and other molecular medicines, as well as methods of early diagnosis for all manner of conditions, including cancer, Alzheimer's, infertility, and genetic defects. Surgeons can apply their acuity to organ disease, severe injuries, and the victims of war. The paradigm can be expanded and refined to its farthest bounds in ecologically safe biotechnology and nanopharmacology. Those who do not want this form of medicine can simply avoid the New York center. Disenfranchising allopathy as the only "scientific" modality will somewhat impede the enthusiasm to attack every malady with heroic methods and to prolong life in its most minimal and devitalized states or by default.

In Toronto and the greater Midwest I will base a school of constitutional and dietary medicine. It will derive from Ayurvedic principles but will also prescribe foods and herbs from all over the world, including Chinese and American Indian formularies, African, Pacific, and Australian ethnobotanies, etc. Culinary schools will teach practitioners how to prepare food, blending ingredients in manners simultaneously health-sustaining and tasteful. It will be, as the name of Denis Cicero's restaurant on Irving Place in New York (twilight blue decor, twinkling fiber-optic stars on the ceiling) is meant to portend, the Galaxy Global Eatery. Everyone will be initiated into food-balancing principles, the relationships of tastes to metabolism and disease, the properties of climate, colors, and seasons, modes of dress and habitats—in other words, general environmental and cosmic cycles in health. Ideally this school can develop a new ecological medicine out of ancient Oriental as well as Western principles and make its teachers available to agribusinesses, ranches, and farms to develop healthy methods for raising food.

In Seattle and the greater Northwest (in lineage with the Indians of the Pacific Basin and the John Bastyr College of Naturopathy) I will

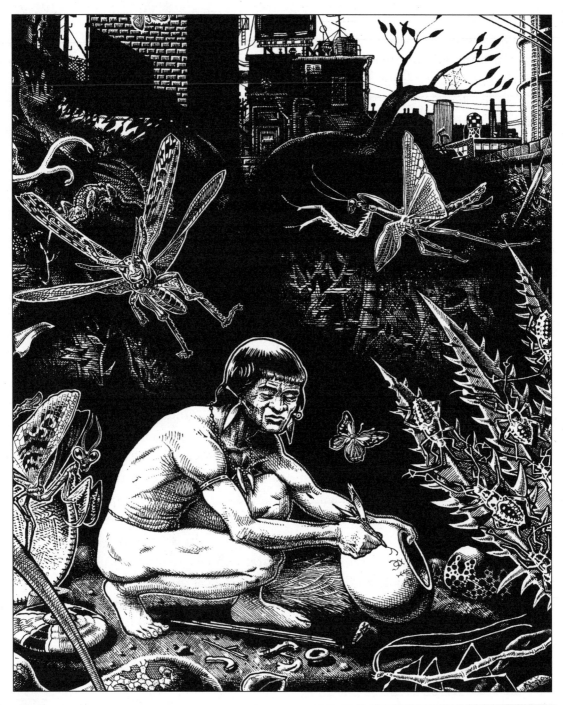

set a center of *chi*-based medicine. Its doctors will teach their students methods of apprehending and moving *chi,* including those of Taoist martial arts and the different levels of *Nei Ching.* This school will also include yoga, acupuncture, moxibustion, Buddhist meditation, and will have its own branches of herbalism and bodywork.

In the San Francisco Bay Area (acknowledging the Hahnemann Clinic already in Berkeley) I will place energy medicine. This will include homeopathy, Bach flower remedies, radionics, Reiki, forms of psychic transmission of cures, *chakra* and color therapies, massage, induction of the different sheaths of the energy body, and faith healing, as well as research into all paraphysical modes of healing. Thus, the laboratory of Kirlian photography will be in the university of this branch. Any mediums who want to channel healers from other dimensions will be able to train and compare information here, too. Jacques Vallee will oversee UFO and crop-circle research from his base in San Francisco (and from the point of view not so much that "they" are aliens—friendly, malicious, etc.—but that they are here and we don't know what they are). Vallee's journal notes upon seeing his first UFO in 1958 could serve as an epigram for this school: "I am left with the single strong impression that we must respond; that human dignity demand[s] an answer, even if it [is] only a symbolic acknowledgment of our lack of understanding. I realized then and there that I would forever be ashamed of the human race if we simply ignored 'their' presence."[2]

In Taos, New Mexico, and the greater borderless Southwest (into Northern Mexico), I will set a shamanic school of medicine. Here students will learn ceremonial sand painting, visualization techniques, healing dances and chants, indigenous and Western art therapy, all modalities of shamanic psychoanalysis (energy transsubstantiation by symbols), the dynamics of abreaction and techniques of reinvoking trauma, vision questing, the uses of hallucinogens in diagnosis and treatment, and methods of finding curative feathers, drums, crystals, amulets, shells, and common stones, and healing with them. This branch will also house a school of world literature and indigenous knowledge and mythology. Shamans—both Third World and industrial—from all over the planet will serve stints on its faculty. Thus, techniques will be pooled and preserved, and each of the traditions—Siberian, Fijian, pan-Australian, native American, African, East Indian, etc.—will have a division within the greater department of shamanic healing. I would think that many Freudian-trained psychoanalysts would prefer to study and practice here (or in Florida) than at the New York school.

In West Palm Beach, Florida, and the greater Southeast into the Caribbean (honoring the Upledger Institute) I will place a school of neo-osteopathy, which will cover all modalities of manipulation, palpation, and attendant methods of psychological investigation and clearing of psychosomatic blocks. This university will have independent departments representing major somatic traditions such as Feldenkrais, Eutony, Body-Mind Centering, Continuum, Rolfing, Zero Balancing, Visceral Manipulation, Aston Patterning, Chiropractic, Reichian, Acupressure, etc. There will also be a research sector studying the relationship among not only these somatic therapies but those practiced at the other regional centers (for instance, Polarity in Toronto and shamanic movement and shape-shifting in New Mexico). Psychotherapists studying here can learn techniques of nonverbal dialogue and means of contacting character and transforming resistance by palpation and words together.

I do not mean to give osteopathy priority over other somatic systems, merely to invoke the underlying osteopathic model of a whole medicine fully equivalent—on the level of palpation, light visceral and cranial "surgery," sensory-motor education, and manipulation—to the competing system of drugs and surgery.

A MEDICAL CULTURE SET UP in this way would inspire a range of flexibility and choice. For instance, a person suffering from any
form of mental disorder (depression, compulsion, multiple personal-

ity, panic attacks) could choose to see a conventional psychoanalyst in New York or a complementary practitioner in any of the other centers. He could engage in a craniosacral dialogue and experience somato-emotional release in Florida. He could learn *chi* movements in the Pacific Northwest. He could go on a guided vision quest in New Mexico. He could also obtain dietary aid in Toronto, potentiated pharmaceuticals in California, Chinese herbs in Seattle, or psychotropics in New York if he preferred to visit the masters in their heartlands.

Not only is such a system both more humane and more profound in how it approaches medical diagnosis and treatment, it is bound to be more cost-effective. Most of the modalities other than allopathy are flat-out less expensive. If even a small percentage of the population elected to use them, the core technological and HMO medical glut would be eased dramatically. Additionally, these modalities tend to favor shorter treatments, the patient taking responsibility for his or her own health, and an acceptance of death in its proper time rather than the employment of Herculean methods to maintain life at all costs. The nonallopathic centers would have their own ethical and ontological orientation and would tend to approach health crises as opportunities of transformation and understanding life rather than as random attacks. Their practitioners would know how to ask a patient, for instance, to practice a *Chi Gung* exercise or meditate regularly or perhaps to prepare for the spiritual metamorphosis of death when that is the "healing" modality needed—instead of just giving a pill, a placation, or a "curtains" prognosis.

When all the other systems fall into their appropriate perspective, allopathy will join "planet medicine" as a necessary partner. The great surgeons with their elite equipment, the laboratory pharmacists and brilliant diagnostic anatomists can take their rightful place at the table of medicine, and all other practitioners, from shamans to homeopaths to Ayurvedic masters and breath-workers, will happily send them those patients who need their craft. Right now the technicians are being asked to do everything, and it is just plain impossible. The heart and spirit and energy fields and karma of every human being are vast, and disease is their foil and dervish. We will finally need the doctors of anatomy for their scrupulous attention to what-is, which is the most powerful manifestation of this incarnation.

Such a medical system would also open the possibility of dealing with a number of other extremely serious, trenchant societal problems not ordinarily associated with medical treatment. For instance, like the women in prison, youth in gangs could be viewed as potential shamanic initiates rather than only as criminals and could be sentenced (medically) to train as samurai, or bodyworkers and herbalists, or be dispatched on vision quests. This may sound ridiculous on the surface, but in fact few people would choose an outlaw existence if there were another option for a fierce, creative life. Plus, society must use the energy at its disposal or be undermined by it in some fashion.

At the turn of the twenty-first century, there are social programs in the United States which place a few selected "youth at risk" on small farms and in urban gardens—they learn about organic agriculture and biodiversity; they prepare food boxes to sell in their neighborhoods and to give away to the poor. They educate their parents and peers about nutrition and wholesome foods. They even teach old-time farmers (stuck with thousands of acres of monocrops) how to diversify to dozens of varieties on just a few acres. In the Central Valley of California they join forces with Hispanic and Filipino family farmers and former migrant workers to reclaim old Mexican and Zuni-Mohave farming traditions. They lead the way back to tribal food rituals with barter of skills and goods.

Other "youth at risk" are enlisted as "big brother" and "big sister" aides to younger kids and serve to "initiate" hardcore members out of gangs.

Many gang members would prefer to play in the National Basketball Association if they had the skills and were given the chance. Many do; only they develop other aspects of their game in order to fit the decorum of the league. Why not enlarge the "National Basketball

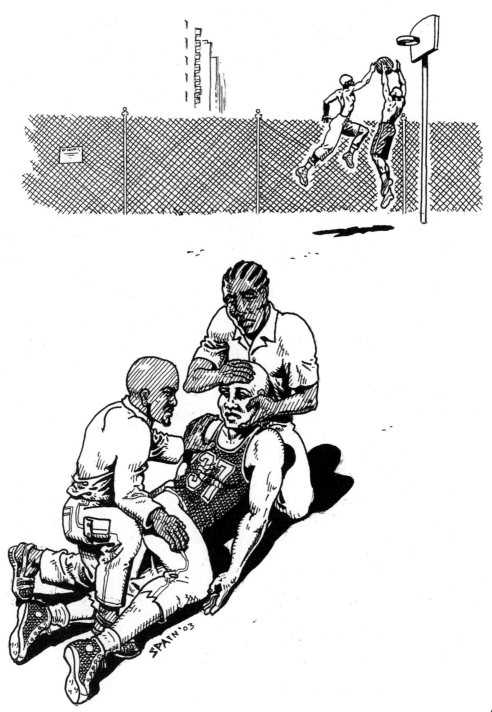

Association" to its full scope, i.e., make its "skills" the skills needed for treating the sick and healing society as well as—with the same aplomb and "badness" as—shakin', bakin', dunking, and sacks. Facials could be replaced by Reiki waves or palpations. Raw ability to heal could be trained in kids who seek something more real than a game and more chivalrous and humanitarian than crime or sterile street battles. To truly serve humanity (and the gods) is everyone's secret desire.

Kumar Frantzis describes being invited through a priest by the prisoners at the New Mexico State Penitentiary in Albuquerque to teach them *t'ai chi* and *Chi Gung*. This was the site of one of the worst prison riots in United States history. Frantzis not only was well received but had dramatic success in improving both the health and the mood of inmates. "The prison is an extremely stressful environment," noted Frantzis; "it's an incredibly violent place. Most of the people who have been in prison a very long time are sick people. I mean they are physically ill in every way that you could possibly imagine. And if you remember the story of Androcles and the lion, when the thorn was taken out of the lion's paw, the lion stopped eating people at random."

One prisoner with extremely high blood pressure had been on medication for eleven years. When interviewed by a television reporter from KNME, he reported not only that his blood pressure was considerably reduced by *Chi Gung* but that he was about to have his medication cut in half. "Everybody is much happier," he added, "much friendlier, jokes more. No one has threatened to kill anybody in six or seven months. So, that's pretty good. I just wish I had found this when I was like eighteen or twenty. I believe it would have made a difference between me going to prison or not."[3]

Gang roles require courage, ingenuity, physical prowess, and leadership. Would it not be better to provide shamanic opportunities for such warriors than to put twenty percent of the population behind bars? Would it not make a healthier society to spread its corporate megabucks among half a million "Michael Jordans" and "Bruce Springsteens" playing neighborhood ball as osteopaths, healers, and curanderos?

The trouble is not with basketball or rap; it is that there are not enough other charismatic, energetic roles—e.g. the teen osteopath as superstar, the *Chi Gung* master as "Big Daddy" or "Big Momma." There is no real shamanic opportunity for inner-city and rural youth or the poor.

Vision quests and Taoist energy trainings lead to martial, shamanic, and magical healing skills. These are more likely to provide stable and sustained prosperity and, finally, life itself than gun-battles, turf wars, and inevitable extortion are; the latter have a quick-fix lure as a method for getting off the bottom of the caste system, but they actually condemn those who become disciples to lives of paranoia, fear, greed, and emptiness. Gangs enforcing prostitution, distributing drugs, running numbers, and committing robbery and violent crimes are the shadows, the ghosts of roving teams of barefoot doctors and "Guardian Angels" we desperately need. Various Jihads and guerrilla armies elsewhere in the world are potential Earth militias and brigades, able to protect life forms from danger and the planet itself from demonic attack and despoliation. That is why they are presently so cruel and fanatic in their causes. Fierceness is required for the true battle—but they are stuck in the global trance, thus fight with utter passion and conviction the wrong war. Prevented from realizing their true selves, they automatically become the enemy (the spirit fire must burn somewhere).

Holistic medicine means to give all people rainbow bodies, or an intuition that rainbow bodies are possible. Gang members and people's armies already understand how tough this world is, how hard it is to get and maintain any kind of "rainbow" in the battle with rival spirits across the anonymous void of the stars, forests, and cities. They have developed some of the prerequisites of power necessary to find and stay with a *chakra,* skills that most civilians would not have.

True healing has more kinship with wild Bear Doctors who maim and kill than it does with the intellectual medicine guilds and academic technicians. And, in any case, many of the patients the gangs would treat at first have already been abandoned by the safety net and are far too cynical to accept medicalized palliatives. They might be willing to look the spirits of healing squarely in the face, for they dwell in the darkness from which such spirits venture.

Gangs and ragtag militias have potentially the same radical power warrior societies did in indigenous cultures. Practicing how to kill, facing their own death regularly from childhood, some gang members know archetypally how to heal many diseases and states of madness medical professionals do not even begin to address. These members do not realize that they have cultivated the prerequisites, if not the techniques, of charismatic healing. And that is their raw talent, without undergoing subsequent retraining in *Chi Gung Tui Na,* barefoot-doctoring, visceral manipulation, cranial osteopathy, etc. This is not to deny that some of their colleagues are trenchantly addicted to violence, but I believe that these are as much the minority in the 'hood as they are in tribes and villages at large.

Can you imagine what this planet could become if terrorist and suicide-attack groups like al-Qaeda and Hamas applied their militant spiritual energy, wiles, and devotion to Allah to healing diseases like AIDS and cancer and restoring ecosystems, economies, and villages?

Maybe the various sports leagues (Major League Baseball, the National Basketball Association, and the National Football League) could donate a portion of the excess profits the players and owners are fighting each other for. They could settle their labor difficulties by contributing all disputed sums to programs training inner-city youth in various modes of healing. Thus, revenue arising from selective media glorification of certain athletic skills could go into developing other skills society more desperately needs (and among just the people most needy). Charisma would spread from victories in games and championships to charismatic acts of life and death in gangs converted to farming and healing guilds. Everyone would be a potential "Big League" participant, not only the stars. The rock music industry and Hollywood could do likewise. All of these "entertainment" businesses that benefit

from making *some people* into ikons could remedy this imbalance by using a portion of their profit to provide roles for *other people.* There would still be so much money left for all parties that few of them could spend it wisely and productively in their lifetimes. The big corporations that hierarchicalize and hoard wealth and resources could then follow suit in a planetary transformation of priorities and values.

We can imagine parallel programs for "criminals" already in jails and homeless people. After all, not everyone requires a formulaic medicine or treatments. Some people merely need jobs. Many violent criminals are potential healers gone totally into the shadow, so deeply that they identify with it and do not even imagine a way out. At that level the shadow requires a puppet show, like a dance of zombies, on its behalf. This is what we oversee in epidemic numbers. But it is only the trance level of a profound energetic shift. Most of these people are not awake, so they don't have the slightest idea how close what they are carrying out, in decadence or predation, is to healing and restoration on another plane.

Viewed from an entirely different perspective, the drug addictions that lie at the source of so much urban misery and crime have their basis partially in the fact that people are so sick they assume they need some kind of medication, and the only drugs (or vision quests) being offered (by many legitimate pharmacies as well as street sellers) are ones making them sicker and more catatonic.

Many homeless people, by the very challenge of living on streets, in alleys, and on various tundras, deserts, and in Third-World scrub wilderness, are on vision quests and have developed shamanic credentials from that. Others are just plain sick and in post-traumatic shock and require treatment from a constitutional-medicine or an osteopathic center.

Chopmaster J, a.k.a. Jimmy Dright of Oakland, former member of the Digital Underground with wildman Tupac Shakur, now runs Herb'n Soul, an organization devoted to replacing drugs with herbs in the ghetto. Selling gingko, ginseng, echinacea, and the like in little bags with spoons, he is telling kids you can use herbs and still be cool. "I want to be the alternative Puff Daddy," he proclaims.

We don't have the slightest idea how many criminals, homeless people, gang members, or simply chronically sick individuals and sufferers of anxiety and depression would regenerate and become productive if they were given homeopathic medicines, Chinese herbs, cranial treatments, Feldenkrais lessons, Reiki, or taught Zen meditation or rebirthing. None of this potential for healing (either way) is cultivated. It is all wasted to the same degree and in the same way that raw materials are squandered in factories producing junk, and farmlands are washed away in pesticide-based, monocrop agriculture.

Fragments of a retribalizing process have been activated in some newly urbanized areas of New Zealand where Maori villages and neighborhoods have been overwhelmed by suburban scourge. In a single generation tribal youth have jumped into modern media culture, forming motorcycle gangs, chanting rap, selling drugs, and killing. Yet, at the same time, they also cover themselves and one another, face and body, with intricate traditional tattoos; they blend Maori songs and verses into their rap; and they invoke Maori warrior rituals and their own ancestors in their combat.

They are not yet hollow automatons like the stricken generations of many other indigenous peoples throughout this planet, rootless and addicted to alcohol, speed, and cargo. As disclosed in the movie *Once Were Warriors,* the Maori are a spiritual fire trapped in a wasteland, burning and condensed at their core, ready to erupt in a pure *toiora* that will consume, destroy, and redeem the world around them. Even though they don't know how to use it, they hold the medicine bundle again in their collective agon—original purveyors of spirit and voodoo and the motility of bone.

Tribal fervor and animal essence—the direct line to Palaeolithic symbols of power and samurai training—must arise in thousands of different contexts in every region of the Earth. It cannot be clan warfare this time or ethnic cleansing. It must touch the deeper ritual at the core where all totems meet and release this planet's great and encum-

bered heart. Waves of compassion, the flow of *wairua* from there, will sweep over seas and jungles like an electromagnetic *prana* field. For now it is too soon and those we rely on are too corrupted, but it represents our best possibility.

The potential role of holistic and energy medicines in transforming civilization is virtually one hundred percent unexplored. Instead, political solutions, dense drugs, and health plans are offered as palliatives, more prisons are financed and stiffer sentences are handed down with blind righteousness. The truly violent are unintentionally trained in greater violence in "correctional" institutions and then set loose, in the sloppiness of bureaucratic arrogance, to kill again. It is almost as though, at the deepest level, we prefer cycles of retribution and revenge to rehabilitation. But it is ourselves we are punishing as deeply as those who bear the physical wounds.

The Big Sleep

WE BLAME OTHER PEOPLE always for the heedless and selfish behavior of our species. We condemn a world in which everyone seems "out for themselves," as if we could individually hide behind superficial and disingenuous screens of innocence we erect in our minds to separate ourselves from "them" who are doing the bad things. In fact, our entire justice system is an attempt to make most crimes seem purely personal (i.e., to assign actionable blame for the outcomes of class structure and other collective deeds). Conversely, our entire medical system is an attempt to make personal destiny institutional (i.e., to redefine diseases and immune responses as universal pathological categories). These twin instances of "misplaced concreteness" combine to crush hope and dehumanize public life.

The bomb in Oklahoma City (April 19, 1995), the shooters at Columbine High (April 20, 1999), the suicide bombers of Palestine and Sri Lanka, the nineteen Muslim hijackers of 9-11-01, carved out precisely the negative space behind the temple of love we have not inhabited and do not know how to inhabit. Look at the rubble where the World Trade Center buildings once stood, culture reduced to molecules of dust. It is like an asteroid colliding with a moon — mute, sterile, antipathetic, millennial. It gives absolutely nothing. It takes away everything. It doesn't even have a reason, not really. Those were acts of destruction in place of the acts of healing we deny in our hearts. Deny them long enough, and the centurions of their antipode will spring up like weeds. Where the cure is depreciated or renounced we can expect explosions of exactly the opposite order, cataclysms in place of *prana* or microdoses because something must occupy the void. Instead of the shaman's transforming chant we hear the muffled shriek of empty souls.

If we will not produce healers, then we must beget killers. If we exile acts of faith, we will get wounds — terrible wounds — that drive us to the bottom where only faith and redemption remain.

Even the worst deeds of recreational killers exist in a collective consciousness. They are the deeds of all of us. In our suicidal civilization there is even some question of how many of us want to transform the poison and go on living. Most people it seems would rather manufacture more and more poison so that they can die more quickly and anonymously, with the least pain. But cure is change; it always involves suffering: separation before new unity. It is far easier to live and die grimly and accept that existence skirts the oblivion of catabolic dissociation.

No doubt part of the attraction of modern science is that it disdains a universe of karma (with all its necessary growth and struggle) and replaces it with a sterile panoply of atoms and molecules. At least those atoms and molecules are under interdict to obey *our* mechanical laws. So the bad news of medical science is always that we are obliterated in the end, but the good news is that at least we get to have "the big sleep," the ultimate disease. We do not have to "get out of here alive."

How can creatures feeding themselves on addictions and adrenaline rushes know their life desires? Until these matters are resolved, it is pointless to ask whether our species as a whole, as it pillages and wastes sentient life everywhere, even has a conscience or a heart.

Some Buddhist groups in Nepal claim that humans have slaughtered so many individual animals—in feedlots as well as in the wild—so swiftly while destroying so many of their genetic templates and habitats that the spirits of these animals have no choice but to come back *as people.* That is why there are too many people. That is why so many of them behave like beasts. They *are* beasts. Which is not to say that beasts act badly, merely that they may not be ready to participate in civil society.

The point is that we are substantially cut off from the qualities that make us sentient, human, and this dilemma is institutional as well as personal.

R EALISTICALLY SPEAKING, it would take a great optimist now to believe that we stand a better chance of healing ourselves than of ending up with a planet-wide Bosnia or a catastrophic environmental meltdown. We tremble before darkness that does not precede a dawn but an apocalyptic rebirth, a radically new order of things. Then perhaps we can start over again with the basics of energy, community, cures, and goods. Men and women alive now have no choice but to work toward solutions that have dignity, humanity, and compassion for other sentient beings. Anything less not only furthers and deepens the pathology but deepens the connection of that person in this lifetime to the pathology, a deepening which tends to vitiate any small rewards and pleasures gained in the process. Our lives themselves are statements of either the impossible or the consciousness of the universe itself. Either way, true gestures we make will not be squandered. We have to understand that. Even if the Sun erupts in a supernova or a pole shift shears the planet with thousand-mile-per-hour winds, nothing is ultimately wasted, nothing is forever incurable, because nothing is fully material without an energy body and a spirit too.

As Vallee put it, "...I would be forever ashamed of the human race if we simply ignored 'their' presence."

Planet
Medicine

To effect anything resembling the restructuring of medicine suggested above would require a massive shifting of resources from not only military and industrial cooption but the transnational corporate superstructure in all the financial giants—the United States, Japan, and Germany—and the rest of the Common Market of Europe, the rising dragons of Asia, and Brazil. It could not be done without also including auto workers in Detroit and Hokkaido, prostitutes in Bangkok, neo-Nazis in Bavaria, war lords in Somalia, shipbuilders in Gdansk, and the descendants of aboriginal Africans, Australians, and Americans. It would require committed participation by Russia, Uzbekistan, Iraq, Sudan, Nigeria, South Africa, India, Pakistan, Afghanistan, Chechnya, Turkey, the Balkans, Mitsubishi, Paramount, Kaiser, Reebok, WalMart, Microsoft, Georgia Pacific, all future Enrons and Taliban brigades, the International Money Fund, a variety of nongovernmental organizations, the National Institutes of Health and their equivalents in other nations, enfranchised scientist-priests upholding a mechanical-molecular world-view as liturgy, megabucks rock stars and athletes (as noted), the Papal establishment, the mullas of Iran, Norwegian fishermen, the various mafias, the Swiss banks, and innumerable other polities, consortia, individuals, indigenous and Third World peoples, and terrorists and Samaritans. That is, it would require everyone, but first those with the most power and equity in the existing order. It would also require at least as much attention to the planet's oceans, forests, soil, insects, birds, fishes, and atmosphere, not in a righteous, ideological fashion, but as part of a general enthusiasm for a larger, more dangerous vision quest and rap.

It can't just be bureaucratic reorganization or a righteously liberal proclamation of a requirement of goodness. That has never worked, and it tends to bring out not only the skinheads and white warriors but the skinhead and fascist elements in everyone. If it can't be raunchy, sassy, and blasphemous, and as multi-layered and many-mooded as humanity is, it won't work. It clearly won't work as any sort of religious fundamentalism or piety. It also won't work from the standpoint of one ethnic superiority or another. We are equally the bad guys in this. We are all jews, niggers, spics, nazis, honkies, hutus, and japs in the way we treat the planet and one another. We are all likewise the only aryan and zulu warriors left that can be counted on to rescue us.

Of course, none of this will come easily. Many people will choose to go down fighting for the status quo, even as they have already. However, a commitment in the direction of planet hygiene will make a big difference just by its intention. After all, the dominant current commitment in the direction of planetary destruction, egoistic greed, antipathetic narcissism, and gross consumptionism is hardly a major conviction or uniform enthusiasm. It is a slight leaning in a particular direction which, because of the trajectory and its encouragement of xenophobic and self-aggrandizing politicians, resembles an intense allegiance, an avalanche. It is maybe an imbalance of 55 percent/45 percent, reinforced by economic imperatives and mass media and maintained mostly in fear—but all it takes is 50.01% (if that) to win each election and declare a mandate. People are truly hypnotized, walking around in low-grade trances like the hum of fluorescent lighting. They think of their trances as mellow living and high times. They think they are awake and conscious and choosing the good life. They have no idea of how deep they go, how much they could feel, how big "this" is, or how much love (power) they actually have. This could all be much more fun, too. A gentle push in another direction may give time for a deeper change to flower over generations. Each of us might contribute .00001 percent to that push.

But it won't begin as long as people are fooled into believing that technology and health plans are going to do it for them, or that it's anybody's responsibility except their own to get well.

T HE MONEY NEEDED to pay for a transformation would be astronomical, but every day on this planet astronomical money pays for something; vast resources go elsewhere. Trillions of gallons of sunlight and orgone and *chi* rain daily unused from interstellar space. Reiki

Epilogue

Planet Medicine

and shamanic gestures flirt idly in the marketplace and evaporate into thin air. Human and psychic energy is trapped in plastics factories, sweatshops, stock exchanges, consumption, envy, greed, and various forms of addiction and prostitution. There is no lack of energy. It is all either stifled or in the wrong places.

It would not cause economic collapse to find ways to direct a little bit of money and real government attention in other directions. Admittedly, by the measures stock markets use, any little bit is a painful little bit off the bottom line and out of investors' profits; 1 percent alone would be gargantuan and would perhaps rescue this planet, enough to give the true depth at the heart of humanity a venue for expressing itself.

Initially the change would mean responding deeply to those on the streets and in jails instead of engaging in a habitual mechanism of blocking out. It would mean new activities, a flicker of hope, and the first inkling that we are not a lost cause (so best enjoy while we can) or God's worst fuck-ups in the universe. It would mean, ultimately, changing to activities that make sense in terms of a possible future for our species. Even a single such sustained global healing gesture could turn around this entire paradigm in a few generations.

Later it will mean facing the truth instead of killing one another and everything else that breathes in hopes of numbing the painful heartbeat. It will mean that those who have been most committed to punishment, retribution, and palliation will have to suffer the pain of awakening. But once they do, they will also experience how vast their life actually is and how long an eternity we all face. They will receive a gift far greater than any concession they make.

* * *

"PLANET MEDICINE" is finally more than a metaphor or even an evolving set of paradigms. It is a statement of the diversity of systems of healing among sentient beings and the continuous generation of those systems from within the depths of unconsciousness. It is a transhistorical link between the elemental dance and the chariots of civilization.

Medicine represents each unique cultural, aesthetic, and intuitive response to the crisis of being alive in a magical (if fragile) situation on a planet of wonders. It is our attempt to reveal texture, express compassion and hope, and respond with dignity to the engines of destruction that epitomize the vast, anonymous nature of which we are clearly offspring. Healing is one of the oldest human guilds, with unbroken roots back into the Ice Age. From the beginning, it was hunting, killing, hexing, and making poisons. It was never as facile as mere fixing and tonifying. The most educated surgeon carries in himself the aura, however faint, of a beast brandishing the horns of another beast and conducting raw spiritual power. Dolphins, birds, felines, insects, spiders, and other creatures likely practice rudiments of "planet medicine": therapeutic touch, psychokinetics, telekinesis, *t'ai chi,* aromatherapy, herbalism, transmutation of sugars and trace minerals, and molecular pharmacology.

Healing originates in the bonds of maternity and sorority, hence of society. In every primary and subsequent form it addresses the gaps and dead spots that separate man and woman from each other and from themselves. It nurtures ravaged bodies and guides lost spirits home, but it also unleashes deadly ghouls and smashes transient artifacts (including other creatures of energy and flesh). It is first and foremost disease itself in another form.

The present enthusiasm for alternative and holistic systems is a response to a primordial flood arising from uncharted depths and changing the Earth and its life forms. In the minds of those creatures who are awakening now, there is a need to know and name the nameless. Thus our new healing imperative is a struggle to shape a metaphor out of forces that are expressing themselves simultaneously in cataclysms, wars, and diseases and in the palliative remediations of these conditions. We call it "medicine" when we reify only its ideological and semantically therapeutic aspect.

These are powerful times. It is no surprise that they spawn remarkable healers and new healing systems.

"Planet medicine" is never a plan to cure or save human beings or the Earth, nor is it lineage of successively more skillful or radical modalities. It is not a doctor in a hospital, but it is likewise not a therapist juggling symbols. It is not a faith healer turning energy into matter. It is solely the impulse, the inarticulate intention to touch and transform what is stagnant.

The Earth doctor is a wild, rabid animal. She is change itself wearing the temporary, eroding mask of a wise Bear. She carries within herself the most devastating forces of destruction as surely as the most miraculous agencies of restoration. This makes her a true shaman, a warrior.

IF THIS BOOK is timely, it is not because medicine has become such a hotly contested topic. It is because we are beginning to see where we fall on a planetary scale of healers and where the current epoch comes in world history. The text ends, rightly, at the moment when medicine returns us to our own inevitability.

Notes

1. The Colorado Board of Medical Examiners vs. W.M. Raemer, D.D.S. Court of Appeals, State of Colorado, Case No. 87CA1589, March 22, 1990. The decision of the Appellate Court in the favor of W.M. Raemer, D.D.S., states, amongst other things, that:

i. temporomandibular joint dysfunction can be treated effectively with cranio-sacral manipulation;

ii. any treatment which relieves pain or corrects a physical condition occurring in the teeth, jaws, or adjacent structures constitutes dentistry (based at least on the Colorado statute);

iii. craniosacral manipulation and the treatment of temporomandibular joint dysfunction constitutes the practice of dentistry.

The ruling was unanimous.

2. Jacques Vallee, *Forbidden Science* (Berkeley, California: North Atlantic Books, 1992), p. 16.

3. Bruce Kumar Frantzis, personal communication and archival videotape, Fairfax, California, 1994.

The Seven Laws of Cure

ALTERNATIVE, HOLISTIC, AND NON-WESTERN MEDICINES implicitly rely on models of the body-mind as metadimensional. We are not solely chemicodynamic events. Pure anatomy is one domain; thoughts and energy matrices (in either the healer or sick person—or both) are another.

This viewpoint is intuitive and epiphenomenal rather than theoretical or systematic. After all, no actual metadimensional or telepathic components have ever been observed, though their hypothetical trajectories lead to manifold, often bizarre medicinal strategies, often on a trial-and-error basis. Working explanations are derived later from *ad hoc* paradigms that could not pass muster inside the castle walls. But just because a modality cannot be programmed does not mean it is not real. If people improve through its practice, it is a medicine. In the absence of any theory for how techniques could succeed, people for millennia have continued to invent ingenious ways to ease pain and sorrow and heal the sick.

Scientists define physical events solely by rational constructs and measurements. Yet witness the transformation of this planet's landscape over thousands of generations by immaterial symbols and their applications. Something is creating and organizing thoughts and words and giving them the energy to materialize and alter reality, something that also organizes cells and tissues. Though any direct link between human

meanings—conscious or unconscious—and molecular or cellular organization eludes us, from this ineffable domain we invent methods of
healing that are not entirely comprised of thoughts, not entirely working through matter, and not energetic in a purely thermodynamic sense.

When practitioners of orthodox medicine confine themselves to
aseptic literalization of sites, they miss the nonlinear hierarchy of forces
binding creatures together. So many different vectors and levels of integration could not be made to oscillate in functional harmony just by
single-tier mechanical effects. There must be a higher-order synergistic influence too, a dynamic agency that distributes information among
layers of anatomy, that transmits vital seeds throughout bodies, that
triggers subcellular and visceral signalling circuits.

In the evolution of biological entities with the capacity to self-
organize and self-heal, systemic intelligence is essential. While genetic
messages underwrite tissue stability and species plan, and enzymes regulate metabolism by biochemical signs, something else, more akin to
what we experience as *chi* fluctuating through meridians, unites genes,
enzymes, and macromolecules in life systems. A form of raw, unminded
omniscience underlies the homeostasis and responsiveness of organisms.

M EDICINAL SHAMANISM is guided by the belief that disembodied
personae can be summoned for good or evil, signs can be turned
into biologically active entities, and agencies can be channeled from
healers to organisms via sympathetic magic and voodoo.

Chinese medicine is rooted in the philosophy of the *Nei Ching* and
other Taoist texts which assert a bioelectric current flowing through
five elements and generating all phenomena of the natural world. It is
activated and sedated in cycles subject to reciprocal balances of yin and
yang.

Contemporary practitioners of **homeopathy** explain the therapeutic effects of microdoses by an interpretation of physics in which water
molecules are pharmaceuticalized with vital effects. Traces of diluted,
succussed tinctures purvey curative power ostensibly as complex, non-

local information about biological design. This theory has been utterly discredited by centuries of research during which potentized-micro-dose influences have failed to be recorded *anywhere* in nature. In fact, there is no basis for presuming the body's molecules are even able to discriminate the molecules of homeopathic medicines (diluted beyond Avogadro's limit) from general background contamination. Yet homeopathy is dispensed with beneficial enough results not only to survive but to emerge as a hot venture-capital item in the twenty-first century.

Aromatherapy, *Chi Gung,* **radionics, Reiki, Polarity,** and **prayer** require not only interchangeability of mind, matter, and energy, but the capacity of life forms to conduct cures from thought into substance.

No ONE CAN TRACK precisely where thought enters cellular nexuses and stimulates neurotransmitters, large proteins, and nucleic acids, but some aspect of molecular intelligence is implicit at the onset of body-mind. Before it is thinkable, thought imbues emergent tissue fields with membranous shape and resilience. We experience thought as cognitive when it germinates in the brain as coherent images and notions; yet it is also atomistic and idiomatic enough to ignite the tiny power stations inside cells.

Primordial codes flow back and forth between the mind of the healer and particles inside the atoms, molecules, and cells of the sick person. These vibrate into one another in a kind of inaudible, atonal cosmic music. Temporal content is "degraded" by energetic jolts, needles, herbal potions, and other transference, as they approach the pagan dialect of "cell." Human designs interact with cellular codices in such a manner that acts of palpation and psychosymbolization are transduced into morphogenetic and psychotherapeutic activity. Reconciling these two tongues is the singular talent of any successful medicine man or woman.

The cell is the root of the mind even as the proton and electron are the basis of the atom. We should not be surprised then that the cell hears the voice of the mind: cells congregate in networks of scalar and neural waves to create mind in the first place. If the unminded thought of nature organizes cells and their tissues, why shouldn't the spiritualized and transpersonalized thought totems of shamans and doctors energize those same tissues?

How to muster archetypal intelligence, how to reempower and transmit it therapeutically, how to give each medicine a signature, how to specify a resonance and destination (so that it arrives inside cell language and tissue matrices in a vital mode) is the mission of all healers. It little matters whether vibrations arise from the chants of a Stone Age priest, the receptive hands of a cranial osteopath, or the cold laser of a modern hospital, as long as they ultimately find their target and catalyze homeostatic activity.

That may seem a pollyanna viewpoint, but I mean it only at the deepest, most nonlinear level. I am not comparing primitive to advanced medicine; I am not comparing quartz crystals to electromagnetic resonance machines. I am talking only about the ultimate invisible resonance behind all life, the consolidating melody at which everyone, no matter his tools, aims blindly and intuitively, because no one can locate its actual instrumentation.

If the medicines described in both volumes of this book are legitimate tools for curing diseases, there must ultimately be some molecular pathway for them in the "real world." Metaphors cannot move cells unless they are more than metaphors, in which case they require either a new science or a revolutionary expansion of existing territory. In this appendix I will propose seven basic principles whereby alternative and holistic medicines might "work." These are not principles by comparison to the axiomatic programs of biology, chemistry, and physics. They represent ways of intuiting factors beyond present knowledge, points of entry into a vast, unknown phenomenal science that we cannot test or codify, perhaps because it is what we are. They include

tropes for the interchangeability of mind, matter, and energy as well as prototypes of post-scientific metaphors for processes which (if they occur at all) skirt traditional understanding of cause and effect, time and space.

In each era scholars select a thought-system into which they indoctrinate themselves and their students. They valorize that system as the sole path to understanding natural phenomena, establish it as an orthodoxy, and censor all noncompliant ideas. Orthodox bureaucratic doctrine presently disputes mind-matter interchangeability because its effects cannot be demonstrated consistently or in the same way that jet propulsion and DNA replication can.

I believe that, despite cosmologists' claims of a near-unified field theory of matter and energy, a great deal more of the dark matter and energy of the universe remains to be uncovered than has yet been identified. The lost branches of science are presently elephants stomping through our midst. As huge as they are, that blind and deaf are we to their existence.

Science unwittingly pretends that mind (and thus it itself) does not exist. As a biochemical artifact and a chimera of random molecular interactions, mind has no basis ontologically. It is the fly in the ointment, but it is more than a fly, it is a whole layer of creation, likely stretching from one end of galactic space to the other. Without it the universe would have no phenomenal properties. And because there is only one universe (not one for physics and another for metaphysics), we are as subject to mind's unexhumed effects as we are to axioms of Newtonian physics and Darwinian evolution.

I have no more idea than the next person of what the real parameters of mind and matter are. In fact, they may not be concretizable in the way other contemporary scientific properties are. They may encompass a radically different sphere of nature and organization through which the imposition of a factor as powerful and weightless as thought can create and transform whole planets. Such a component must fall along the cutting edge of being and nothingness, where we exist and hardly exist, where we turn to try to see ourselves turning to see.

IN THE FORESEEABLE future, mind must remain outside the equation, an epiphenomenon of neural activity. However, if weightless intelligence can target and conduct discrete physical information out of the molecular space of individual minds, then it can transmit imaginal effects to other organisms. This would mean that mind requires a new ontological status within physics, chemistry, and medicine.

We also cannot presume telekinesis just because it is the simplest catch-all explanation. Even if we do, we cannot dismiss the possibility that raw telekinesis (like any energy) requires polymorphous applications, tagging itself idiosyncratically in visualization, breath, movement, palpation, microdoses, sounds, and needles. That way, molecular effects are signified and channeled.

Electricity doesn't simply flow from the natural world into lights and motors; it needs engineers and engines. This analogy might explain why so many different modalities have arisen for conveying healing energy.

True doctors and healers of all persuasions, if they have subliminal and telepathic power, can adapt more than one paradigm or modality to their mode of transmission. As they create rituals for what they are doing, they employ cover stories for the paraphysical transmission of cures from one body-mind to another. Healing itself remains the singular modality.

MY CHOICE OF the popular number seven and my laws of cure are devices for helping the reader to understand abstruse and meta-concrete healing systems. There are not seven laws of cure any more than there is one law or 256 laws. These represent seven models for understanding much the same thing, either from different perspectives or as aspects nested in one synergistic whole. If holistic medicines "work," all seven-plus laws must contribute to cures in all systems. Most likely they do, for they are not laws so much as putative attributes of the relationship between mind and matter, or ways to understand mind-body systems. Actual medicines are complex, dimensionless, culturally adorned homeostases combining rituals and beliefs and not reducible to formulae anyway.

My "laws" resemble other quasi-scientific crypto-objects and sympathetic cause-and-effect actions proposed all the way from the European Renaissance to the twentieth-century New Age. Mesmerism, vital energy, ectoplasm, etheric projection, pyramid (and spheroid) power, lei lines, morphic resonance, and alchemical transmutation of minerals and elements represent outsider phenomena that have been thoroughly debunked by science. Committees of technocratic skeptics continue to stamp them out wherever they rear up lizard heads under new rubrics and names.

The difference between the above-mentioned paraphysical aliases and my principles is that I am not proposing mine even remotely as laws or as things; in fact, my use of the word "law" is ironical. Laws are axioms considered compulsory by those who believe in them.

Couching therapeutic rules in exaggerated neo-etymologies such as "hologrammaticization" and "iconicization" is a way of toying with both scientific nomenclature and New Age pretend-science, e.g. by coining a slightly archaic language to distinguish actual medical acts from allegories and metaphors. My terminology is archaicized and twisted out of usual word forms. Although I have chosen common terms for some of my mock laws, for others I have either made up names or added syllables (representing quanta of action) to more familiar names in order to distinguish the event I am intuiting from some other, more common activity (iconicization is different from iconization, and hologrammaticization is an octave up from holograms). I have also listed alternate words after each "law" to give other ways of conceptualizing their territory.

Do not be intimidated by these aggrandized terms and models. They are no more real than Lewis Carroll's mock turtles, vorpal blades, or frumious bandersnatches, or for that matter the charmed quarks, superstrings, and buckyballs of fairytale physics.

Remember also that this Appendix is an attempt to invent a terminology for hypothetical events. All of what follows may be little more than posturing about the unknowable.

Embryogenesis (catalysis/enzymaticization)

THE EMBRYOGENIC PRINCIPLE recruiting molecules into organs and creatures is an elusive force behind life. Its transcendent properties are why pathologies often cannot be assigned to mechanical causes. How can sickness and health be explained if body-mind itself is a mystery?

We exist because of an infinitesimalized guiding template, not through quantifications of mass effects and dense fabrics. Billions of discrete chemical interactions honor morphogenetic grids binding them and their phenomena together. This embryogenic force in nature metabolizes thermokinetic energy in membranes and cell layers and puts it at the service of autonomous agencies.

We were made once by fluctuations of protein molecules, organelles, and cells, and we exist solely as their oscillating community. Modes of primal tissue organization in the fetus resolve into contemporary fields with properties of motility, mutability, and potentiation. Cell layers that folded in gastrulation to carve our central axis, nervous system, and gut continue to resonate along an invisible therapeutic channel from the pineal gland/third eye of our forehead up over the peak of our crown down our vertebralized nerve cord to our tailbone. Its elixirs are potent enough that an eclectic range of healers can invigorate their seeds.

Healing must respect the gestation and self-manufacture of living organisms from inanimate matter and their sustenance by the same esoteric principle. We do not know how dynamic, energy-transmitting systems coalesce out of molecular configurations and operate in bodies so successfully for so long, but a nonlinear set of events daringly skirts the thermodynamic zone that medicine honors.

Embryogenesis embraces all other factors—synergistic, holo-

grammatic, metabolic, genetic, nucleic, and iconic—that contribute to the self-organization of life forms. Hence, embryogenic intelligence is the single force that must be tripped or unleashed by physicians of all persuasions.

PATHOLOGY IS A DEVIATION of embryogenesis, a birth defect after parturition. It shows up in body-mind not at its point of origin in a proximally damaged organ but (from the standpoint of holistic medicine) as a wrinkle in the embryogenic field, where homeostasis is most at risk of losing its capacity to compensate. If life is morphogenetic coordination of separate signals, disease is a gap in that transmission.

This is why skillfully blended pharmaceuticals and MRI-perfect surgeries may fail to do their jobs, why they may even activate pathological forces as destructive as the ailment they are enlisted to treat. As precise and refined as they may be, at the level of organismal integrity they are paws groping inside a hornet's nest. How can crude laboratory drugs accurately strike the delicate embryogenic fields generating vital activity; how can they avoid disturbing the choir of electrons and electrolytes among cells? How can even the sharpest blade cut away the sick from the healthy inside a mutable wave of fluctuating energies? How can any sort of physicomechanical activity—pharmaceutical, radioactive, or surgical—pin itself onto the synergizing force inside a creature?

A doctor treating manifest tissue shapes may well misgauge the systemic depth of the effect before him.

SOMETHING BEYOND THERMODYNAMICS, heat, and gravitational effects is generating the temporal appearance of body-mind—and it is that coaction which must be energized by a cure in order to restore a sick person's matrix and reactive the seeds that guided his underlying blastula of stem cells into tissues and coherent organs.

The ember that made tissue alive in the first place must be fanned and stirred into fresh consignments. An intelligence beyond mere thermochemical hierarchies must be stimulated to do its magical cellular dance, bluffed into remumbling abracadabra syllables leading to bio-logical cohesion. A healer must sound the topokinetic bugle and per-suade tissues made of carbon, hydrogen, oxygen, and phosphorus that they are somehow vital and still want to thrive in bodies and exchange and convert energies for the same mysterious reason that they requited in the first place.

Doctors must be shamans, for they bribe cells to reenact the self-organizing power of their genesis and herd unruly molecules anew into orderly, interdependent collocations of tissues.

Doctors must speak the ancient, forgotten language of "cell."

Therapeutic palpation initiates the embryogenic force by acti-vating inertial and lethargic tissue states. Manipulation rouses embryogenic axes of organ motility. To be effective it must orient toward primordial tissue freedom rather than some idealized resting state.

Herbs function as morphogens, enzymaticizing cellular shifts and tissue agglutinations.

Traditional Chinese Medicine is a vintage embryogenic system; its needles and herbs catalyze the vectors underlying mature tissue com-plexes. In this context acupuncture is a form of primal induction. If its needles stimulate therapeutic reconfiguration, it is because they provide precise, discrete signals that impel tissues to reenact embryogenic tra-jectories. Treating a liver or a heart by energetic points is not a matter of penetrating and repairing the literal space of these organs; it is an energizing of the viscerocellular dynamics that led to their formation in the first place. The acupuncturist's filaments tap into not the spaces of organs *per se* as much as their contrails and developmental paths emer-gent from the fetus. Flowing in currents to and from adult tissue nodes, these morphogenetic vestiges begin and end at some geographical dis-tance from their ultimate consolidations. In the embryogenic process they have expanded and reorganized as scalar, electromagnetic fields and liquid waves radiating from organ chrysalides.

Osteopaths enact an energetic version of surgery, for they ply the grains and embryogenic tissue pattern established during fetal development. By palpating at the level at which the tissues are innately disposed, the healing hand reads and supports organs' primal self-organizing principles. Embryogenic pathways of liver, lungs, stomach, and spleen embody their implicit vital throb and motile range. These organ masses each have an innate pulsation, range, tropismic identity, and characteristic patterns of oscillation, all of which can be stabilized or enhanced by treatment, even when the actuating touch is conducted through clothing, skin, musculoskeleton, and other organs.

The lungs, gathered up in fascia, muscles, ribs, and pleura, are rocked tenderly until they regain their innate comfort level and natural cycle. The liver is lifted and molded gelatinously back toward its embryogenic state. The heart and its valves and arteries are tuned by hands-on vibrations.

Craniosacral therapy addresses the resonant fields and fluids of body-mind as a quantum super-system beyond ordinary anatomy. According to William Sutherland, a universal and archetypal intelligence is imprinted in cerebrospinal fluid with the first germ cells and transmits its organizing hologram into the blastula. Conducted through bioelectromagnetic crystals, young cerebrospinal nectar becomes a configuring ambrosia. Vibrating its pulse against the wetsuit of the meninges and dural tube, this organizing stream invisibly beats the Breath of Life into all the tissues and cells of the body. Respiration, heart-pumping, lymphatic current, cerebrospinal flush, and craniosacral orbits of flexion and extension scald a unitary flow of "liquid light" through skeletal and cellular space. While oscillating between its own long and short tidal phase states, it folds and unfolds from something into nothing, from implicate stillness and void into explicate creature existence.

Potentization (succussion, synergization)

POTENTIZATION MEANS IMPARTING a vital, active property to a substance, image, sound, etc. A potentized remedy is one that has had its channel of manifestation and transmission exponentialized. A moderately medicinal substance becomes a powerfully transformational one with new attributes and effects.

Potentization is presumed to raise or subtilize dormant forces so that they express new traits with the potential to facilitate the body in discrete and intricate ways. It is a beneficent network disruptor.

A potentized boost coincides paradoxically with serial reductions in molecular substance (dilution)—the less substance: the more healing vitality, the greater its specificity. The presumption is that potentization of a molecularly coarse substance not only cleanses and submolecularizes but medicinalizes the properties of the underlying remedy.

A potentized cure's subsequent dispersal and globalization is synergistic, establishing a momentum by which specified nano or micro events are incorporated into larger systems that enhance one another and induce large-scale change, constantly recombining initial agencies with their after-effects. A potentized herb, charm, or magic word essentializes and radiates information beyond its denotative or physical molecular state throughout body-mind and its cellular matrices. A cognitive meaning ultimately becomes a biological meaning.

THE MOST WELL-KNOWN example of potentization is the supposed transformation—alchemization or spiritualization—of molecules in the preparation of **homeopathic medicines**; in fact, "potentization" is a generic homeopathic term. Ground herbs or other substances are medicinalized by dilution with succussion. The intended result is a change in state of matter even more profound than that from a liquid to a solid or gas.

After being dissolved and diluted many times in decimal ratios (or their exponents) with hard shaking each cut, what is left of a tincture of homeopathic sulphur has totally different qualities from the raw sulphur at its source. Homeopathic sepia, bryonia, chestnut, gold, aluminum, salt, and the diluted and succussed tinctures of spores of various bacteria, viruses, etc., are all transformed from either simple pharmaceuticals (or toxins) into submolecular phase states in which a hibernating molecular vitality is released while any pathologizing properties are expelled. The sublimation of negative effects demonstrates how a hyper-specified dilution can neutralize or convert poisons into medicines. Perhaps even strong pollutants like DDT and spent nuclear fuel can someday be potentized into wide-acting environmental medicines.

In homeopathic microdoses, succussion is usually conceived in decimal-type stages (centesimal, millesimal, etc.); these represent jumps in capacity from tens to hundreds to thousands and millions. There is no reason that tens alone should guide the successive scale; octaves, sevens, twenties, and twelves each trigger ratios of therapeutic force in systems in one or another non-Western culture.

On occasion, potencies may also cause diseases and/or symptoms because of their strong actions, but these are not toxic effects, i.e., poisonings or injuries, so much as secondary disruptive offshoots from a change in an organized phase state or meta-stable level of organization. After all, a shift in homeostasis will be curative only if the body-mind responds to it in a positive fashion. Some microbiologists believe that cancer is primarily a phase-state perturbation among a body of cells provoked by aneuploidy, the transmission of irregular quantities of chromosomes to daughter cells.

S UPERCHARGING A REMEDY by a reduction and hyperconcentration of substance or information is a paradox that lies at the heart of systems of healing as remote from one another as Bach's flower-petal remedies are from Ainu chanting and craniosacral therapy. Quantal permutation of vibrations occurs in wavelengths of hues in photic stimulation and other color therapies; tonal and chord shifts in chants, mantras, and shamanic commands; and exponential scales of aromatic essences. Potentization also describes the charging of meaning in ordinary syllables and words, the stacking of cellular forces and tissue layers in palpation, and the activation of biological energy by metallic filaments in acupuncture.

Convinced that there is no such thing as potentization of matter, mainstream scientists attribute any positive results from such therapies to placebo effects.

Submolecularization (nanopharmacology, particularization, vibration)

WE ARE A UNIFIED, semi-fluid colloid—a dynamic set of matrices reverberating and synapsing with gross states of matter, from the wormlike movements of our viscera to DNA helices vibrating atomically inside the nuclei of our cells. Life decisions inside us are made within carbon rings and proteins fluctuating through metadimensional uncertainty states with probabilistic expressions. These translate millionfold networks of signals and psychosomatic noise into intelligent, energy-modulating creatures. They must have submolecular as well as molecular expressions.

All energy-based healing modalities, from Reiki to rebirthing, from Body Electronics to aromatherapy, depend to some degree or another on pre-atomic or nanopharmacological characteristics of substances. The more submolecular the potency invested in a configuration or modality, the deeper and more wide-ranging its ripples and the more subeffects, supereffects, and networks radiate from them.

MOLECULARIZATION IS THE protocol of standard pharmacology; submolecularization is a meta-pharmacological process by which alternative medicines attempt to arouse dormant properties of matter from below the molecular level. It denotes actions of deep cures by fractal parameters.

Submolecularization requires particularization (the homeopathic

"Similar"): the less gross material there is to a substance or nodule of information, the more precise and recognizable that minute trace has to be. Otherwise, its effects dissipate into the noisy, chaotic biochemical background. Medicinalization is not just a matter of achieving the functional equivalents of micro or nano phase states but of the correct pitch in a precisely resonant plane of meaning, morphology, or vibration. Healing is, in a certain sense, a method of matching the subtle vibration of a disease or character state with the quite separately originating vibration of a remedy.

Everything exists by vibration. At a submolecular level vibrations hold the universe together. The right medicine is a vibration. Cell signalling is another vibration. Herbs are chemical vibrations. Skilled palpation is vibratory. Of course, pathologies are vibrations too.

This is perhaps how systems like curative eurhythmy, Haitian voodoo, Applied Kinesiology, and Haida shamanism function equivalently as medicines. A Tibetan turquoise pill can be the functional and energetic equivalent of a *kum nye* exercise or a chiropractic adjustment. They are all, at their common nucleus, vibrations.

Submolecular medicines—whether substances, sounds, colors, or meanings—must not only be particularized but singular (the homeopathic "single dose"). For microdoses, plant essences, visualizations, directed breath, pulse diagnoses, and most modes of palpation, more is almost never better. When a reading or remedy is repeated during its active phase, an overuse syndrome sets in and the revelatory or curative effect is underspecified or deadened. In a sense the message becomes redundant, hence tautological. It is important not to presume that if a little is good, more is better, or if once is effective, again and again are "the cat's meow." The singular shock or activating effect of a particularized, similarized signal, sensation, or submolecularization *is* its homeostatic motif, the nonequilibrium basis of its psychosomatic effects. Repetition of the signal at best has no effect, at worst antidotes the original message.

Submolecularization and iconicization form a pair in the sense that all codes and medicinal signs (DNA, RNA, neurological, linguistic, totemic, metalinguistic) resonate among alternate energetic versions of one another at the subliminal level at which matter approaches energy—and being, nothingness.

Iconicization
(symbolic resonance, archetypalization)

COMPLEX CHAINS OF ciphers lie at the heart of nature and are the means by which one sort of form or substance becomes another (see transduction, below). Biological codes negotiate the iconic essences linking inanimate matter and life.

We think and communicate in phonetic and voltaic alphabets. As electro-organic forms comprised of protein configurations become potentized and particularized anew, they reembody and retransmit their iconicized states in different dialects. These phenomena surge synaptically and hieroglyphically through circuit breakers and transformers of the body. Signals activating curative states pass into cells and organs.

Iconicization is the first step toward the establishment of a curative modality on a purely archetypal level. It makes possible the transfer of information between a mind-symbol form like a muscle test or sand painting and a physical state. It converts potential healing elements to sigilized forms whereby they resonate into proteins. These pathways serve as unconscious commuters of effects from one modality and level of manifestation into another. Their intermediate status could be breath octaves, cerebrospinal light fluctuations, electrolytic currents, electromagnetic crystals, morphogenetic inductions, and/or reverse DNA transcription.

THE DISCOVERY THAT a sequence of ciphers generates biological form in a developmental relationship between genes and amino acids, amino acids and protein molecules, proteins and protein-based tissues, is no less than an insight into the iconic basis of form/meaning itself. How biomolecular and symbolic activity—ciphers in different domains of reality—can be spontaneously linked by medicinal signals speaks to the original mystery whereby cells could arise from bubbles of sea spume and make a biosphere. Healing metaphors and bionucleic ciphers may be preposterously disparate texts written in unrelated mediums, but they are both lodged in and emergent from biomolecular crystals where all deep syntax strings begin. Biological and semantic codes represent the same elementary system, albeit that one kind of rune is presently emergent inside a cell and another in thought bursts of creatures made of such cells. Fundamentally and primally, they are interintelligible.

We are held together not by a genetic formula—though we could not exist without DNA—but by iconicized resonances passing through tissue-webs in diaphanous fields. Language is an aspect of the biological field. A subtilized potentiation of cell organizational principles is transmitted in animal howls, mantras, and chants. "Cell" and Hopi are both nucleic languages—equally defective, equally invocatory. The formation of life was never confined by semantic barriers anyway, for all biological, cognitive, and therapeutic codes arise from a common source. Human talk and cell talk are *both cell talk.*

I CONICIZATION IS THE basic immune-system mode for DNA-based forms. Perennial diseases from the legacy of the Earth's genomes matriculate unstably in phase states beneath surface ciphers of genes and immunity globules. Strings of junk DNA along with remnants of endogenous retroviruses and lysogenic phages molecularly craft proteins to solve their emerging crises. Writing icons and transmitting symbolic fields, they transmute one set of information (DOS) into another, and then another, and so on indefinitely.

Any organ can hypothetically recover the aspect of itself that stores the primordial stem cells from which its *anlage* arose. Such templates are dormant throughout inactivated strands of DNA and other vestigial languages in our cell nuclei. There is no need to clone and harvest tissues to obtain the raw material of organs. Invoking totemic entities, medicine men and women enlist cells to reprise their initial embryogenic act. Our bodies specify and assemble tissues as we need them. Miraculous healing may require only breaking through networks of protein suppressors and telling cells what we need them to do at the level of gastrulation and organogenesis.

If human-to-cell talk were not possible, nothing could ever be cured and we would probably not live very long (or at all). Entropy and molecular degradation would rule nature.

That people get healthier and tissues are repaired suggests that the simple intention to turn mind into matter (symbol into tissue, germ cell into medicine) in fact accesses a link between presignified realms of form and substance.

Transduction (transsubstantiation, decoherence, alchemical projection)

ICONICIZATION FORESHADOWS TRANSDUCTION. Transduction is the change of one entire state (homeostatic organization) into another. It is the physical means whereby informational units (organized icons) of one discrete code or vibration are translated into a different one. While iconicization imprints information in one or another cipher or bio-runic system, transduction reorganizes it as a new phase state in a different hierarchy. A variety of runes can thus transduce biological action via touch, chants, images, etc., and equally through insights (abreaction) provided by a therapist/shaman. Touch and vision literally become energy.

Viewed in terms of iconicized sets, the goal of any medicine is to create a translation field that disrupts (makes decoherent) the fixed symbols of a pathology on both physical and mental planes. Thus, ritualized meaning becomes newly active, transformable, and reintegrative. Tissue states recoil, at least partially, to formative basins of attraction.

PALPATION TRANSDUCES THE physical effects of iconicized touch into morphogenetic counterparts. **Words, images, sounds, smells, microdoses,** etc., resonate at molecular points of contact into psychosomatic activity. **Continuum, Body-Mind Centering, vipassana meditation, *Chi Gung,* and kriya yoga** send charged decoherence patterns to the roots of biological configurations.

The molecular substance of a **homeopathic potency** is transduced through dilution and succussion into biochemical activity. The sensation of a **color** or **mandala** is transduced psychosomatically into beats of breath and visceral rhythm. These transitions resemble the quantum chemistry whereby matter is turned into energy in the chloroplasts of plant cells, and a blastula becomes an organism via the selective resignification of its cells. Though **alchemy** may be the vintage transductional system (for it transmutes toxic or inert metals into medicinal products), in fact any herbal potion transduces and synergizes its elements into new curative modes streaming through chemical lattices.

A striking instance of medical transduction is the internalizations, gyrations, and breath patternings of ***Chi Gung,*** as breath and image orchestrate tissue changes at different scales in the body. The physical movements themselves, like comic gesticulations and mod dance steps, are at best loosely oriented toward neuromuscular or visceral change. If they cause deeper healing activity, it is because they are transduced and then globalized.

Hologrammaticization (crystallization, holism)

HOLOGRAMMATICIZATION IS AN esoteric though fundamental process in nature whereby information and templates manifest in identical shape-states in many places simultaneously or harmonically sequenced with one another. Iterization with scalar dissemination is more or less instantaneous in biological systems, hypothetically resembling laserlike patternings of magnetic atoms mirrored among foci of elliptical rings.

The hologram is a phase in the development of every multicellular life form on Earth. The trademark instance of hologrammaticization is the blastula stage of mammalian development during which each separate blastomere is fully potentiated to become a complete mature organism; yet those holograms will each eventually specialize into only a single aspect of an actual creature—a nerve, an intestinal goblet, a kidney morsel, a hair or nail, etc. Thus, an entire organism preexists in some fashion at millions of separate sites; every part of us was once capable of fissioning and becoming all of us; every cell retains that capacity at some level, even if its potentiation is enzymatically masked. The body is a hologram of crystals in which even mind is a dynamic crystalline projection.

Healing can occur much in the way development did in the blastula, by specifying which cells are to congregate in which tissues and at what level of intrinsic dynamic tension. This is the inductive matrix to which therapeutic touch, mantra, and breath then address themselves vibrationally. Pathologies are cured in the way nodules of separate information were syncretized into a functional creature.

Hologrammaticization suggests that healing information introduced at one level or in one region of the body-mind becomes transmitted to other levels, other regions, and to the organismic entirety, not simply as a linear chronological residue of chemical seepage or a ladder of neural synapsing but as an intrinsic, irreducible, scalar principle, transcending thermodynamics and gravity while fusing them along the curve of space-time. Not only is each part remanifested throughout the whole but every specified bit of information, no matter how insubstantial physically, is available and potentially active everywhere.

The act of cure is not limited to the transposition of form or data (as in surgery or pharmacy) but distributes itself as a hologrammaticization of unconscious signs.

Transduction and iconicization are equivalent principles of the healing process, for without automatic translation of codes between levels, it is hard to conceive of how, for instance, touch could be hologrammaticized and turned into enzymatic activity, or mantras and breath

into cellular activity, etc.

Hologrammaticization is also more or less how information is stored in the cerebral subcrystals of the organism. The brain does not form picture-perfect replicas of events that constitute individual acts of learning and memory; it distributes memory redundantly and hologrammatically. Information precipitates in many places simultaneously. When portions of brain tissue are elided or damaged by disease, accident, or surgery, other brain tissue continues to retain some version of it, perhaps in a different configuration, and is capable of constructing new pathways to access it.

Educational techniques like those taught by Alexander, Bates, and Feldenkrais rely on the fact that somatic repatterning transmits lessons through a hologrammatic core. An exercise practiced by the right hip or shoulder or right eye is instantaneously conveyed to its left counterpart, not merely by the brain learning and then reapplying it, but as patterning imprinted in tissue and then globalized.

Despite holograms, information does not simply put itself everywhere equally; the result would be total mush. Instead, once potentized and exponentialized (decimalized), signals are specified and sublimated before they are retransmitted in such a way that, although they can appear anywhere at any time, they are only used in a manner that restores tissue locally to vital functioning.

A **homeopathic medicine** hypothetically initials (iconicizes) morphogenetic information in molecules or even electrons of water (by submolecularization), transduces it into other states of matter while potentizing it, and hologrammaticizes it as a Similar (a precise replica of the disease's symptomatic action without its pathological grip); then it radiates (resonates) this patterning throughout the body-mind.

Polarity Therapy, **Body Electronics, Reiki, and holotropic and transformative breathing** all rely on a principle of instantaneous scalar transmission, as if the body-mind were a crystal of crystals made up of the electromagnetized cells and thought waves. Upon saturation of the organism with enzymes and trace minerals (in **Body Electronics**), meridian-based pressure points are palpated and released; then the organism exudes its toxins and chemical surpluses as well as its neuroses and other psychopathologies into tiny, hard crystals which are eliminated with other bodily wastes. At least, this is the goal, whether such crystals are actual or metaphysical.

The same principle of simultaneous multiplication and transmission may be observed in most, if not all, systems of somatics and physical therapy. Resonant touch has effects that distribute themselves beyond the immediate impact of manipulation or stacking. Palpation, chiropractic adjustment, visceral massage, and other hands-on transmissions are (on the one hand) mechanical operations with specific kinetic goals and (on the other) morphogenetic reactivations of the field states in which their forerunners—holograms of developing, embryonic tissue complexes—were initially responsive to induction and organization by other complexes and thus coalesced holistically into a body-mind.

The presumption is that synergistic contact at a precise resonant visceral and neural level hologrammaticizes throughout the body's tissues and phase states, causing them to reenact something like their original embryogenic situations. Trajectories of palpation convey unique messages to the vitalized nodes and granules of tissue through which they pass that become particular to each structure and vibrate with its quantum state.

By this model, healing touch is simultaneously kinetic, chemicomechanical, biochemical, neural, phenomenological, and even nucleic in transferring information (in Lamarckian fashion) from soma into DNA.

The diagnostic system of **iridology**, based on the sympathetic transmission of field states between crystals of different sizes and shapes within an organism, relies on a vestige of the multipotentiality of the cells of the blastula. Tissue of the whole is projected through each part, so a region or organ takes on the organism in miniature. More sensitive organs acquire stigmata of energy patterning from the entirety. The phase states of the body—their relative health by region—fission into replica components in the flecks, hues, and pools of the irides of the eyes, likewise in the separate fleshy and hued regions of the tongue, the furrowed geography of the palm, the grid of the face, and the spiral pygmies of the ear. In tribute to the transdimensional profundity of this principle, some spiritual systems seek the source of past-lifetime diseases and deaths in the birthmarks and defects of people's present bodies.

The hologrammatic principle in healing has been newly confirmed by Frank Lowen's connective-tissue regulators. This previously unknown—or only vaguely conceptualized—anatomical network was discovered by Lowen in the early 2000s. The network's full scope and therapeutic import remain substantially unexplored to date, but its capacity for information storage and transfer could turn out to be paradigmatic.

Lowen describes a series of morphodynamic centers (or homunculi) throughout the body. At each one, information is hologrammaticized. With their own depths, planes, countours, and angles, these discrete homuncular shapes represent organized tissue states as well as anatomical relationships and movements. They also startlingly resemble small human people, with spines, fronts and backs of skulls, arms, shoulders, legs, etc. Some of the humanoid shapes (e.g. those in the brain) are distorted by the necessities of their proportional placement in the anatomy.

A homunculus and its representative tissue comprise simultaneous patterns of activity (energy). For locating dysfunction, one can utilize the homunculus itself interpretively like an iris or tongue, though on an energetic, tensional, rhythmic (rather than cartographic) basis, sensing its multidimensional layers manually.

Zones represented microcosmically respond and normalize as the appropriate pattern within their hologram is engaged. While tissue areas contain equivalent patterns, the concentrated homunculus is always the impetus. The sacral homunculus is a pivot of transference for a range of bodily forces, notably those involving ligaments—not surprising given the diverse complexes stored and synopsized in the sacrum. A homunculus in the sternum serves as a fascial regulator, and one in the vicinity of the trachea helps balance gas and liquid pressures. Homunculi around the hara or umbilicus express muscle units.

For treatment, the homunculus is used reflexively with the region of tissue that it represents (the left wrist, the right eye, the smooth muscle of the gall bladder, the limbic system, etc.) in the discrete way in which it represents it. If one palpates an area on the homunculus and its respective nexus in the body simultaneously in a manner that supports their congruence, the hands will be guided along specific tensional outlines that generate therapeutic ripples. When both sites are engaged at their own scales, the practitioner reaps the strongest response, for the homunculus functions like a fulcrum. Gathering tension in a site-specific way, the therapist grasps each hologram and interacts with it, neither pushing nor pulling. A heightened impulse is triggered from the hologram to the peripheral tissue, surging as palpation itself leans into its own movement. A barrier is attained; i.e., a pressurized urging accumulates until its tension suddenly holds. Then it reorganizes, and a curative flush billows, aikido-like, through the tissue.

Transference
(telekinesis, the physics of love)

HEALERS DO NOT ultimately treat tissues or organs, or even neuroses, but fluctuations of holograms. The doctor's meaning field and vibration and the vibration of his medicine interact with the field of the patient. As the disease is represented and projected symbolically and psychosomatically, its icons respond to the icons being proposed to it. That is how chants, Reiki runes, breath phonemes, and charismatic prayers become cell-dynamic activities. Tissue complexes reenact some aspect of the protolinguistic stem cells from which their rudiments arose.

Modern science has proven that emotional responses to both soothing and stressful events produce changes in blood pressure, heart rate, degree of stomach acidity, digestive capacity, levels of hormonal activity, etc., so words, emotions, and touch have immediate effects in sympathetic and parasympathetic nervous systems. If telekinesis is possible, then these same words, acts of empathy (or antipathy), and healing touch can have major impact on cell movements and the intrinsic condition and vitality of tissues.

Transference acknowledges the persona of the healer (apart from his or her technique) as a conduit of energy or a focal point for iconicization and transduction. The presentation of an "other" to the sick person or disease empowers the remedy. Transference in the most general sense is the capacity of a therapist to impose himself or herself as an alternative to the pathologized state in the patient—to substitute one wave-length, one vibration, one pulse for another.

The physics of love is shorthand for the notion that healing intention can be molecularized, channeled, and given energetic and cellular form. This is not just a case of benignly conducted healing power but also a feature of the most deadly voodoo and curses. The danger of negative transference, as discussed earlier in this volume, is that the malefic, incompetent, or inflated physician equally transmits his or her unrealized complexes in the guise of molecularized intention, with the result that the patient is further hexed and pathologized rather than healed.

Unrealized complexes must become sublimated through curative iconicization and transduction before they are medicinalized in a client. When they are unconscious shamanic weapons before they are medicines, they become the precise opposites of medicines.

Telekinesis is one possible avenue of transference but not a prerequisite for transference, as energy can travel emotionally, by personality resonance, by herbal and sensual vibration, and through the holograms of palpation. Whatever the medium in which he or she is transmitting, an experienced healer can then feel the actual tissue changes fluctuating under his or her fingers.

THE RELATIONSHIP BETWEEN DNA and therapies of language, touch, and sensation contains within its mystery a clue to the present void between orthodox and alternative healing systems. That gap is the major obstacle to a radically different medical profession in the twenty-first century. In a fully holistic modality, healing would transcend not only the phenomenal world formed by synapses of light and sound-vibrations into meaning systems, but all nexuses and rules made of phonemes and syllables. It would speak directly from "molecules" of herbs, palpations, needles, potentizations, etc., into molecules of cells and tissues, transmitting potentials that are simultaneously linguistic and metalinguistic. Needles, aroma essences, herbs, faith-based transmissions of cosmic energy, mandalas, palpation techniques, and even surgical operations would ultimately translate signs into other signs within a living syntax of organism and meaning. Such a system of transformation and transference would forge its own accommodation with modern science.

The medicine of the future must evolve past not only concretization of organs but commoditization of cells and chromosomes; it may reap new stem cells by inspiring communications between Golgi bodies and mitochondria, providing a basis for fresh tissue. A modern synthesis of shamanic resonance and biological alchemy may retranscribe icons, therapeutic palpations, herbal potions, aroma essences, and photic wavelengths into fresh heart tissue, cell lining for intestines, retinal cells, and other needed differentiations.

RESOURCE GUIDE

THE GOAL OF this guide is to share with interested readers my sources for some of the practices that lie behind *Planet Medicine.* It is limited to the modalities and practitioners discussed in the text. It is also limited to institutions and people with whom I have had direct experience (though in a few cases I have listed national organizations or people whose work I know reliably secondhand). It should also be regarded as subjective and theoretical rather than concrete, literal advice. If in doubt about any of the applications of practices, practitioners, or products mentioned on the following pages, please consult a doctor or other health professional. This guide is not a substitute for experienced advice.

A complete resource guide would be an enormous undertaking of its own, well beyond the scope of this book. To be useful to the majority of readers, it would have to include major urban areas and rural communities in at least the English-speaking world. It would also have to be researched and corrected on a regular basis. Too many directories are simply copied from one source to another and are untested, out of date, or both.

Most readers will not be able to use this guide with regard to actual practitioners, but they may be able to find equivalent local options by reading practitioner directories (usually free at alternative bookstores and markets), querying natural-foods markets and health-food stores, checking community bulletin boards, asking friends for referrals, doing Internet searches, and contacting national organizations (in the case of some modalities) for listings in their area.

I will try to update this section from edition to edition. However, individual practitioners may move or may elect not to take on new clients.

Acupuncture

(See also American College of Traditional Chinese Medicine, Chinese Medicine, Amini Peller, Paul Pitchford)

Ching-Chun Ou
3091 Grand Avenue
Oakland, California 94610
Phone: 510-547-6798

Robert Zeiger
3031 Telegraph Avenue
Berkeley, California 94710
Phone: 510-843-7397

Alexander Technique

Jerry Sontag
The Art of Learning
2547 8th Street/Studio 39
Berkeley, California 94710
Phone: 510-486-1317

The Alexander Educational Center (TAEC)
Giora Pinkas and John Baron, Directors
2727 College Avenue
Berkeley, California 94705
Phone: 925-933-0602

American Society for the Alexander Technique
30 North Maple
Florence, Massachusetts 01062
Phone: 800-473-0620
website: www.alexandertech.org

American College of Traditional Chinese Medicine

455 Arkansas Street
San Francisco, California 94107
Phone: 415-282-7600 or 415-282-9603 (clinic)
The American College of Traditional Chinese Medicine serves as a training institution for people wanting to practice acupuncture and moxibustion and to prepare and prescribe Chinese herbs. It also emphasizes methods of diagnosis and treatment, the study of classical texts, and Chinese approaches to nutrition and massage. For more advanced students, work in the clinic provides an opportunity to develop skills in differential diagnosis and observing the progressive manifestations of disease and cure. The four-year graduate degree providing a Master of Science in Traditional Chinese Medicine may be completed in three years. A number of students from a variety of professions (mostly but not exclusively health-related) attend this and equivalent schools in order to make mid-life career changes.

Aromatherapy

Joni Loughran
1001 Samuel Drive
Petaluma, California 94952
Phone and Fax: 707-765-6986
website: www.light-touched.com
email: jonitk@sonic.net
Aromatherapist specializing in the practical and esoteric uses of essential oils and aromatherapy skin care.

Ayurveda

Vijaya Stallings, M.A.
Dhanvantari Ayurvedic Center
11847 Canon Blvd. Suite 8
Newport News, Virginia 23606
Phone: 757-595-7757 / 873-3900
website: www.ayurveda-virginia.com

California Association of Ayurvedic
Medicine
Post Office Box 3116
Santa Rosa, California 95402
Phone: 800-292-4882
Fax: 707-284-3052
website: www.ayurveda-caam.org

Bates Method

Thomas R. Quackenbush
Natural Vision Center
Post Office Box 986
Ashland, Oregon 97520
Phone: 541-512-2525
website:
www.NaturalVisionCenter.com
email:
TomQ@NaturalVisionCenter.com

Body Electronics

Douglas Morrison
Phone: 717-774-6707
website: www.bodyelectronics.net

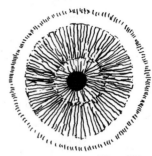

Mineral Ring

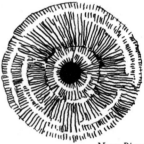

Nerve Rings

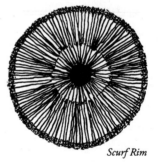

Scurf Rim

Body-Mind Centering

Bonnie Bainbridge Cohen
189 Pondview Drive
Amherst, Massachusetts 01002-3230
Phone: 413-256-8615
Fax: 413-256-8239
website: www.bodymindcentering.com
email: info@bodymindcentering.com

Breema

The Institute for Health Improvement
6076 Claremont Avenue
Oakland, California 94618
Phone: 510-428-0937
Fax: 510-428-9235
IHI is the source of information for courses and intensives taught by
Manocher Movlai and others, free-treatment evenings, and names of
practitioners.
website: www.breema.com
email: center@breema.com

Manocher Movlai
The Institute for Health Improvement
6076 Claremont Avenue
Oakland, California 94618
Phone: 510-428-0937
Fax: 510-428-9235

Jon Schreiber
6201 Florio Street
Oakland, California 94618
Phone: 510-428-1234

California Institute of Integral Studies Somatics Program

This is a M.A. program with a degree either in Somatics itself or in Psychology with a specialization in Body-Oriented Family Therapy. The course of study includes an integration of Western and non-Western approaches to the human body in relation to psychology, the healing arts, and spiritual practice. It is derived from methods created at the turn of the century by such people as Sigmund Freud, Elsa Gindler, F. Matthias Alexander, Wilhelm Reich, and Moshe Feldenkrais, who challenged the splitting of body, mind, and spirit into the rigid categories that have dominated Western theory and practice. Among contemporary modalities studied in this program are Authentic Movement, Focusing, The Lomi School, Continuum, Body-Mind Centering, Process-Oriented Psychology, Aston Patterning, Gestalt Therapy, Sensory Awareness, Hakomi, Trager, Rolfing, and the various branches of Reichian psychotherapy. This program does not train students in the practice of these methods but provides a groundwork in the theories, strategies, and transformational attitudes that are required in any somatics training.

Randy Cherner
Deer Run House
15 Deer Run
Corte Madera, California 94925
Phone: 415-924-2685
Somatic work oriented around Feldenkrais, craniosacral therapy, Lomi technique, and aikido.

Chi Gung

Bruce Kumar Frantzis
Post Office Box 99
Fairfax, California 94978-0099
Phone: 415-454-5243
Fax: 415-454-0907

website: www.energyarts.com
e-mail: askthemaster@energyarts.com
Frantzis teaches *Chi Gung* in a beginners' program (Dragon and Tiger *Chi Gung*) and an intermediate program (Spine *Chi Gung*—Bend the Bow). He also teaches Wu and Yang style *T'ai Chi Ch'uan, Ba Gua* Form Work and Self-Defense, *Hsing-I Ch'uan,* and Eight Drunken Immortals (a martial art composed of extremely flexible reeling, lurching, drunken movements and a playful fighting style). Although most of his training is done in Northern California, he runs workshops worldwide.

Chinese Medicine (see also acupuncture)

Robert Zeiger
3031 Telegraph Avenue, Suite 106
Berkeley, California 94710
510-843-7397

Chiropractic

Tom Hendrickson
406 Berkeley Park Boulevard
Kensington, California 90706
Phone: 510-524-8256
Fax: 510-524-8242
website: www.orthopedicmassage.com

Linda Mayo
1301 Solano Avenue
Albany, California 94706
510-524-5800

Continuum

Emilie Conrad
1629 18th Street
Santa Monica, California 90404
Phone: 310-453-4402
website: www.continuummovement.com
email: office@continuummovement.com

Suzanne Scurlock-Durana
2230 Wakerobin Lane
Reston, Virginia 22091
Phone: 703-620-4509
Hands-on healing, transformation, and rejuvenation, specialty also in CranioSacral Therapy.

Craniosacral Biodynamics

The Karuna Institute
Maura and Franklyn Sills
Natsworthy Manor, Natsworthy, Widecombe In The Moor,
Devon, England, TQ13 7TR
Phone: in UK: 01647 221 457; International: 0044 1647 221 457
website: www.karuna-institute.co.uk
email: office@karuna-institute.co.uk
The Karuna Institute offers accredited training programs and advanced courses in Core Process Psychotherapy, a Buddhist-influenced therapy form, and Craniosacral Biodynamics, a craniosacral approach pioneered at the Institute.

CranioSacral Therapy (See Upledger Institute)

Feldenkrais Method

Feldenkrais Resources Center
830 Bancroft Way
Berkeley, California 94710
Phone: 510-540-7600
Feldenkrais Resources provides tools, literature, and lists of practitioners for the Feldenkrais Method.

Food

All of the companies and individuals in the Food section have a variety of nutritional, herbal, and medicinal products. One can contact them for complete lists through the information given below.

Enzymes International
Post Office Box 157
Manitowish Waters, Wisconsin 54545
Phone and Fax: 715-543-8401
e-mail: enzymes@centurytel.net
One recommendation I have been given is to take this company's Super Food-n-Zymes with every meal and their Green Papaya tablets during meals that include meat, dairy products, or other digestively challenging items. Enzymes International also provides co-enzyme minerals in both tablet and liquid form. My source says that the liquid form is better and that if one wants their bottled trace minerals in steamed form that tastes fairly neutral (like slightly muddy water instead of rusty water), they can try Silverado Nutritionals (see below).

HealthComm, Inc.
5800 Soundview Drive
Gig Harbor, Washington 98335
Phone: 800-648-5883
HealthComm, Inc., is the provider of a nutritional product (UltraClear Sustain) for digestive problems and immune difficulties based on changes

in the thin lining that separates the intestinal tract from the rest of the body. This product requires physician supervision for purchase and use.

Microlight Nutritional Products
124 Rhodesia Beach Road
Bay Center, Washington 98527
Phone: 800-338-2821
Source for high-quality blue-green algae and bee pollen.

Omega Nutrition
6515 Aldrich Road
Bellingham, Washington 98226
Phone: 604-253-4228
website: www.omegaflo.com
e-mail: info@omegaflo.com

I have purchased various nutritional and cooking oils from this highly recommended company. Flax-seed and hemp-seed oils are drunk (or taken in gel-cap form) for their essential fatty acids, high omega-3 and other omega contents, and phytochemicals. Ingested herbally, they are decidedly not for cooking. Other herbal oils include borage, canola, soy, and walnut. None of these are meant for cooking, no matter how and where they are marketed otherwise; they should be heated only up to 120 degrees F.

The only oils recommended for high-heat cooking (including stir-frying and other browning and frying) are coconut oil and ghee (separated butter). However, this does not mean *any* coconut oil. Cosmetic-grade coconut oil, often rancid on store shelves, is for external use only. Industrial coconut oil (like industrial palm oil) is considered a major contributor to heart disease and other serious degenerative conditions. These oils are used universally in candies, cakes, and other food products and are best avoided (read the labels). They have little in common with unrefined coconut oil, a serious food which has the additional benefit of containing 43-53 percent lauric acid (an ingredient in mother's milk). Fry with coconut oil or ghee. Do not mind that these generally arrive in solid form (they are especially hard when refrigerated). That is one indication of the correct chemical balance for high-heat cooking. Liquefying at 75 degrees F, coconut oil is easily extracted and has a strong resistance to chemical change, even when heated. By contrast, corn oil, which is derived from grain with some difficulty (does corn seem particularly oily?), is not recommended for high-heat cooking. Coconut oil *is* especially vulnerable to light and air and thus should be packaged in containers that are as dark and airtight as coconuts.

Despite common usage, such oils as safflower, sunflower, pumpkin, and the like can be heated only up to 212 degrees F before breeding isomers and free radicals that have serious adverse health effects. These oils can be baked at high temperatures (up to 325 degrees F) because the moisture inside bread, muffins, and cakes keeps the temperature under 212 degrees F. Sesame, olive, pistachio, hazelnut, and other nut oils can be heated up to 325 degrees F (light sautéing) without adverse effects.

Hydrogenated and refined oils and saturated fats (including many of the above oils manufactured commercially and even by so-called health-food corporations and subsidiaries of industrial food conglomerates) have health liabilities and nutritional deficiencies. Though they are widely used and considered relatively benign (compared to Crisco, other lard, refined coconut and palm products, and the like), they are quite different from the unrefined organic oils produced by Omega and a few other companies. In fact, some commercial oils widely available at natural markets are apparently derived (unethically) from large batches of culinary oils industrially produced at high heat for the general supermarket trade.

Paul Pitchford
Heartwood Institute
220 Harmony Lane
Garberville, California 95542
Phone: 707-923-9292

website: www.healingwithwholefoods.com
email: wpaul3@aol.com

Silverado Nutritionals (for trace-mineral water)
150 South State Street
Orem, Utah 84058
Phone: 800-887-4583 or 541-512-2525
email: silverado11@mindspring.com

Heartwood Institute

220 Harmony Lane
Garberville, California 95542
Phone: 877-936-WOOD (9663)
website: www.heartwoodinstitute.com
email: hello@heartwoodinstitute.com
Heartwood Institute offers an environment of immersion in learning
and healing in a retreat-like mountain setting with organic food. Its
residential trainings are preparations for careers in the healing arts and
growth experiences, with vocational education in holistic health, therapeutic massage, Polarity Therapy, and bodywork. A curriculum in
Asian healing arts and integrative nutrition is taught by Paul Pitchford.
All programs are accredited.

Homeopathy

Homeopathic Educational Services
2036 Blake Street
Berkeley, California 94704
Phone: 510-649-0294
Fax: 510-649-1955
website: www.homeopathic.com
email: mail@homeopathic.com
For publications, medicines, and supplies.

National Center for Homeopathy

801 North Fairfax Street, Suite 306
Alexandria, Virginia 22314
Phone: 703-548-7790
website: www.homeopathic.org
For referrals and general information.

Martial Arts

Aikido of Tamalpais

76 East Blythedale
Mill Valley, California 94941
Phone: 415-383-9474
Richard Heckler, Wendy Palmer, and George Leonard teach here.

Richard Strozzi Heckler

Rancho Strozzi Institute
Center for Leadership and Mastery
4101 Middle Two Rock Road
Petaluma, California 94952
Phone: 707-778-6505
Fax: 707-778-0306
website: www.ranchostrozzi.com
email: richard@ranchostrozzi.com

Peter Ralston

Post Office Box 63080
Pipe Creek, Texas 78063
website: www.chenghsin.com
As well as his own form and workshops in ontology, Ralston teaches *Hsing-I Ch'uan, T'ai Chi Ch'uan,* and *Ba Gua,* sword forms, boxing, and general self-defense.

"It is the freedom, power, and clarity attained by the warrior when he has truly adopted the state in which he as an individual is already dead. This is not seen in a morbid or noble sense. It is a complete and total surrender (sacrifice) of the self-identity, the individual, the illusion of an independent self. Only when this is so is there no more tendency to be distracted by, trapped in, or confused with any particular form. However, this must be so every moment. It must be so beyond time."

Ron Sieh
Wu Wei School
Old Arizona Building
2821 Nicolet Avenue South
Minneapolis, Minnesota 55406
Phone: 612-722-8664
T'ai Chi Chu'an, Hsing-I, Ba Gua, Escrima, *Chi Gung.* Sieh is especially good with children and teenagers.
Ron Sieh's basic precepts:

1. Unless you train yourself in violent situations, how you'll act if you find yourself in one will be no more than a guess.

2. See advantage in disaster. A punch toward my head is either an opportunity or something disastrous.

3. The more control I have over the situation, the less damage I have to do.

4. The more control I have over my internal experience, the less damage I will do to myself and others.

5. It's the people closest to you who have the potential to hurt you the most. The double meaning here is intentional.

Meditation

Vipassana
S.N. Goenka
website: www.dhamma.org

The Middendorf Breath Institute

Jürg Roffler
198 Mississippi
San Francisco, California 94107
Phone: 415-255-2174

Naturopathy

Andrew Lange

3011 Broadway, Suite 14
Boulder, Colorado 80304
Phone: 303-443-8163
website: www.andrewlange.com
Specializes in getting at the root of disease, with an emphasis on the
"laws of cure" and the homeopathic approach.

Amini Peller

2150 White Oak Way
San Carlos, California 94070
Phone: 650-593-6914
Cross-cultural approaches to somatic therapies that relink the "felt
sense" disrupted by trauma. Also Somatic Experiencing, CranioSacral
Therapy, Lymphatic Drainage, Pilates, Zero Balancing, Breema, spir-
itual counseling, energy work. Amini Peller works with Wazir Peller,
acupuncturist, Somatic Experiencing practitioner, Zero Balancer, Vis-
ceral and CranioSacral Therapist, and Chinese herbalist.
Phone: 650-637-8014

Polarity Therapy (see Heartwood Institute)

Prison Integrated Health Program

Wendy Palmer
809 Vendola Drive
San Rafael, California 94903
Phone: 415-472-1619
The Prison Integrated Health Program is a sponsored project of the San Francisco Women's Centers. The program needs qualified volunteers and donations. The *Gateways Newsletter* is available.

Rebirthing

Bob Frissell

Post Office Box 1191
Inverness, California 94937
Phone: 415-669-1442
website: www.bobfrissell.com
email: bob@bobfrissell.com
Bob Frissell offers both Rebirthing and Flower of Life workshops.

Rolfing

International Rolf Institute

Post Office Box 1868
Boulder, Colorado 80306
Phone: 800-530-8875
The International Rolf Institute will provide a list of accredited practitioners in your area.

Michael Salveson
Structural Integration
1430 Leroy Avenue
Berkeley, California 94708
Phone: 510-548-8270

Jeffrey Maitland
8300 North Hayden Road, Suite 104
Scottsdale, Arizona 85258
Phone: 800-934-7189

Sexuality

More University
1507 Purson Lane
Lafayette, California 94549
Phone: 510-930-9244

T'ai Chi Ch'uan (See Peter Ralston, Ron Sieh, Paul Pitchford, and Bruce Kumar Frantzis)

Trauma

Peter A. Levine
Foundation for Human Enrichment
Post Office Box 110
Lyons, Colorado 80540
Phone: 303-823-9524
website: www.traumahealing.com
email: ergos1@earthlink.net
Work in healing trauma individually and socially.

The Upledger Institute, Inc.

11211 Prosperity Farms Road, D-325
Palm Beach Gardens, Florida 33410-3487
Educational Services: 561-622-4334 or 1-800-233-5880
Fax: 561-622-4771
website: www.upledger.com
email: upledger@upledger.com

The Upledger Institute (UI) is a health resource center dedicated to the advancement of innovative techniques that complement conventional care. It provides continuing-education programs, clinical research, and therapeutic services. Founded in 1985 by John E. Upledger, DO, OMM, UI has trained more than 50,000 practitioners in fifty-six different countries in CranioSacral Therapy and other modalities, such as Visceral Manipulation, Mechanical Link, and Lymph Drainage Therapy. Today it conducts hundreds of workshops each year educating healthcare professionals of diverse disciplines in cities throughout the world. Check their website for sites and dates.

Upledger Institute HealthPlex Clinical Services

11211 Prosperity Farms Road, D-325
Palm Beach Gardens, Florida 33410-3487
Phone: 561-622-4334

The Upledger Institute HealthPlex Clinical Services staffs physicians and therapists educated in a wide range of conventional and complementary methods. In addition to private CranioSacral Therapy sessions, the clinic offers a series of intensive therapy programs addressing concerns such as brain and spinal cord dysfunction, learning disabilities, autism, therapist rejuvenation, and post-traumatic stress disorder. UI HealthPlex also provides infancy to preschool evaluations, and helpful one-day ShareCare® seminars designed for the general public.

Upledger Institute Europe

Postbus 86
6880 AB Velp
The Netherlands

Visceral Manipulation (See also Upledger Institute)

Marilyn Radojcich
4546 El Camino Real, Suite A 15
Los Altos, California 94022
Phone: 415-327-6536

Frank Lowen
Threshold Therapeutics
8338 Comanche North East
Albuquerque, New Mexico 87116
Phone: 505-291-8100
website: www.biovalentsystems.com

Michael Wagner
Phone: 415-457-6392
e-mail: vatalink@yahoo.com

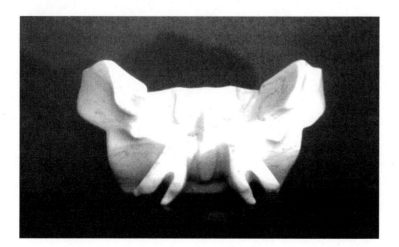

BIBLIOGRAPHY

The Academy of Traditional Chinese Medicine. *An Outline of Chinese Acupuncture.* Peking: Foreign Languages Press, 1975.

Ackerknecht, Erwin H. "Problems of Primitive Medicine," *Bulletin of the History of Medicine,* Volume XI, 1942.

Alexander, Gerda. *Eutony: The Holistic Discovery of the Total Person.* Great Neck, New York: Felix Morrow, 1985.

Alon, Ruthy. *Mindful Spontaneity: Lessons in the Feldenkrais Method.* Berkeley, California: North Atlantic Books, 1995.

Amaringo, Pablo, and Luis Eduardo Luna. *Ayahuasca Visions: The Religious Iconography of a Peruvian Shaman.* Berkeley, California: North Atlantic Books, 1991.

Aston, Judith. "Three Perceptions and One Compulsion," in *Bone, Breath, and Gesture: Practices of Embodiment.* Don Hanlon Johnson, ed. Berkeley, California: North Atlantic Books, 1995.

Bach, Edward. *Heal Thyself.* London: C. W. Daniel, 1931.

Baginski, Bodo J., and Shalila Sharamon. *Reiki: Universal Life Energy: A Holistic Method of Treatment for the Professional Practice/Absentee Healing and Self-Treatment of Mind, Body, and Soul.* Mendocino, California: Life Rhythm, 1988.

Baker, Courtney, Robert Dew, Michael Ganz, and Louisa Lance. "Wound Healing in Mice (Part I)," in *Annual of the Institute of Orgonomic Science,* Vol. 1, No. 1, September 1984.

Baker, Wyrth P., Allen C. Neiswander, and W. W. Young. *Introduction to Homeotherapeutics.* Washington, DC: American Institute of Homeopathy, 1974.

Barfield, Owen. *Unancestral Voice.* Middleton, Connecticut: Wesleyan University Press, 1965.

Barral, Jean-Pierre, and Pierre Mercier. *Visceral Manipulation.* Seattle, Washington: Eastland Press, 1988.

Barrett, S. A. *Pomo Bear Doctors,* University of California Publications in American Archaeology and Ethnology, Vol. 12, No. 11, July 11, 1917. Berkeley, California: University of California Press, 1917.

Bateson, Gregory. "Restructuring the Ecology of a Great City," *Io #14, Earth Geography Booklet No. 3, Imago Mundi,* Cape Elizabeth, Maine, 1972.

Bauman, Edward, Armand Ian Brint, Lorin Piper, and Pamela Amelia Wright, eds. *The Holistic Health Handbook.* Berkeley, California: And/Or Press, 1978.

Bennett, J. G. *Gurdjieff: Making a New World.* New York: Harper/ Colophon, 1973.

Binik, Alexander. "The Polarity System," in *The Holistic Health Handbook.* Bauman, et al., eds. Berkeley, California: And/Or Press, 1978.

Boas, Franz. *The Religion of the Kwakiutl Indians, Part II: Translations.* New York: Columbia University Press, 1930.

Böhm, Karl. *The Life of Some Island People of New Guinea: A Missionary's Observations of the Volcanic Islands of Manam, Boesa, Biem, and Ubrub.* Berlin: Dietrich Reimer Verlag, 1983.

Bookchin, Murray. *The Ecology of Freedom: The Emergence and Dissolution of Hierarchy.* Palo Alto, California: Cheshire Books, 1982.

Bordeu, Théophile. *Oeuvres.* Paris: Caille & Ravier, 1818.

Brennan, Richard. *The Alexander Technique Workbook.* Rockport, Massachusetts: Element Books, Ltd., 1992.

Britton, Nathanial, Lord, and Hon. Addison Brown. *An Illustrated Flora of the Northern United States, Canada, and the British Possesions.* New York: Charles Scribner's Sons, 1913.

Brooks, Rachel, ed. *The Stillness of Life: The Osteopathic Philosophy of Rollin E. Becker, D.O.* Portland, Oregon: Stillness Press, 2000.

Buckley, Mary. "Feng Shui: The Art of Grace in Place," in *New Dimensions Journal,* Spring 1993.

Burger, Bruce. *Esoteric Anatomy: The Body as Consciousness.* Berkeley,

California: North Atlantic Books, 1998.

Calderón, Eduardo, Richard Cowan, Douglas Sharon, and F. Kaye Sharon. *Eduardo el Curandero: The Words of a Peruvian Healer.* Berkeley, California, North Atlantic Books, 1982.

Cannon, Walter B. "'Voodoo' Death," in *American Anthropologist,* XLIV, 1942.

Carroll, Jon. "The Odd Saga of Marlo Morgan," *San Francisco Chronicle,* September 7, 1994, p. E8, and September 8, 1994, p. E10.

Castaneda, Carlos. *The Teachings of Don Juan: A Yaqui Way of Knowledge.* Berkeley, California: University of California Press, 1969.

——. *A Separate Reality.* New York: Simon & Schuster, 1971.

——. *Journey to Ixtlan.* New York: Simon & Schuster, 1972.

——. *Tales of Power.* New York: Simon & Schuster, 1974.

Caufield, Charles R., with Billi Goldberg. *The Anarchist AIDS Medical Formulary: A Guide to Guerrilla Immunology.* Berkeley, California: North Atlantic Books, 1994.

Celsus, Aulus Cornelius. *De Medicina.* Three Volumes. Translated by W. G. Spencer. Cambridge, Massachusetts: Loeb Classical Library, Harvard University Press.

Chancellor, Philip M. *Handbook of the Bach Flower Remedies.* London: C. W. Daniel Co., 1971.

Chopra, Deepak. *Quantum Healing: Exploring the Frontiers of Mind/Body Medicine.* New York: Bantam Books, 1989.

Codere, Helen. *Fighting with Property: A Study of Kwakiutl Potlatching and Warfare, 1792–1930.* Monographs of the American Ethnological Society, Volume XVIII. New York: J. J. Augustin, 1950. Reprinted in *Indians of the Northwest Coast.* Tom McFeat, ed. Seattle, Washington: University of Washington Press, 1966.

Cohen, Bonnie Bainbridge. "Research in the Field of Somatics," California Institute of Integral Studies, San Francisco, November 1992.

——. *Sensing, Feeling, and Action: The Experiential Anatomy of Body-Mind Centering.* Northampton, Massachusetts: Contact Editions, 1993.

Bibliography

Cohen, Don. *An Introduction to Craniosacral Therapy*. Berkeley, California: North Atlantic Books, 1995.

Coles, William. "Adam in Eden, or The Paradise of Plants," republished in *Io #5*, *Doctrine of Signatures*, Ann Arbor, Michigan, 1968.

Collin, Rodney. *The Theory of Celestial Influence*. London: Stuart & Watkins, Ltd., 1954.

Conger, John P. *The Body in Recovery: Somatic Psychotherapy and the Self*. Berkeley, California: Frog, Ltd., 1994.

———. *Jung & Reich: The Body as Shadow*. Berkeley, California: North Atlantic Books, 1988.

Cook, James. *The Journals of James Cook: The Voyage 1776–1780*. London: Hakluyt Society, Vol. I, No. 36, extra series.

Corbin, Henry. *Creative Imagination in the Sufism of Ibn 'Arabi*. Translated from the French by Ralph Manheim. Princeton, New Jersey: Bollingen Foundation, Princeton University Press, 1969.

Coulter, Harris Livermore. *Divided Legacy, A History of the Schism in Medical Thought, Vol. I: The Patterns Emerge: Hippocrates to Paracelsus*. Washington, DC: Weehawken Book Company, 1975.

———. *Divided Legacy, Vol. II: The Origins of Modern Western Medicine: J. B. Van Helmont to Claude Bernard*. Berkeley, California: North Atlantic Books, 1977.

———. *Divided Legacy, Vol. III: The Conflict Between Homeopathy and the American Medical Association: Science and Ethics in American Medicine 1800–1914*. Berkeley, California: North Atlantic Books, 1982.

———. *Divided Legacy, Vol. IV: Twentieth-Century Medicine, The Bacteriological Era*. Berkeley, California: North Atlantic Books, 1994.

———. *Homeopathic Science and Modern Medicine: The Physics of Healing with Microdoses*. Berkeley, California: North Atlantic Books, 1981.

Cousins, Norman. "The Mysterious Placebo," in *Saturday Review*, October 1977.

Covarrubias, Miguel. *Island of Bali*. New York: Alfred Knopf, 1938.

Cowan, Richard, and Douglas Sharon. *Eduardo the Healer.* Oakland, California: Serious Business Company, 1978.

Crews, Frederick. "The Revenge of the Repressed, Part II," in *The New York Review of Books,* Vol. XLI, No. 20, December 1, 1994.

Croft, William, C. S. T. "Light Energy Practices (Yoga/Qi-gong/Aikido) and *Working with Light*—A Synergy," flyer, 1993.

Crowley, Aleister. *The Confessions of Aleister Crowley.* John Symonds and Kenneth Grant, eds. New York: Hill & Wang, 1969.

———. *Magick in Theory and Practice.* New York: Castle Books, n.d.

Das, Baba Hari, and Dharma Sara Satang. "Ayurveda: The Yoga of Health," in *The Holistic Health Handbook.* Bauman, et al., eds. Berkeley, California: And/Or Press, 1978.

de Berval, Réné. *Kingdom of Laos.* Saigon, Vietnam: France-Asie, 1956.

de Langre, Jacques. *Dō-In 2: The Ancient Art of Rejuvenation Through Self-Massage.* Magalia, California: Happiness Press, 1978.

DeMeo, James, Richard Blasband, and Robert Morris. "Breaking the 1986 Drought in the Eastern United States," in *The Journal of Orgonomy,* Vol. 21.

Derrida, Jacques. "Freud and the Scene of Writing." Translated from the French by Jeffery Mehlman. *Yale French Studies.* New Haven, Connecticut: Yale University Press, n.d.

———. *Of Grammatology.* Translated from the French by Gayatri Chakravorty Spivak. Baltimore, Maryland: Johns Hopkins University Press, 1976.

Dhalla, Maneckji N. *Zoroastrian Civilization.* Cambridge, England: Oxford University Press, 1922.

Dickens, Charles. *A Tale of Two Cities.* New York: Charles Scribner's Sons, 1898.

Diderot, Denis. *Encyclopedié ou Dictionnaire Raisoneé des Sciences des Arts et des Métiers.* Paris: Edition Garniere Frères, 1765.

Dodé Kalpa Zangpo, quoted by Sogyal Rinpoche in *Dzogchen and Padmasambhava.* Berkeley, California: Rigpa Fellowship of California, 1990.

Dorn, Edward. *Recollections of Gran Apachería.* Berkeley, California: Turtle Island, 1974.

Dorn, Edward, and Gordon Brotherstone, "The Aztec Priest's Reply," in *New World Journal,* Berkeley, California, Vol. I, Nos. 2/3, 1977.

Douillard, John. "Ayurveda and Reaching Mainstream America," talk at Ayurveda International Symposium, California Association of Ayurvedic Medicine. Berkeley, California, May 4, 2002.

Drury, Neville. *The Healing Power: A Handbook of Alternative Medicines and Natural Health.* London: Frederick Muller Ltd., 1981.

Duesberg, Peter. *Infectious AIDS: Stretching the Germ Theory Beyond Its Limits.* Berkeley, California: North Atlantic Books, 1995.

Eisenbud, Jule. Interview conducted by Richard Grossinger, January 8, 1972, originally published in *Io #14, Earth Geography Booklet #3, Imago Mundi.* Republished in *Ecology and Consciousness: Traditional Wisdom on the Environment.* Richard Grossinger, ed. Berkeley, California, 1978. Revised second edition, 1992.

——. *Paranormal Foreknowledge: Problems and Perplexities.* New York: Human Sciences Press, 1982.

Elkin, A. P. *Aboriginal Men of High Degree.* Sydney: Australasian Publishing, 1944.

Emerson, Barbara. *Self-Healing Reiki: Freeing the Symbols, Attunements, and Techniques.* Berkeley, California: North Atlantic Books, 2001.

Emmons, George Thornton. *The Tlingit Indians.* Seattle, Washington: University of Washington Press, 1991.

Enslin, Theodore. "Journal Note," in *The Alchemical Tradition in the Late Twentieth Century.* Richard Grossinger, ed. Berkeley, California: North Atlantic Books, 1979.

Espanca, Jutta. "The Effect of Orgone on Plant Life (Part 7)," in *Offshoots of Orgonomy,* No. 12, Spring 1986.

Faraday, Michael. *The Chemical History of a Candle: A course of lectures delivered before a juvenile audience at the Royal Institution.* New York: Viking Press, 1960.

Feldenkrais, Moshe. *The Case of Nora: Body Awareness as Healing Ther-*

apy. 1977. Berkeley, California: Frog, Ltd., 1993.

———. *The Potent Self: A Guide to Spontaneity.* New York: Harper & Row, 1985.

Ferenczi, Sandor. *Thalassa: A Theory of Genitality.* Translated from the German by Henry Alden Bunker. New York: Norton, 1968.

Fields, Rick. *How the Swans Came to the Lake: A Narrative History of Buddhism in America.* Boulder, Colorado: Shambhala Publications, 1981.

Fiore, Edith. *The Unquiet Dead.* New York: Ballantine Books, 1988.

Flammonde, Paris. *The Mystic Healers.* New York: Stein & Day, 1974.

Foucault, Michel. *The Birth of the Clinic.* Translated from the French by A. M. Sheridan Smith. New York: Pantheon Books, 1973.

Fox, R. B. "The Pinatubo Negritos: Their Useful Plants and Material Culture," in *The Philippine Journal of Science,* Vol. 81, Nos. 3-4, 1953.

Frantzis, Bruce Kumar. *Opening the Energy Gates of Your Body.* Berkeley, California: North Atlantic Books, 1993.

———. *The Tao in Action: The Personal Practice of the I Ching and Taoism in Daily Life.* Unpublished manuscript at the time of publication. Berkeley, California: North Atlantic Books, 1996.

Freud, Sigmund. *An Outline of Psychoanalysis.* Translated from the German by James Strachey. New York: Norton, 1949.

———. *The Interpretation of Dreams.* Translated from the German by James Strachey. New York: Basic Books, 1955.

Frissell, Bob. *Nothing in This Book Is True, But It's Exactly How Things Are.* Berkeley, California: Frog, Ltd., 1994.

From Bindu to Ojas. San Cristobal, New Mexico: Lama Foundation, 1970.

Frost, Robert. *Applied Kinesiology.* Berkeley, California: North Atlantic Books, 2002.

Fulder, Stephen. *The Root of Being: Ginseng and the Pharmacology of Harmony.* London: Hutchison Publishing Group, 1980.

Fuller, John G. *Arigo: Surgeon of the Rusty Knife.* New York: Crowell, 1974; Pocket Books, 1975.

Gelfand, Michael. *Medicine and Custom in Africa.* Edinburgh: Livingstone, 1964.

Gillispie, Charles Coulston. "Lamarck and Darwin in the History of Science," in *Forerunners of Darwin, 1745–1859.* Bentley Glass, Owsei Temkin, and William L. Straus, Jr., eds. Baltimore: The Johns Hopkins University Press, 1959.

Ginzberg, Jeremy. "Pharmaco-Hell Calling," in *East Bay Express,* Berkeley, California, January 21, 1994.

Golden, Stephanie. "Body-Mind Centering," in *Yoga Journal,* Berkeley, California, September/October 1993.

Goodwin, Kathleen. "Alternative Medicine: A Note of Caution," in *City Miner,* Berkeley, California, Vol. 3, No. 3, 1978.

Grey, Alex. *Sacred Mirrors.* Rochester, Vermont: Inner Traditions, 1990.

Groddeck, Georg. *The Book of the It.* Translated from the German by V. M. E. Collins. New York: Funk & Wagnalls, 1950.

——. "Psychic Conditioning and the Psychoanalytic Treatment of Organic Disorders," in *The Meaning of Illness.* M. Masud R. Khan, ed. London: The Hogarth Press, 1977.

Grossinger, Richard. "Alchemy: Pre-Egyptian Legacy, Millennial Promise," in *The Alchemical Tradition in the Late Twentieth Century.* Richard Grossinger, ed. Berkeley, California: North Atlantic Books, 1979.

——. "Cross-Cultural and Historical Models of Energy in Healing," paper delivered at the conference *Conceptualizing Energy Medicine: An Emerging Model of Healing,* University Extension and School of Public Health, University of California, Berkeley, California, March 28, 1981.

——. "The Dream Work," in *Dreams are Wiser Than Men.* Richard A. Russo, ed. Berkeley, California: North Atlantic Books, 1987.

——. *Embryogenesis: Species, Gender, and Identity.* North Atlantic Books, 2000.

——. *Embryos, Galaxies, and Sentient Beings: How the Universe Makes Life.* Berkeley, California: North Atlantic Books, 2003.

——. *Homeopathy: The Great Riddle.* Berkeley, California: North Atlantic Books, 1998.

——. "A Phenomenology of Panic," in *Panic: Origins, Insight, and Treatment.* Leonard J. Schmidt, M.D., and Brooke Warner, ed. Berkeley, California: North Atlantic Books, 2002.

——. "Why Somatic Therapies Deserve As Much Attention as Psychoanalysis in *The New York Review of Books* and Why Bodyworkers Treating Neuroses Should Study Psychoanalysis," in *The Body in Psychotherapy: Inquiries in Somatic Psychology.* Don Hanlon Johnson and Ian J. Grand, ed. Berkeley, California: North Atlantic Books, 1999.

——, ed. *An Olson-Melville Sourcebook, Vol. I: North America. Vol. II: The Mediterranean.* Plainfield, Vermont: North Atlantic Books, 1976.

——, ed. *Ecology and Consciousness: Traditional Wisdom on the Environment.* Berkeley, California: North Atlantic Books, 1978. Revised second edition, 1992.

——, ed. *Io,* 1964–79. Amherst, Massachusetts; Ann Arbor, Michigan; Cape Elizabeth, Maine; Mount Desert, Maine; Oakland, California; Plainfield, Vermont; and Richmond, California.

Gurdjieff, G. I. *Views from the Real World: Early Talks.* New York: Dutton, 1975.

Haehl, Richard. *Samuel Hahnemann: His Life and Work,* Vol. I. London: Homeopathic Publishing Co., 1922.

Hahnemann, Samuel. *The Chronic Diseases, Their Peculiar Nature and Their Homeopathic Cure.* Translated by Louis H. Tale from the second enlarged German edition, 1835. Philadelphia: Boericke and Tafel, 1904.

——. *The Lesser Writings of Samuel Hahnemann.* Collected and translated by R. E. Dudgeon. New York: Radde, 1952.

——. *The Organon of Medicine,* Sixth Edition. Translated by William Boericke, M.D. Calcutta, India: Roysingh, 1962.

Handy, E. S. Craighill, Mary Kawena Pukui, and Katherine Livermore. *Outline of Hawaiian Physical Therapeutics.* Honolulu, Hawaii: Bernice P. Bishop Museum, Bulletin 126, 1934.

Bibliography

Harley, George Way. *Native African Medicine.* Cambridge, Massachusetts: Harvard University Press, 1941.

Harman, Robert. "Current Research with SAPA Bions," in *The Journal of Orgonomy,* Vol. 21.

Harner, Michael J. *The Jívaro.* Garden City, New Jersey: Doubleday/Natural History Press, 1972.

Harvey, Andrew. *Hidden Journey: A Spiritual Awakening.* New York: Henry Holt & Co., Inc., 1991.

Hauschka, Rudolf. *The Nature of Substance.* Translated from the German by Mary T. Richards and Marjorie Spock. London: Stuart & Watkins, 1966.

———. *Nutrition.* Translated from the German by Marjorie Spock and Mary T. Richards. London: Stuart & Watkins, 1967.

Heckler, Richard Strozzi. *In Search of the Warrior Spirit: Teaching Awareness Disciplines to the Green Berets.* Berkeley, California: North Atlantic Books, 1989.

Heisenberg, Werner. "The Relationship Between Biology, Physics, and Chemistry," in *Physics and Beyond.* Translated from the German by Arnold J. Pomerans. New York: Harper & Row, 1971.

Heller, Joseph, and William Henkin. *Bodywise: Introduction to Hellerwork.* Oakland, California: Wingbow Press, 1986.

Herbert, Frank. *Dune.* New York: Berkley, 1965.

———. *Whipping Star.* New York: Berkley, 1977.

Herriot, Eva M. "Ayurvedic Sense Therapy," in *Yoga Journal,* Berkeley, California, January/February 1992.

Hickey, Gerald Cannon. *Village in Vietnam.* New Haven, Connecticut: Yale University Press, 1964.

Higgins, Mary, and Chester M. Raphael, eds. *Reich Speaks of Freud.* New York: Farrar, Straus and Giroux, 1967.

Hillman, James. *The Myth of Analysis.* Evanston, Illinois: Northwestern University Press, 1972.

Hippocrates. *Medical Works.* Four Volumes. Translated by W. H. S. Jones. Cambridge, Massachusetts: Loeb Classical Library, Harvard

University Press.

Hoagland, Richard C. *The Monuments of Mars: A City on the Edge of Forever.* Berkeley, California: North Atlantic Books, 1986.

Hodosi, Oskar. *Tantra Partnerschaft: Neue Dimensionen der Liebe Durch Eine Jahrtausendealte Kultur.* Munich: Mosaik Verlag, 1992.

Holbrook, Bruce. *The Stone Monkey: An Alternative Chinese-Scientific Reality.* New York: Morrow, 1981.

Hsu, Hong-Yen. *How to Heal Yourself with Chinese Herbs.* Los Angeles: Oriental Healing Arts Institute, 1980.

Inglis, Brian. *A History of Medicine.* Cleveland: World Publishing Company, 1965.

———. *The Case for Unorthodox Medicine.* New York: Putnam, 1965.

Jarrell, David G. *Reiki Plus: Professional Practitioner's Manual for Second Degree.* Celina, Tennessee: Hibernia West, 1992.

Jenness, D. "The Carrier Indians of the Bulkley River," in *Bulletin No. 133.* Washington, DC: Bureau of American Ethnology, 1943.

John, Bubba Free (Da Free John). *The Eating Gorilla Comes in Peace: The Transcendental Principle of Life Applied to Diet and the Regenerative Discipline of True Health.* Middletown, California: The Dawn Horse Press, 1979.

Johnson, Don Hanlon. *Body, Spirit and Democracy.* Berkeley, California: North Atlantic Books, 1993.

———. *The Protean Body.* New York: Harper & Row, 1977.

———. "The Way of the Flesh: A Brief History of the Somatics Movement," in *Bone, Breath, and Gesture: Practices of Embodiment.* Don Hanlon Johnson, ed. Berkeley, California: North Atlantic Books, 1995.

——— and Ian Grand, ed. *The Body in Psychotherapy: Inquiries in Somatic Psychology.* Berkeley, California: North Atlantic Books, 1999.

———, ed. *Bone, Breath, and Gesture: Practices of Embodiment.* Berkeley, California: North Atlantic Books, 1995.

Jung, Carl. *Archetypes of the Collective Unconscious.* Translated by R. F. C. Hull. Bollingen Series XX. New York: Pantheon Books, 1959.

———. *Psychological Reflections.* Jolande Jacobi, ed. New York: Harper & Row, 1953.

———. *Psychology and Alchemy.* Translated from the German by R. F. C. Hull. London: Routledge & Kegan Paul, 1953.

Kahn, Morton C. *Djuka: The Bush Negroes of Dutch Guiana.* New York: Viking Press, 1931.

Katz, R. "Education for Transcendence: Lessons from the !Kung Zhu Twasi," in *Journal of Transpersonal Psychology,* November 2, 1973.

Keleman, Stanley. *Living Your Dying.* New York: Random House, 1974.

———. "Professional Colloquium," in *Ecology and Consciousness: Traditional Wisdom on the Environment.* Richard Grossinger, ed. Berkeley, California: North Atlantic Books, 1978. Revised second edition, 1992.

Kelly, Lolette. "Faith and the Placebo Effect." *Ions: Noetic Sciences Review,* March-May, 2002, #59.

Kent, James Tyler. *Lectures on Homeopathic Philosophy.* 1900. Berkeley, California: North Atlantic Books, 1979.

Kerouac, Jack. *The Dharma Bums.* New York: Viking Press, 1958.

Khan, M. Masud R., ed. *The Meaning of Illness.* London: The Hogarth Press, 1977.

Kroeber, A. L. *Ethnology of the Gros Ventre.* Anthropological Papers of the American Museum of Natural History, Vol. I, Part IV, New York, 1908.

Kushi, Michio. *The Book of Dō-In: Exercise for Physical and Spiritual Development.* Tokyo: Japan Publications, 1979.

Lade, A., and R. Svoboda. *Tao & Dharma—A Comparison of Ayurveda and Chinese Medicine.* Unpublished manuscript at the time of publication.

Lamb, F. Bruce. *Rio Tigre and Beyond: The Amazon Jungle Medicine of Manuel Córdova-Rios.* Berkeley, California: North Atlantic Books, 1985.

Lansing, Gerrit. "Fundamentals of Indian Medical Theory," from *Notes on Structure and Sign in Ayurveda.* Unpublished manuscript, 1981.

Lawlor, Robert. *Voices of the First Day: Awakening in the Aboriginal Dreamtime.* Rochester, Vermont: Inner Traditions, 1991.

Le Guin, Ursula K. *A Wizard of Earthsea.* New York: Bantam Books, 1975.

Leigh, William S. *Bodytherapy.* Coquitlam, British Columbia: Water Margin Press, 1989.

Leri, Dennis. "Learning How to Learn," unpublished manuscript.

Lessa, William A., and Evon Z. Vogt. *Reader in Comparative Religion.* New York: Harper & Row, 1958.

Lévi-Strauss, Claude. *From Honey to Ashes.* Translated from the French by John and Doreen Weightman. New York: Harper & Row, 1973.

——. *The Raw and the Cooked.* Translated from the French by John and Doreen Weightman. New York: Harper & Row, 1969.

——. *The Savage Mind.* Chicago: University of Chicago Press, 1966.

——. "The Sorcerer and His Magic," in *Structural Anthropology.* Translated from the French by Claire Jacobson and Brooke Grundfest Schoepf. Garden City, New Jersey: Doubleday/Anchor, 1967.

——. *Totemism.* Translated from the French by Rodney Needham. Boston: Beacon Press, 1963.

Leviton, Richard. "The Healing Energies of Color," in *Yoga Journal,* Berkeley, California, January/February 1992

——. "Healing Vibrations," in *Yoga Journal,* Berkeley, California, January/February 1994.

Lewis, C. S. *The Magician's Nephew.* 1951. New York: Collier Books, 1970.

Lindner, Robert. *The Fifty-Minute Hour.* New York: Bantam Books, 1956.

Liu, Qingshan. *Qi Gong: Der chinesische Weg für ein gesundes langes Leben.* Munich: Hugendubel, 1992.

Lo, Pang Jeng, Martin Inn, Susan Foe, and Robert Amacker. *The Essence of T'ai Chi Ch'uan: The Literary Tradition.* Berkeley, California: North Atlantic Books, 1979.

Maitland, Jeffrey. *Spacious Body: Explorations in Somatic Ontology.* Berkeley, California: North Atlantic Books, 1995.

Bibliography

Makavejev, Dussan. *WR: Mysteries of the Organism.* New York: Avon Books, 1972.

Mann, Felix. *Acupuncture: The Ancient Chinese Art of Healing and How It Works Scientifically.* New York: Random House, 1973.

Mann, W. Edward. *Orgone, Reich and Eros: Wilhelm Reich's Theory of Life Energy.* New York: Simon & Schuster, 1973.

Mars, Louis. *The Crisis of Possession in Voodoo.* Translated from the French by Kathleen Collins. Berkeley, California: Reed, Cannon & Johnson Co., 1977.

Marshack, Alexander. *The Roots of Civilization.* New York: McGraw-Hill, 1972.

Max, Otto. Review of *Planet Medicine,* in *East West Journal,* Boston, Massachusetts, August 1981.

McKenna, Terence. *The Archaic Revival: Speculations on Psychedelic Mushrooms, the Amazon, Virtual Reality, Evolution, Shamanism, the Rebellion of the Goddess, and the End of History.* San Francisco: Harper-Collins, 1993.

Meek, George W. *Healers and the Healing Process.* Wheaton, Illinois: Theosophical Publishing House, 1977.

Melchizedek, Drunvalo. "Flower of Life Workshop," Dallas, February 14–17, 1992. Video recording.

Melville, Herman. *Moby Dick; or the Whale.* 1851. Berkeley, California: University of California Press, 1979.

Middendorf, Ilse. *The Perceptible Breath: A Breathing Science.* Paderborn, Germany: Junferman-Verlag, 1990.

Milne, Hugh. *The Heart of Listening: A Visionary Approach to Craniosacral Work.* Berkeley, California: North Atlantic Books, 1995.

Mitchell, Faith. *Hoodoo Medicine: Sea Island Herbal Remedies.* Berkeley, California: Reed, Cannon & Johnson, 1978.

Moore, Omar Khayyam. "Divination—A New Perspective," in *American Anthropologist,* LIX, 1957.

Morrison, Douglas. *How We Heal: Nutritional, Emotional, and Spiritual Fundamentals.* Berkeley, California: North Atlantic Books, 2001.

Moss, Thelma. "Kirlian Photograph and the Aura," interview with Roy L. Walford, in *Io #19, Mind Memory Psyche*, Plainfield, Vermont, 1974.

Muldoon, Sylvan, and Hereward Carrington. *The Projection of the Astral Body.* New York: Samuel Weiser, Inc., 1970.

Müller, Brigitte, and Horst Günther. *A Complete Book of Reiki Healing.* Mendocino, California: Life Rhythm, 1995.

Murdock, George Peter. "Tenino Shamanism," in *Culture and Society: Twenty-Four Essays.* George Peter Murdock, ed. Pittsburgh, Pennsylvania: University of Pittsburgh Press, 1965.

Nicoll, Maurice. *Psychological Commentaries on the Teaching of Gurdjieff & Ouspensky.* London: Robinson & Watkins, 1952.

Norbu, Chögyal Namkhai, and Adriano Clemente. *The Supreme Source* (The Kunjed Gyalpo): *The Fundamental Tantra of Dzogchen Semde.* Translated from Italian by Andrew Lukianowicz. Ithaca, New York: Snow Lion Publications, 1999.

Olschak, Blanche Christine. *Mystic Art of Ancient Tibet.* Translated by George Allen. New York: McGraw-Hill, 1973.

Olsen, Stanley J. *Mammal Remains from Archaeological Sites, Part I: Southeastern and Southwestern United States.* Cambridge, Massachusetts: The Peabody Museum, 1964.

Olson, Charles. *The Maximus Poems.* 1950. Berkeley, California: University of California Press, 1979.

———. *Muthologos,* Vol. I. Bolinas, California: Four Seasons Foundation, 1978.

Oracion, Timoteo S. "The Bais Forest Preserve Negritos: Some Notes on Their Rituals and Ceremonies," in *Studies in Philippine Anthropology.* Mario D. Zamora, ed. Quezon City, Philippines: Alemar-Phoenix, 1967.

Orr, Leonard. *Bhartriji: Immortal Yogi of 2000 Years.* Chico, California: Inspiration University, 1992.

———. *Breaking the Death Habit: The Science of Everlasting Life.* Berkeley, California: Frog, Ltd., 1998.

Bibliography

Ouspensky, P. D. *In Search of the Miraculous: Fragments of an Unknown Teaching.* New York: Harcourt, Brace, & World, 1949.

Oyle, Irving. *The New American Medicine Show.* Santa Cruz, California: Unity Press, 1979.

Palmer, Wendy. *The Intuitive Body: Aikido as a Clairsentient Practice.* Berkeley, California: North Atlantic Books, 1994.

Paracelsus. *The Hermetic and Alchemical Writings of Paracelsus the Great.* Translated by A. E. Waite. London: James Elliott, 1894.

Perlman, David. "Controversial AIDS Theories Debated at Forum in S.F.," *San Francisco Chronicle,* June 22, 1994.

Phillips, Wendell. *Unknown Oman.* New York: David McKay Company, Inc., 1966.

Pitchford, Paul. *Healing with Whole Foods: Oriental Traditions and Modern Nutrition.* Berkeley, California: North Atlantic Books, 1993.

Poncé, Charles. *The Archetype of the Unconscious and the Transfiguration of Therapy: Reflections on Jungian Psychology.* Berkeley, California: North Atlantic Books, 1990.

Post-Traumatic Stress Disorder in Vietnam Veterans: An Intensive CranioSacral Treatment Program. Palm Beach Gardens, Florida: The Upledger Foundation (VHS video format), 2000.

The Private Life of Chairman Mao: The Memories of Mao's Personal Physician, Dr. Li Zhisui. Translated by Tai Hung-chao. New York: Random House, 1994.

Ptashek, Alan. "The Moving Body: An Integrated Movement Course," in *Contact Quarterly,* Northampton, Massachusetts, Winter 1992.

Pujols, Lee, and Gary Richman. *Miracles & Other Realities.* San Francisco: Omega Press, 1990.

Quindlen, Anna. "Gulf War's Killing Legacy," *San Francisco Chronicle,* October 10, 1994.

Radcliffe-Brown, A. R. *The Andaman Islanders.* Glencoe, Illinois: Free Press, 1948.

Rappaport, Roy A. "Sanctity and Adaptation," in *Io #7, Oecology Issue,* 1970; reprinted in *Ecology and Consciousness: Traditional Wisdom on*

the Environment. Richard Grossinger, ed. Berkeley, California: North Atlantic Books, 1978. Revised second edition, 1992.

Rasmussen, Knud. *Intellectual Culture of the Iglulik Eskimos: Report of the Fifth Thule Expedition to Arctic North America.* Copenhagen, Denmark: Gyldendalske Boghandel, Nordisk Forlag, 1929.

Rechung, Ven. Rinpoche Jampal Kunzang. *Tibetan Medicine.* Berkeley, California: University of California Press, 1973.

Reese, Mark. "Moshe Feldenkrais' Verbal Approach to Somatic Education: Parallels to Milton Erickson's Use of Language," in *Somatics,* Novato, California, Autumn/Winter 1985–86.

Regardie, Israel. *The Eye in the Triangle.* Llewellyn Publications, St. Paul, Minnesota, 1970.

Reich, Peter. *A Book of Dreams.* New York: Harper & Row, 1973.

Reich, Wilhelm. *Character Analysis.* Third Edition. Translated from the German by Vincent R. Carfagno. New York: Farrar, Straus and Giroux, 1972.

———. *Cosmic Superimposition.* Translated from the German by Therese Pol. New York: Farrar, Straus and Giroux, 1973.

———. *The Emotional Plague of Mankind: Volume 1, The Murder of Christ.* Rangeley, Maine: Orgone Institute Press, 1953.

———. *Ether, God & Devil—Cosmic Superimposition.* Translated from the German by Therese Pol. New York: Farrar, Straus and Giroux, 1973.

———. *The Function of the Orgasm.* Translated from the German by Vincent R. Carfagno. New York: Farrar, Straus and Giroux, 1973.

Reichard, Gladys A. *Navaho Religion.* New York, Bollingen Foundation, Pantheon Books, 1950.

Reif, A. Veronica. "Eurhythmy and Curative Eurhythmy," essay accompanying lecture at the Berkeley Anthroposophical Society, 1978.

Ros, Frank. *The Lost Secrets of Ayurvedic Acupuncture: An Ayurvedic Guide to Acupuncture.* Twin Lakes, Wisconsin: Lotus Press, 1994.

Roberts, Jane. *The Seth Material.* Englewood Cliffs, New Jersey: Prentice-Hall, 1970.

Rolf, Ida. *Ida Rolf Talks About Rolfing and Physical Reality.* New York:

Harper & Row, 1978.

——. *Rolfing: The Integration of Human Structures.* New York: Harper & Row, 1977.

Rose, Jeanne. *The Aromatherapy Book: Applications & Inhalations.* Berkeley, California: North Atlantic Books, 1992.

Rubenfeld, Ilana. "Alexander: The Use of the Self," in *Wholistic Dimensions in Healing: A Resource Guide.* Leslie J. Kaslof, ed. New York: Doubleday & Company, Inc., 1978.

Rush, Benjamin. *Medical Inquiries and Observations.* Philadelphia: Pritchard and Hall, 1789.

Rutkow, Ira M. *Surgery: An Illustrated History.* St. Louis: Mosby-Year Book, 1993.

Sahlins, Marshall. *Stone Age Economics.* Chicago: Aldine-Atherton, 1972.

Sannella, Lee. *Kundalini—Psychosis or Transcendence?* San Francisco: Dakin, 1976.

Schaffer, Carolyn. "An Interview with Emilie Conrad-Da'oud," in *Yoga Journal,* Berkeley, California, No. 77, November/December 1987.

Schiotz, Eiler H., and James Cyriax. *Manipulation Past and Present.* London: William Heinemann Medical Books, Ltd., 1975.

Schmidt, M.D., Leonard J., and Brooke Warner. *Panic: Origins, Insight, and Treatment.* Berkeley, California: North Atlantic Books, 2002.

Schreiber, Jon. *Touching the Mountain: The Self-Breema Handbook— Ancient Exercises for the Modern World.* Oakland, California: California Health Publications, 1989.

Schultz, Barbara L. "New Age Shiatsu," in *The Holistic Health Handbook.* Bauman, et al., eds. Berkeley, California: And/Or Press, 1978.

Schultz, R. Louis. *Out in the Open: The Complete Male Pelvis.* Berkeley, California: North Atlantic Books, 1999.

Schwartz, Jesse. "Some Experiments with Seed Sprouts and Energetic Fields," in *Living Tree Journal,* Bolinas, California, 1986.

——. "Science vs. Scientism," in *Brain/Mind,* Vol. 18, No. 5.

Segal, Mia. Interview in *Somatics,* Novato, California, Autumn/Winter 1985–86.

"Sex Between Therapist and Patient," transcript of the June 21, 1976, meeting of the American Psychiatric Association, in *Psychiatry*, Vol. 5, No. 12.

Sharaf, Myron. *Fury on Earth: A Biography of Wilhelm Reich.* New York: St. Martin's Press, 1983.

Shklovskii, I. S., and Carl Sagan. *Intelligent Life in the Universe.* Translated from the Russian by Paula Fern. New York: Delta Books, 1967.

Siegel, Bernie. "Letter to the Editor," in *Common Boundary*, Bethesda, Maryland, September-October, 1994.

Sieh, Ron. *T'ai Chi Ch'uan: The Internal Tradition.* Berkeley, California: North Atlantic Books, 1993.

Sills, Franklyn. *Craniosacral Biodynamics (Volume One): The Breath of Life, Biodynamics, and Fundamental Skills.* Berkeley, California: North Atlantic Books, 2001.

———. *The Polarity Process: Energy as a Healing Art.* Berkeley: California: North Atlantic Books, 2002.

Smith, Harvey H. *Area Handbook for Iran.* Washington, DC: United States Government Printing Office, Foreign Area Studies, American University, 1971.

Sogyal Rinpoche. *The Tibetan Book of Living and Dying.* San Francisco: HarperSanFrancisco, 1992.

Speck, Frank G. *A Study of the Delaware Indian Big House Ceremony*, Vol. II. Harrisburg, Pennsylvania: Publications of the Pennsylvania Historical Commission, 1931.

Spencer, Dorothy M. *Disease, Religion and Society in the Fiji Islands.* New York: Augustin, 1941.

Stewart, Daniel Blair. *Akhunaton: The Extraterrestrial King.* Berkeley, California: Frog, Ltd., 1995.

Still, A. T. *Osteopathy: Research & Practice.* 1910. Seattle, Washington: Eastland Press, 1992.

Stone, Randolph. *Polarity Therapy*, Vol. I. Sebastopol, California: CRCS Publications, 1986.

———. *Polarity Therapy*, Vol. II. Sebastopol, California: CRCS Publi-

Bibliography

cations, 1987.

Suzuki, Shunryu. *Zen Mind, Beginner's Mind.* New York: Weatherhill, 1970.

Swadesh, Morris. "Diffusional Cumulation and Archaic Residue as Historical Explanations," in *Language in Culture & Society: A Reader in Linguistics and Anthropology.* Dell Hymes, ed. New York: Harper & Row, 1964.

Swanton, John R. *Religious Beliefs and Medical Practices of the Creek Indians,* 42nd Annual Report to the Bureau of American Ethnology, 1924–25. Washington, DC: Smithsonian Institution, 1928.

Tait, David. "Konkomba Sorcery," in *Magic, Witchcraft, and Curing.* John Middleton, ed. New York: The Natural History Press, 1967.

Tantaquidgeon, Gladys. *Folk Medicine of the Delaware and Related Algonkian Indians.* Harrisburg, Pennsylvania: Pennsylvania Historical and Museum Commission, 1972.

Teilhard de Chardin, Pierre. *The Phenomenon of Man.* Translated from the French by Bernard Wall. New York: Harper & Row, 1959.

Temple, Robert K. G. *The Sirius Mystery.* New York: St. Martin's Press, 1976.

Tenen, Stan. *Hebrew—First Hand.* San Anselmo, California: Meru Foundation, 1994.

——. *The Matrix of Meaning for Sacred Alphabets.* San Anselmo, California: Meru Foundation, 1991. Video recording.

Thakkur, Chandrashekhar G. *Ayurveda: The Indian Art & Science of Medicine.* New York: ASI Publishers, Inc., 1974.

Thera, Nyanaponika. *The Heart of Buddhist Meditation.* New York: Samuel Weiser, Inc., 1969.

Tierra, Michael. *The Way of Herbs.* New York: Simon & Schuster, 1994.

Tomlinson, Cybèle. "Breema Bodywork," in *Yoga Journal,* Berkeley, California, November/December 1994.

Tompkins, Peter, and Christopher Bird. *The Secret Life of Plants.* New York: Harper & Row, 1973.

Trungpa, Chögyam. *Cutting Through Spiritual Materialism.* Berkeley,

California: Shambhala Publications, 1973.

Turner, Victor W. *Lunda Medicine and the Treatment of Disease.* Occasional Papers of the Rhodes-Livingstone Museum, No. 15. Northern Rhodesia, Zambia: Livingstone, 1964.

Tyler, M. L. *Homeopathic Drug Pictures.* Holsworthy, Devon, England: Health Science Press, 1942.

Upledger, John E. *CranioSacral Therapy II: Beyond the Dura.* Seattle, Washington: Eastland Press, 1987.

———. *SomatoEmotional Release: Deciphering the Language of Life.* Berkeley, California: North Atlantic Books, 2002.

———. *SomatoEmotional Release and Beyond.* Palm Beach Gardens, Florida: UI Publishing, 1990.

Upledger, John E., and Jon D. Vredevoogd. *CranioSacral Therapy.* Seattle, Washington: Eastland Press, 1983.

Urquhart, David. *Manual of the Turkish Bath.* Sir John Fife, M.D., ed. London: Churchill, 1865.

Vallee, Jacques. *Forbidden Science.* Berkeley, California: North Atlantic Books, 1992.

Van Helmont, Jan Baptista. *Oriatrike, or Physick Refined.* London, 1662.

Vithoulkas, George. *The Science of Homeopathy: A Modern Textbook,* Vol. I. Athens, Greece: A.S.O.H.M., 1978.

Vlamis, Gregory. "Interview with Pierre Pannetier," in *Well-Being Magazine,* No. 28, 1978.

Waite, A. E. *See* Paracelsus, above.

Watson, James. *The Double Helix.* New York: Atheneum, 1968.

Westlake, Aubrey T. *The Pattern of Health.* Berkeley, California: Shambhala Publications, 1973.

Wheelwright, Philip, ed. *The Presocratics.* Indianapolis, Indiana: Odyssey Press, 1966.

Whicher, Olive. *Projective Geometry: Creative Polarities in Space and Time.* London: Rudolph Steiner Press, 1971.

Whitehead, Alfred North. *Process and Reality.* Toronto: Macmillan, 1929.

Whiting, Alfred F. *Ethnobotany of the Hopi*. Northern Arizona Society of Science and Art, Bulletin 15. Flagstaff, Arizona: Museum of Northern Arizona, 1939.

Whitmont, Edward. *The Alchemy of Healing: Psyche and Soma*. Berkeley, California: North Atlantic Books, 1993.

——. *Psyche and Substance: Essays on Homeopathy in the Light of Jungian Psychology*. Berkeley, California: North Atlantic Books, 1979.

Wildschut, William. *Crow Indian Medicine Bundles*. John C. Ewers, ed. New York: Museum of the American Indian, Heye Foundation, 1975.

Williams, William Carlos. *Pictures from Brueghel and Other Poems*. New York: New Directions, 1962.

Wilson, Robert Anton. *Cosmic Trigger*. Berkeley, California: And/Or Press, 1977.

Wisdom, Charles. *The Chorti Indians of Guatemala*. Chicago: University of Chicago Press, 1940.

Wyman, Leland C. *Beautyway: A Navaho Ceremonial*. Recorded and translated by Father Berard Haile. New York: Bollingen Foundation, Pantheon Books, 1957.

Wyvell, Lois. "Orgone and You," in *Living Tree Journal*, Bolinas, California, 1986.

Yates, Frances. *Giordano Bruno and the Hermetic Tradition*. Chicago: University of Chicago Press, 1964.

——. *The Rosicrucian Enlightenment*. London: Routledge & Kegan Paul, 1972.

The Yellow Emperor's Classic of Internal Medicine (Huang Ti Nei Ching Su Wên). Translated from the Chinese by Ilza Veith. Berkeley, California: University of California Press, 1966.

Yoe, Shway. *The Burman*. London: Macmillan, 1910.

Yogananda, Paramahansa. *Autobiography of a Yogi*. Los Angeles: Self-Realization Fellowship, 1946.

INDEX

This is a cumulative index for *Planet Medicine: Origins* and *Planet Medicine: Modalities* or Volume 1 and Volume 2, respectively. Accordingly, the page references for each volume are identified as follows: Vol. 1 *(Origins)* page references are listed first in each entry, with a 1 preceding that list. Page references for Vol. 2 *(Modalities)* are listed second in each entry, with a 2 preceding that list. Where both Vol. 1 and Vol. 2 references appear, the lists are separated by a semicolon (;). For example:

planet medicine
    changes necessary for, 1.527–30; 2.8–10, 11, 450–53

entry Vol. 1 *(Origins)*   Vol. 2 *(Modalities)*

Page references in **bold** refer to illustrations or photographs. The term *passim* refers to a discontinuous discussion of a topic over several pages. The terms *above* and *below* refer to subentries within the main category. The letter "n" attached to a page reference refers to a note on that page.

Index

Chinese medicine compared to, 1.296–297, 345
conventional medicine, acceptance by, 1.473
as energy medicine, 2.341–342
esoteric aspects of, 1.297
herbal medicine, 2.468
holistic themes applying to, 1.476–477
homeopathy and, 1.537
humoral types, 1.316–317, 324–325
as language system, 2.83
overview, 1.305–310, 326
prana, 1.232, 234, 311, 318, 324, 325–326
resources for, 2.608
subtle body of, 1.318
theory, 1.310–317; 2.84, 435, 457, **457**
as Tibetan influence, 1.326–327, 332
treatments, 1.323–326
Azande, 1.257
AZT, 1.54
Aztec Indians, 1.123–124

Babaji, 2.38, 51, 61–62, 85
Baba, Meher, 1.511
Babbit, Edwin, 2.452
baboon troop organization, 1.72
Babylonian medicine, 1.292–293
Bach, Edward, 1.89n, 253–254, 255
Bach Flower Remedies, 1.253–255
Baglivi, Giorgio, 1.286
ba gua see *pa gua ch'ang*
Bainbridge Cohen, Bonnie, 1.481; 2.174–175, 385–386, 390–403, **401**, 609
Baker, Courtney, 1.460

Bali, medicine of, 1.144–145, 164, 194–195; 2.92
barbarism, social and humanitarian, 1.118
Barfield, Owen, 1.14, 128
Barker, Herbert, 2.36
Barral, Jean-Pierre, 2.295, 299–301, 302, 303, 304
Bates Method, 2.165, 194–209, 608
Bateson, Gregory, 1.17
baths, 1.99, 153–154, 474
Baughman, John Lee, 2.38
bear doctors *see* Pomo Indian bear doctors
Becker, Rollin E., 2.272, 362
behavior
    interrelationships of, 1.394–396
    modification, 1.410–411, 413; 2.143
    return of the repressed, 1.386
Bennett, T. J., 2.290–291
Beringer, Elizabeth, 2.214
Berry, Lauren, 2.286–287
Bhartriji, 2.65
Big and Small Louse Gravel, 1.326
biological vitalism, 1.231–234, 238–239, 259, 261, 449
Blind Lemon, 2.539
bliss, 2.83–84
Blondlot, Prosper, 1.232
bloodletting, 1.165
Blue and Sun-Lights (Pleasanton), 2.452
blue oils, 1.532
Boas, Franz, 1.169, 172
Bobath, Karl and Berta, 2.393–394
body
    accepting disease and cure, 1.180, 202

Index

Index

striving for higher, 1.508

consent to healing, 2.28, 66, 380

Constructive Conscious Control
(Alexander), 2.183

contact improvisation, 1.481–483

Continuum Therapy, 2.403–409, 597,
612

contraries, law of, 1.279, 286, 297, 325

conventional medicine (technological
medicine)

 acceptable for most, 2.426–427

 alternatives to

  case against, 1.63–65

  Chinese medicine *see* Chinese
   medicine: allopathy

  critical distinction between,
   2.12–13, 19

  homeopathy distinguished
   from, 1.267, 287

  naturopathy, 1.474–475

  origins compared, 1.469–476

  osteopathy and, 1.472–473;
   2.255, 257, 261–264,
   265–268, 279–280,
   287–288, 306–307,
   308–309

  recognition of, 1.473; 2.37,
   265–268, 277, 306–307

  scorn for *see* hegemony of, *below*

  success of, vs. failure of
   conventional, 2.555–557

 anesthesia and, 2.471, 474

 art of healing vs., 1.4–5, 131–132; 2.3

 and character, 2.97–98

 clinical environment, 2.124

 commoditization *see* commoditization

 complementary medicine and, 1.10

context of healing, 1.85

and curative message, 2.81–82, 97

definition of, 1.4

and disease *see* disease:
 conventional view of

doctors *see* doctors (conventional
 medicine)

egalitarian influence of, 2.503

and environmental destruction,
 1.485–486

as externalizing medicine,
 2.421–427

eyesight and, 2.194–197, 197, 199

failures of, 2.487, 488–492, 555–557

fragmentation and specialization
 of, 1.22–23, 485–486; 2.84–85

hegemony of, 1.11, 63, 134, 148–149,
 469–476; 2.3, 4, 13–20, 197,
 552–554

 see also American Medical
  Association

hospitals *see* hospitals

iatrogenic disease *see* pathology:
 healers and doctors creating

inexplicable cures and, 1.23–24

and intelligence of system,
 2.579–580

invasiveness of, 2.262–264

method as focus of, 2.122

as mirror, 1.485–486, 488, 490–491,
 492; 2.130

muscle testing used in, 2.288–289,
 294–295

mythology of, 1.70, 84, 266

neglect of mind/spirit, 1.288

origins

 elementalism, 1.261, 265–266,
  269, 299

Index

dentistry, osteopathy and, 2.556
Derrida, Jacques, 1.383, 392
desire to be well, 2.347–348, 510–516,
    538
destiny, 1.200–201
detachment, 2.515
Detwiller, Henry, 1.471
"developing" world, 2.176
Dewey, John, 2.190, 228
Dhanvantari Ayurvedic Center,
    2.608
diagnosis
    complexity of, 1.63, 65
    health insurance and, 2.89
    systems avoiding, 2.382–383
    touch vs. technology, 2.490
Dickens, Charles, 2.535–536
diet
    addiction to consumption,
        2.459–460, 461–463
    Ayurvedic, 1.312, 314–316, 321, 324,
        325
    Chinese, 1.345; 2.95
    color therapy and, 2.453
    enzyme and mineral therapies,
        2.468–471, 613–615
    foods as herbs, 2.459, 460–461
    herbs as foods, 2.464
    importance of, 2.457–459
    and industrialization, 1.488
    naturopathy and, 1.474, 475, 476
    oils, cooking and nutritional,
        2.614–615
    osteopathy/chiropractic and, 1.472
    Polarity Therapy, 2.355–356
    in process of healing, 2.486
    raw foods, 2.469
    resources for work on, 2.613–616

separated from disease treatment,
    1.487
and spectrum of healing, 2.**423**,
    471
Tibetan, 1.328–329
vegetarianism, 1.487; 2.460, 486
differentiation, 2.219–220, 224
Dimon Institute, 2.607
di Prima, Diane, 2.539
disabilities and sexuality, 2.115
disease
    archetypes, understood through,
        1.497–508
    awareness and, 1.511–513
    blaming the sick person, 2.504–506
    categories as subjective, 1.44–57
    choosing risk of, 1.66
    collective *see* collective disease
    conventional medicine and
        collective hygiene and, 1.21
        external causes sought, 1.24–25,
            280, 293; 2.14–15, 16–17,
            19, 262
        incurable, 1.23
        legal treatments, 1.24–25
        native society as inherently
            diseased, 1.112
        unrecognized diseases,
            2.279–280
    as created, 1.183–185, 201; 2.348
    definitions of
        absence of clear mind and
            natural breath, 2.428
        ambition, 2.515
        blocked libidinal energy, 1.385,
            393–394, 396, 436, 440
        disorder of meaning and spirit,
            1.121, 201

Index

Index

empiricism and, 2.5
food and, 2.459, 460–461, 464
lineage of, 1.494, 495
overview, 1.132–138, 530–533;
    2.464–468
of Paracelsus, 1.284
preparation and administration,
    1.136–138, 141–147; 2.464–468
shamanic, 1.138–141, 197–198
and spectrum of healing, 2.**423**,
    471
Thomsonian, 1.470
vitalism and, 1.229–230
see also pharmaceutical medicine
Herbert, Frank, 1.163
Herb'n Soul, 2.569
Hering, Constantine, 1.471
hermetic vitalism, 1.231–234, 232, 259
Herodotus, 1.290
heterosexual biases, 2.116–117
Higher Self, affirming self, 2.57
Hillman, James, 1.500–501
Hindus
    medicine of *see* India, medicine of
    philosophy of, 1.308
Hippocratic medicine and principles,
    1.249, 265–269, 275, 283, 477;
    2.239, 257, 261
Hirschberg, Gerald, 2.288
Hitler, Adolf, 2.502
HIV, 1.48–55
holism
    blaming the sick person in,
        2.504–506
    caricatures and delusions of,
        2.492–499, **494, 497, 499**
    competing ideologies of, 1.32–35;
        2.425–426, 477–478

definition of, 1.10, 476–477; 2.152
errors in treatment, 2.85–86
and Freudian influence, 1.388–389,
    402, 422
Jung and, 1.497, 501, 503; 2.499
linguistic and metalinguistic
    potentials of, 2.603
native indifference to, 1.83, 190–191
nostalgia of, 1.83
and origins of disease, 1.388
Reich's description of, 1.429
synthesis of modern, 1.477–478,
    502–504, 522–523, 525
two movements of, 2.497
whole, treatment of, 2.84–85
holistic medicine *see* alternative medi-
    cine
hologrammatic medicine, 1.533–534
hologrammaticization, 2.597–602
Holy Order of Mans, 1.511
home and homelessness, 2.520–521,
    536–537
Homeopathic Educational Services,
    2.616
homeopathy
    allopathy distinguished from,
        1.267, 287–288
    clinical success of, 1.252
    complementary systems and,
        2.478, 479, 482, 483
    depleted by scientism, 1.214–215,
        281
    Hippocratic healing and, 1.268
    holistic by default, 1.477
    and Jungian archetypes, 1.502
    as language system, 2.83
    Law of Similars in, 1.250–251, 495,
        496

PLANET
MEDICINE

MODALITIES

id, the
    Freud and, 1.385, 386, 390, **391**, 448
    the It and, 1.421–422
    Reich and, 1.427–428, 448
imaginal as real, 1.221–222, 382–383
immortality, 2.60–66
incest, 1.73; 2.330, 336
incisions, flesh, 1.91, 100, 164–165
India, medicine of
    acupuncture, 1.161–162
    Ayurveda *see* Ayurvedic medicine
    bone-setting, 1.160
    invasion of medieval institutions,
        1.308–309
    and memory, 2.443
    pancultural aspects, 1.289,
        298–299, 299–301
    Paracelsus and, 1.282
Indians *see* American Indians
indigenous societies
    ethnographic bias about, 1.110–112,
        114–116, 122–124
    New Age cultural imperialism and,
        2.496–497, 521
    restraints on healers in, 2.500,
        501–502
    spirituality as power in, 1.85–86
    world views, 1.121–122
    see also culture; native medicine;
        individual tribes and groups
industrialism *see* technology
industrial medicine *see* conventional
    medicine
information, increase of, 1.113–114,
    118; 2.601–602
initiation
    current rites, 2.492–493
    of Reiki healers, 2.46, 51–52

of shamans, 1.211–214; 2.92
    and psychoanalysts, compared,
        1.179–180
inner child, 1.180–181
insanity, 1.71, 382
inside *see* interior; internalization
insight therapy *see* psychological
    medicine
Institute for Health Improvement,
    2.609
Intelligence, 1.189–193, 202; 2.81, 352,
    355
    laws of cure (proposed) and,
        2.579–603
Intelligent Life in the Universe
    (Shklovskii), 1.236–237
interior
    as anterior, 1.14–15
    dreams as revealing, 1.401–409
    martial arts and, 1.368
    omission of, 1.15–16
internalization
    of cynicism, 2.59
    of martial arts, 2.100
    medicines of, and spectrum,
        2.421–427, **423**
    shamanic healing and, 2.94–95
    see also Chi Gung Tui Na; transference
International Rolf Institute, 2.620
Interpretation of Dreams, The (Freud),
    1.398, 400
intersexuals, 2.117
intuition, 1.135–136, 358
iridology, 1.533–535; 2.600–601
Iroquois Indians, 1.119, **201**
Islamic medicine, 1.282, 293, 294, 295,
    298
It, the, 1.421–422

Index

metamorphosis, 1.533

metaphysical healing, 2.442–445

methodology
    as culturally based, 1.56–57
    as focus, vs. individual healer,
        2.122, 158–159
    psychoanalysis and failure to
        produce, 1.409–417, 426–429

Mexico, Indian medicine of, 1.161

microdoses *see* homeopathy

Microlight Nutritional Products, 2.614

micromovements, 2.404–407

Middendorf Breath Institute, 2.619

Middendorf, Ilse, 2.143, 149, 150–151

Middle Eastern medicine, survey of,
    1.290–295

middle ground, 1.444–446

midwifery, 1.91, 147

migration, forced, 2.520–521

military *see* war

mind
    body, finding mind through,
        2.134–135
    in *Chi Gung Tui Na,* 2.429
    and creative power of body,
        2.147–149
    dualistic semantics examined,
        1.189–191
    energy basis of, 1.382–383, 386–389;
        2.64–65
    imaginal as real, 1.221–222, 382–383
    Intelligence, 1.189–193, 202; 2.81,
        352, 355, 579–603
    laws of cure (proposed) and,
        2.579–603
    in meditation, 1.520–521;
        2.428–429
    modern view of, 1.40–41
    movements of, natural, 2.410–411
    negative thoughts of, 2.62–64,
        533–534
    the objectifying, 1.95
    and Polarity Therapy, 2.352, 355
    see also consciousness; dreams and
        dreaming; psychological
        medicine; visions;
        visualization

mind/body
    dualistic semantics examined,
        1.189–191
    split
        as limiting perception, 1.189–191
        native medicine not resolving,
            1.182
        validity of, 1.251; 2.147–149
    unity
        Buddhism and, 1.518–519
        disease origin in *see under*
            disease
        ego and, 1.189
        language deficit for, 1.41
    see also somatic systems

mineral therapy, 2.468–471

miracles, 1.222

Mitchell, Faith, 1.470

Miwok Indians *see* Pomo Indian bear
    doctors

mob rule, 2.501–503, 535–536

Moby Dick, 1.198–199, 200; 2.539

Molière, 1.63

money, 2.52–53, 510 *see also* economics

Moore, Omar Khayyam, 1.207

More University, 2.117–122

Morrison, Douglas, 2.515, 608

mortality rate, 1.112

Moss, Thelma, 2.32

Index

Index

Index

Index

White, Leslie, 1.115
Whiting, Alfred, 1.195
Whitman, Walt, 1.516
Whitmont, Edward
  blaming the sick person, 2.504,
      505–506
  botanical morphology, 1.208
  healer's illness, cure through,
      2.130–131
  healing defined by, 1.34
  homeopathy, 1.250, 251, 506–507
  meaning of medicine and disease,
      1.140
  pathogenic healer, 2.124, 125, 126,
      128–129, 483
  and placebo effect, 2.30–31
  therapeutic relationship, 1.213–214
  transmutations, 1.506–507
Whorf, Benjamin Lee, 1.391
Wildschut, William, 1.104
Williams, William Carlos, 2.539–540
will to live, 2.510–516, 538
wish fulfillment, 1.407–408
witchcraft
  black, 1.257
  see also magic; voodoo
Wizard of Earthsea, A (Le Guin),
      1.216–217
women
  alternative sexualities and,
      2.119–120
  gender, 1.424, 440; 2.116–117
  genital Rolfing of, 2.242
  matriarchal lineage, 2.400, 402
  as natural healers, 2.114–115
wounds, as initiatory requirement,
      1.212–213, 214
Wyvell, Lois, 1.458

X-rays, 2.266, 290–291

Yaqui Indians *see* Don Juan Matus
      (Castaneda)
Yellow Emperor, system of the, 1.339,
      386; 2.88–89
  character and, 2.91, 95, 97
Yellow Emperor, The (Veith, trans.),
      1.333, 345; 2.97
Yin-Yang, 1.342–344, 347, 349,
      357–358, 371
yoga
  in Ayurveda, 1.265, 297, 299, 307,
      319, 324
  as exercise, 2.287
  and food, 2.462
  as lineage, 1.478, 511
  rebirthing as, 2.61
  tantra, 2.108, 113, 117
  transduction and, 2.597
Yogananda, Paramahansa, 1.509, 510;
      2.34
youth, pursuing mirage of, 2.555–556
Yugoslavia, 2.310

Zaporah, Ruth, 1.481
zazen, 1.519, **519, 520**, 522, 523, 525;
      2.332
Zeiger, Robert, 2.424, 606
Zen *see* Buddhism
Zenji, Dogen, 1.518–519
Zero Balancing, 1.528; 2.254, 385–390,
      386
zoology, native classifications of,
      1.107, 110
Zoroastrian medicine, 1.293–294, **293**

Index